Technologies of Sex Selection and Prenatal Diagnosis

Volume 14 of the
Research Studies

Royal Commission on
New Reproductive Technologies

This volume is available in both official languages. Each volume is individually priced, but is also available as part of a complete set containing all 15 volumes.

Available in Canada through your local bookseller
or by mail from
Canada Communications Group — Publishing
Ottawa, Canada K1A 0S9

CANADIAN CATALOGUING IN PUBLICATION DATA

Main entry under title:

Technologies of sex selection and prenatal diagnosis

(Research studies ; no. 14)
Issued also in French under title: Les techniques de choix du sexe et le diagnostic prénatal.
Includes bibliographical references.
ISBN 0-662-21388-2
Cat. no. Z1-1989/3-41-27E

1. Prenatal diagnosis. 2. Fetus — Diseases — Diagnosis. 3. Obstetrics — Diagnosis. 4. Sex preselection. I. Canada. Royal Commission on New Reproductive Technologies. II. Series: Research studies (Canada. Royal Commission on New Reproductive Technologies) ; 14.

RG628.P73 1993   618.2'2   C94-980081-3

The Royal Commission on New Reproductive Technologies and the publishers wish to acknowledge with gratitude the following:

- Canada Communications Group, Printing Services
- Canada Communications Group, Graphics

Consistent with the Commission's commitment to full equality between men and women, care has been taken throughout this volume to use gender-neutral language wherever possible.

Contents

⟨1⟩ **Ethical Issues of Prenatal Diagnosis for Predictive Testing for Genetic Disorders of Late Onset**

Michael Cooke

⟨2⟩ **Prenatal Testing for Huntington Disease: Psychosocial Aspects**

Shelin Adam and Michael R. Hayden

◇3◇ Screening for Genetic Susceptibilities to Common Diseases

Lynn Prior

Preference for the Sex of One's Children and the Prospective Use of Sex Selection

Martin Thomas

Tables

Bibliography on Preferences for the Sex of One's Children, and Attitudes Concerning Sex Preselection

Martin Thomas

Attitudes of Genetic Counsellors with Respect to Prenatal Diagnosis of Sex for Non-Medical Reasons

Z.G. Miller and F.C. Fraser

Preimplantation Diagnosis

F. Clarke Fraser

⟨8⟩ Somatic and Germ Line Gene Therapy: Current Status and Prospects

Lynn Prior

Preface from the Chairperson

As Canadians living in the last decade of the twentieth century, we face unprecedented choices about procreation. Our responses to those choices — as individuals and as a society — say much about what we value and what our priorities are. Some technologies, such as those for assisted reproduction, are unlikely to become a common means of having a family — although the number of children born as a result of these techniques is greater than the number of infants placed for adoption in Canada. Others, such as ultrasound during pregnancy, are already generally accepted, and half of all pregnant women aged 35 and over undergo prenatal diagnostic procedures. Still other technologies, such as fetal tissue research, have little to do with reproduction as such, but may be of benefit to people suffering from diseases such as Parkinson's; they raise important ethical issues in the use and handling of reproductive tissues.

It is clear that opportunities for technological intervention raise issues that affect all of society; in addition, access to the technologies depends on the existence of public structures and policies to provide them. The values and priorities of society, as expressed through its institutions, laws, and funding arrangements, will affect individual options and choices.

As Canadians became more aware of these technologies throughout the 1980s, there was a growing awareness that there was an unacceptably large gap between the rapid pace of technological change and the policy development needed to guide decisions about whether and how to use such powerful technologies. There was also a realization of how little reliable information was available to make the needed policy decisions. In addition, many of the attitudes and assumptions underlying the way in which technologies were being developed and made available did not reflect the profound changes that have been transforming Canada in recent decades. Individual cases were being dealt with in isolation, and often in the absence of informed social consensus. At the same time, Canadians were looking more critically at the role of science and technology in their lives in general, becoming more aware of their limited capacity to solve society's problems.

These concerns came together in the creation of the Royal Commission on New Reproductive Technologies. The Commission was established by the federal government in October 1989, with a wide-ranging and complex mandate. It is important to understand that the Commission was asked to consider the technologies' impact not only on society, but also on specific groups in society, particularly women and children. It was asked to consider not only the technologies' scientific and medical aspects, but also their ethical, legal, social, economic, and health implications. Its mandate was extensive, as it was directed to examine not only current developments in the area of new reproductive technologies, but also potential ones; not only techniques related to assisted conception, but also those of prenatal diagnosis; not only the condition of infertility, but also its causes and prevention; not only applications of technology, but also research, particularly embryo and fetal tissue research.

The appointment of a Royal Commission provided an opportunity to collect much-needed information, to foster public awareness and public debate, and to provide a principled framework for Canadian public policy on the use or restriction of these technologies.

The Commission set three broad goals for its work: to provide direction for public policy by making sound, practical, and principled recommendations; to leave a legacy of increased knowledge to benefit Canadian and international experience with new reproductive technologies; and to enhance public awareness and understanding of the issues surrounding new reproductive technologies to facilitate public participation in determining the future of the technologies and their place in Canadian society.

To fulfil these goals, the Commission held extensive public consultations, including private sessions for people with personal experiences of the technologies that they did not want to discuss in a public forum, and it developed an interdisciplinary research program to ensure that its recommendations would be informed by rigorous and wide-ranging research. In fact, the Commission published some of that research in advance of the Final Report to assist those working in the field of reproductive health and new reproductive technologies and to help inform the public.

The results of the research program are presented in these volumes. In all, the Commission developed and gathered an enormous body of information and analysis on which to base its recommendations, much of it available in Canada for the first time. This solid base of research findings helped to clarify the issues and produce practical and useful recommendations based on reliable data about the reality of the situation, not on speculation.

The Commission sought the involvement of the most qualified researchers to help develop its research projects. In total, more than 300 scholars and academics representing more than 70 disciplines — including the social sciences, humanities, medicine, genetics, life sciences, law, ethics, philosophy, and theology — at some 21 Canadian universities and 13 hospitals, clinics, and other institutions were involved in the research program.

The Commission was committed to a research process with high standards and a protocol that included internal and external peer review for content and methodology, first at the design stage and later at the report stage. Authors were asked to respond to these reviews, and the process resulted in the achievement of a high standard of work. The protocol was completed before the publication of the studies in this series of research volumes. Researchers using human subjects were required to comply with appropriate ethical review standards.

These volumes of research studies reflect the Commission's wide mandate. We believe the findings and analysis contained in these volumes will be useful for many people, both in this country and elsewhere.

Along with the other Commissioners, I would like to take this opportunity to extend my appreciation and thanks to the researchers and external reviewers who have given tremendous amounts of time and thought to the Commission. I would also like to acknowledge the entire Commission staff for their hard work, dedication, and commitment over the life of the Commission. Finally, I would like to thank the more than 40 000 Canadians who were involved in the many facets of the Commission's work. Their contribution has been invaluable.

Patricia A. Baird

Patricia Baird, M.D., C.M., FRCPC, F.C.C.M.G.

Introduction

Prenatal diagnosis, as it has so far been used and as discussed in the previous two volumes, is a means of providing information to women and couples who are at higher risk for a serious disorder — either a congenital anomaly or genetic disease — in their children. As the studies in this volume demonstrate, however, new developments already, or will soon, make it possible to detect prenatally a growing range of attributes, including sex, late-onset single-gene disorders, and susceptibility to some common diseases. This raises important issues for individuals, physicians, and society as a whole to address if potential harms are to be avoided.

Prenatal diagnosis can now be applied to conditions that will not manifest themselves until adulthood. Similarly, recent developments in DNA technology mean that it is now possible to identify genes that create susceptibilities to common diseases, that is, genes whose presence indicates that there is a somewhat increased probability of that person becoming ill. It is also possible to use prenatal diagnosis for non-medical reasons, such as to discern the sex of a fetus for a couple who wish to have a child of a given sex. Another application of genetic knowledge is focussed on how DNA technology may allow treatment of individuals with a genetic disease by adding the normal gene to their body cells. Other possibilities are being raised too — for example, the possibility of using DNA technology to alter genes in the eggs or sperm or to alter genes to "improve" people.

The Studies

Huntington disease is probably the best known late-onset single-gene disorder for which predictive (that is, presymptomatic) testing is possible. Because the disease does not manifest itself until later in life, and because of the complexity of the testing procedure, which, until recently, has required testing of other family members, the testing raises additional ethical issues to be considered. Many of these issues are not specific to

Huntington disease, but are relevant to all late-onset single-gene disorders for which prenatal testing is possible.

Michael Cooke examines the ethical aspects of using prenatal diagnosis to identify Huntington disease in the absence of any known cure for the condition. He examines the question of individual rights to information and availability of the technology, and highlights the importance of counselling to assist parents in exercising informed choice. He notes that, in cases where parents do not intend to consider terminating an affected pregnancy, there are deep ethical concerns about giving birth to a child whose likelihood of developing a condition as severe and debilitating as Huntington disease will be known to both the child and others to be almost certain. There are also wider social implications in the availability of this type of prenatal testing for late-onset disorders, and Mr. Cooke examines these too, focussing particularly on issues relating to attitudes toward the disabled, to freely chosen or mandatory genetic testing, and to the meaning of fully informed choice.

Shelin Adam and Michael Hayden focus on the decisions about prenatal testing of pregnant couples at risk for passing Huntington disease to their children, to gain a better understanding of why they chose to use testing or not. The couples were all participants in the Canadian Collaborative Study of Predictive Testing for Huntington Disease. Only 7 of the 38 couples (18 percent) eligible for prenatal testing wanted it, a lower demand than was anticipated by earlier survey data.

The most common reason for refusing prenatal testing was the belief that, even if a couple had a child with the gene for Huntington disease, a cure would be found in the lifetime of the child. Some felt that, even if a cure were not found, it was likely that some form of therapy effective enough to halt the progression of the disease would be developed. Many of the couples who declined prenatal testing already had children and appeared unwilling to create a situation where some of their children would be aware of their likelihood of developing Huntington disease, while others would not. The study's findings about patients' understanding of the complex nature of exclusion testing, and the need for careful counselling for at-risk couples confirm Mr. Cooke's more theoretical analysis.

Another application of DNA technology is screening for genetic susceptibility to common diseases. These diseases have genetic determinants to them, but environmental factors are also involved in the pathway to illness. As Lynn Prior outlines, testing for genes that increase susceptibility to some common illnesses is a difficult technical undertaking. This, together with the ethical issues raised and the potential for harm, makes it an area for great caution. While there may be benefits from susceptibility testing (for example, allowing individuals to take preventive measures or to benefit from early diagnosis), there are also potential harms. Some of these harms are to the individual, such as harm to self-image and happiness or adverse effects on the parent-child relationship. Others are societal in scope: discrimination against carriers by employers, insurance companies, or peers, or possible societal stigmatization.

Ms. Prior outlines the criteria that she feels must be met before a population screening program for genetic susceptibility is set up, and she points out that for none of the susceptibility genes identified to date are these criteria fulfilled. This, coupled with the fact that some fetuses that might never have developed the disorder could be terminated, leads Ms. Prior to conclude that prenatal susceptibility testing is not justified.

A possible use of increasing genetic knowledge is to apply it to select the sex of offspring. This topic is examined in the next three studies of this volume. In the first study, Martin Thomas presents an exhaustive review of the three main methods of selecting the sex of a fetus. In the first, sex-selective abortion, prenatal diagnosis is used to determine the sex of a fetus, followed by termination if the fetus is not of the desired sex. In the second method, X- or Y-bearing sperm cells are enhanced through treatment of the sperm, and in the third, the sex-chromosome makeup of zygotes created through *in vitro* fertilization (IVF) is diagnosed and only those zygotes of the desired sex are implanted. Dr. Thomas combines this review with the results of an extensive national survey aimed at measuring Canadians' preferences for the sex of their children and their willingness to use different methods of sex selection and preselection to obtain their preference.

Dr. Thomas found that the most widely held desire among Canadians is to have at least one child of each sex. Overall, his survey found no appreciable sex bias among women and a very slight pro-son bias among men. Almost no respondents would use abortion after prenatal diagnosis to select sex. Only 21 percent of respondents would be willing to use a sex preselection procedure to increase the probabilities of having a fetus of the desired sex, even if a method existed that was as easy as taking a pill. Those who would be willing would do so to try to have at least one child of each sex. Dr. Thomas found that the sex ratio in Canada would be unlikely to change even if such sex preselection technologies were available.

This extensive review is complemented by the next study, which reviews publications dealing with preference for the sex of one's children and with the social science or ethical aspects of sex preselection. This bibliography will be of value both to scholars seeking in-depth information on this issue and to the layperson who seeks more information about the issues raised in this volume. Dr. Thomas's commitment to maintaining the bibliography enhances its value for many years to come.

In the last study related to sex selection, Gail Miller and Clarke Fraser report the results of their survey of 200 genetic counsellors associated with centres providing prenatal diagnosis in Canada. Genetic counsellors were asked about their willingness to provide information about the sex of a fetus to patients receiving prenatal diagnosis when there was no medical indication (that is, there was no increased risk that a child of one sex would be affected by a disorder). The survey found that very few geneticists

(2 percent) personally approved of prenatal diagnosis simply for diagnosis of sex. It also found that, in spite of this, geneticists were more willing either to test for sex preference or to refer to a centre that would when they were given the detailed circumstances surrounding the request. These involved a pregnant immigrant woman with three daughters and under intense pressure from her husband to have a son. Overall, however, geneticists in Canada, like those in other countries who have responded to similar surveys, rejected the idea of using prenatal diagnosis for sex preference.

The findings of these studies provide data that suggest there is no increasing demand for or acceptance of the use of prenatal diagnosis for non-medical reasons such as sex selection or preselection. They demonstrate that neither couples having children nor geneticists providing prenatal diagnosis believe that this is an appropriate use of prenatal diagnosis.

Identification of the sex of the zygote before implantation is but one possible application in the new and developing field of preimplantation diagnosis. For this diagnosis to be possible, the zygote must be accessible for testing and, therefore, the procedure requires the use of IVF. Clarke Fraser examines preimplantation diagnosis and concludes that, because of the difficulties involved, it is likely to remain limited to a small percentage of couples at identified high risk for having offspring with a specific genetic disorder. He examines ethical issues raised by this particular use of technology, finding that, in essence, they are similar to the issues raised by conventional prenatal diagnosis and by IVF. In addition, the high costs of both IVF and preimplantation diagnosis and the low implantation rate raise ethical questions about whether it is a good use of scarce medical resources to pursue this use of technology further.

The final study in this volume moves beyond the diagnosis of genetic disorders to their treatment. Lynn Prior examines the current status of, and research into, gene therapy, a process whereby genetic material (DNA) is introduced into humans for the purpose of correcting a genetic disorder. She looks at three uses of DNA technology: somatic cell gene therapy, in which gene insertion is used to ameliorate diseases caused by recessive genetic mutations; gene alteration for enhancement of "superior" traits; and germ line gene alteration. The last is not yet technically possible in humans, but it has been the object of increasing speculation. Somatic cell gene therapy does not present unique ethical or legal problems, but rather raises issues that apply to all new human therapeutic treatments. Ms. Prior finds that genetic enhancement and germ line gene alteration, on the other hand, present serious ethical concerns.

Conclusion

The overall conclusion that one reaches from the studies in this volume is that a very cautious approach is indicated to new developments that expand the boundaries of prenatal diagnosis away from its traditional function of providing information to women and couples who are at higher risk for either a congenital anomaly or genetic disease. It is important to assess and differentiate carefully between such new developments and uses.

Some, such as predictive testing for late-onset disorders, are technically complex, and it is demanding for both providers and patients to ensure fully informed choice. However, these developments still may be of value to those at-risk couples who wish to take advantage of them. Screening for susceptibility genes is also complex in technical terms, but proves on closer examination to be of much more limited use at this time. Sex selection is revealed as being even further away from the core aim of prenatal diagnosis. While preimplantation diagnosis as currently proposed shares the goals of conventional prenatal diagnosis, it is very costly and of limited applicability. Finally, examination of the possibilities of applying knowledge about altering human DNA indicates that there are some valid uses that allow movement from diagnosis to treatment in somatic cell gene therapy. Other uses of the capacity to alter DNA, such as genetic enhancement and germ line gene alteration, are extremely problematic in terms of the ethical and practical issues they raise.

Another point that emerges from a careful reading of the studies in this volume is the importance of an "early warning system." Some of the techniques described are based on recent discoveries in genetics and are many years away from introduction into the health care system or application in clinical care. However, they underline the need to examine carefully new developments, especially their ethical aspects and implications, while they are still at the experimental stage. The issues to be assessed and moral reasoning to be carried out will take time, and it is important to do this in advance. Finally, it becomes clear that the basic tenets of prenatal diagnosis — individual autonomy and counselling to support informed choice — should also apply to new developments in this area.

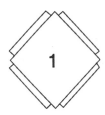

Ethical Issues of Prenatal Diagnosis for Predictive Testing for Genetic Disorders of Late Onset

Michael Cooke

Executive Summary

The use of new technologies to diagnose disorders before birth raises issues such as abortion, reproductive autonomy, right to life, and questions of wrongful life or birth. In late-onset disorders, such as Huntington's disease, these issues may be particularly difficult to assess because the disease, although severe, is not manifest during childhood, and the methods involved in diagnosis are complicated.

Two levels of discussion coexist in the literature. One level addresses the question of individual rights to information and availability of the technology. The right to complete reproductive freedom is weighed (in the courts) against the claims and rights of others, including the right not to be born. Genetic counselling must take these issues into account and also must explain the technology in ways that permit truly informed choice.

In the second level of analysis, the very use of the technology is questioned, because of the social change it may bring about. Opposing points of view highlight the issues of autonomy, problems and concerns about attitudes toward the disabled, the question of mandatory genetic screening, and the meaning of fully informed choice.

This paper was completed for the Royal Commission on New Reproductive Technologies in March 1992.

There are implications that may affect individuals and future society. The need to protect the principle of fully informed choice, awareness of social costs, and requirements for accountable resource allocation demand an informed public and government attention.

Introduction

The discovery of numerous polymorphic DNA markers linked to the mutant gene causing Huntington's disease has made predictive testing for this disorder possible (Gusella et al. 1983; Hayden et al. 1987; Meissen and Berchek 1987; Wasmuth et al. 1988; Brandt et al. 1989). In Canada, predictive testing for Huntington's disease has been offered under the auspices of the Canadian Collaborative Study of Predictive Testing for Huntington's Disease (CSHD), involving centres across the country. The guidelines of this research project have provided for predictive testing for adults at 50 percent risk for Huntington's disease and for prenatal testing for at-risk individuals.

This project has encountered compelling ethical dilemmas relating to Huntington's disease's status as a late-onset disorder for which predictive testing requires marker analysis within families rather than direct analysis for specific mutations. Other ethical issues related to prenatal diagnosis also apply to prenatal predictive testing for Huntington's disease. As befits its role as part of an inquiry into reproductive technology, the present report will focus mainly on issues closely related to prenatal testing. Because some of the issues such as claims of third parties that relate to predictive testing of adults strongly influence the context within which prenatal predictive testing may be sought, these issues will also be considered.

This report finds that there are basically two areas of ethical discourse surrounding the development of prenatal diagnosis and predictive testing. Although these areas are interrelated, it is possible and useful to conceptualize them as two levels of inquiry. The first level deals with the relationship between those providing the service and those seeking to avail themselves of it. Discussions centre around traditional principles of medical ethics such as autonomy, beneficence, confidentiality, and justice (see for instance Huggins et al. 1990). These principles are central to the 1990 *Ethical Issues Policy Statement on Huntington's Disease Molecular Genetics Predictive Test* prepared by the Committee of the International Huntington Association (IHA) and the World Federation of Neurology (WFN) (Went 1990). Essentially, the focus is on questions such as when, how, and to whom should this technology be offered.

The second level of discussion is concerned with the relationship of reproductive technology to society. Unlike the ethical approach of physicians, which accepts implicitly that prenatal diagnosis should be available, commentators find the development of prenatal diagnosis itself to be problematic, and they address themselves to the more basic question: Should this be done at all?

In general, discourse in the second area draws attention to the possible long-term social effects of the development of prenatal diagnosis of any kind. Concerns raised include those relating to the reproductive freedom of women, the position of the disabled in society, and the possible contribution of prenatal diagnosis to the development of eugenic ideology. Implicitly contributing to the context of this discussion is the question of resource allocation. Many of these issues have been presented to the Royal Commission on New Reproductive Technologies in other forums but will be discussed in this report, since the social and ethical issues relating to Huntington's disease must be considered within the broader social context.

Individual Rights and Conflicts of Rights

With respect to the first area of discussion, some of the ethical dilemmas encountered in the CSHD have been unique and are related to Huntington's disease's status as a late-onset, terminal disorder for which there is no cure. Bloch and Hayden point out: "In contrast to the more usual DNA analyses, persons at risk for HD may learn about the possibility that they will develop a devastating disease sometime in the future. They will also learn that there is no treatment which can modify this outcome. Such testing is fundamentally different from assessment of risk for other dominant genetic disorders, such as familial hypercholesterolemia, where individuals at high risk may, with diet or drugs, modify the course of the illness" (Bloch and Hayden 1990, 1).

The CSHD has provided extensive descriptions of some of the dilemmas faced (Huggins et al. 1990). These situations are compelling for the individuals involved — for example, the issue of obtaining blood, which is essential to diagnosis, from unwilling or incompetent relatives; or relating a serendipitously discovered decrease in risk status to an individual whose expressed wish is to obtain no information regarding his/her status. However, they would not appear to present the need for reformulation of current approaches.

There have, however, been issues that become more problematic if predictive testing for Huntington's disease becomes offered as a service funded by the health care system. Perhaps the most obvious of these relates to prenatal testing. The CSHD specifically states that predictive testing should not be performed for minor children, nor prenatally in cases where parents do not consider termination of pregnancy an option. This differs significantly from the usual practice of genetic counselling, which attempts to be non-directive and does not make suggestions regarding parents' decisions about the pregnancy. The CSHD practice, which is supported by the IHA and WFN, relates to Huntington's disease's status as a late-onset disorder with no known cure.

The underlying rationale for the CSHD position is rooted in concern for the well-being of children identified as being at increased risk, and it is based upon the principle of autonomy that has been accorded explicit primacy by the CSHD and elsewhere. The rationale is explained by two leaders of the Canadian study:

> Children clearly cannot make an informed decision about whether to participate in predictive testing. The request is made by a third party, in this instance a parent. The only justification for doing predictive testing in childhood is if an advantage can clearly be demonstrated for the child. There is currently no known treatment which might prevent or delay the age of onset for HD. Such testing may be disadvantageous for the child, either because of possible distortion of parent/child or sib/sib relationships or because of limitation of resources for the child shown to be at increased risk. The self-esteem and sense of worth of a developing child may be profoundly and negatively affected. The attitude of society and its agencies toward high-risk individuals has not yet been clarified. Since no treatment is available and there is the possibility of harm, we oppose the testing of children. (Bloch and Hayden 1990, 2)

Because testing of parents who do not plan to terminate a high-risk pregnancy could result in the birth of a child identified as having a high risk for Huntington's disease, the same reasoning also has been applied to prenatal testing. The obvious drawback in this situation is that such parents do not have the opportunity of having their anxiety lessened by obtaining information that their fetus is at low risk for having inherited the gene for Huntington's disease.

Although this position has generally been supported (Went 1990; Tyler and Morris 1990; Harper et al. 1990), it has been challenged in the literature (Pelias 1991). The challenge has been based upon American legal precedent and theory and includes the expressed concern that withholding full disclosure may result in litigation that will damage the credibility of the profession. In terms of its ethical aspect, it somewhat ironically refers to the protection of autonomy — in this case that of the parents to make decisions regarding their own children.

The argument made by Pelias in favour of full disclosure follows three steps. The first of these is the argument that the definition of parents as third parties is contrary to the historical judicial recognition of parental prerogative in making medical decisions for minor children (Bowen v. American Hospital Association 1986). Second, it is argued that the practice of withholding prenatal testing under the conditions stated by Bloch and Hayden may result in successful actions regarding wrongful birth. Given that the basis of wrongful birth tort actions is the failure of a health care professional to provide information that would have enabled parents to avoid the undesired birth of a disabled child, it is somewhat unclear how this relates to the case at hand, in which information is withheld on the basis of parents' expressed stance against termination.

Perhaps more worthy of consideration is the argument that "parents deprived of complete information about the genetic status of their children will assert that their parental autonomy was compromised when they were deprived of the chance to explore every available opportunity for their child with a deleterious gene" (Pelias 1986, 350). There would seem to be greater grounds for parental action in this context, assuming that prenatal prediction of increased risk would allow for financial planning, etc., in preparation for the future onset of symptoms. This position has received support in the legal literature (e.g., Becker 1988).

The position of the CSHD would become more difficult to maintain if predictive testing for Huntington's disease is offered as a service provided by a government-funded health care system rather than within a research program, when it would appear that clinician discretion in this matter may be more defensible.

The IHA and WFN policy statement recommends that "any couple requesting prenatal diagnosis must be made aware of the fact that if they intend to complete the pregnancy whatever the result, there is little point in taking the test." It goes on to say that "the primary object in requesting a prenatal test is to avoid giving birth to a child who carries the HD gene" (Went 1990, Article 6.1).

Individuals who feel that free choice in light of prenatal diagnostic information involves the right to choose options other than termination may disagree with the policy. This relates to Pelias's objection, stated above (1986, 350). If the position is considered tenable that the primary goal of prenatal testing for Huntington's disease is to avoid giving birth to a child who carries the Huntington's disease gene, it would seem that the health care system would have ethical justification to consider prenatal assessment of a late-onset disorder to have low priority when termination is not an option.

Whatever the legal issues involved, the ethical requirement of adequate counselling is obvious. Also, it has been the experience in the Canadian study that such issues can be dealt with through adequate exploration of the problems raised seeking access to the technology.

The question of predictive testing for minor children and the related concerns about prenatal predictive testing may raise legal issues regarding the right of clinicians to refuse testing that seems inappropriate. In addition to legal issues, the complexity of such situations creates a compelling illustration of the need for counselling services that may exceed those normally provided in prenatal genetic counselling.

The need for extensive pre-test counselling is underscored by findings that individuals have difficulty understanding the technical and ethical aspects of assessments — particularly in the case of exclusion testing. In this procedure a fetus may be assigned a low risk of carrying the Huntington's disease gene or a risk similar to that of its parent, without identifying the status of the parent (Tyler et al. 1990). Given the goal of informed choice espoused by genetic counselling, more extensive and in-depth counselling for conditions such as Huntington's disease is needed, because the prenatal identification of these conditions depends on marker analysis, and this has resource implications.

In contrast to the strong emphasis placed on individual autonomy by the CSHD, other commentators have proposed that certain limitations of individual autonomy may be ethically defensible. Arguments concerning predictive testing for Huntington's disease have referred to the fiduciary claims of family members and future offspring (Lamport 1987) and are often placed in the context of reproductive issues. Smurl and Weaver argue: "Spouses, especially if they are parents as well, and the children of presymptomatic or asymptomatic persons have a *prima facie* right to know the results of tests in order to make informed decisions about their own reproductive ... futures" (Smurl and Weaver 1987, 252).

Lamport argues that in the context of reproductive planning individual autonomy is outweighed by the principle of beneficence as it applies to future offspring. She argues that "autonomy may be exercised only so long as ... actions are not detrimental to others and do not infringe upon their own autonomous actions. By passing on a fatal disease, a parent has, in effect, harmed his [or her] offspring and has interfered with [the] ability to behave in an autonomous manner. In this case, the benefit to the child outweighs the claim for exemption from testing through the right to autonomy" (Lamport 1987, 309).

The arguments presented by these commentators, though advanced from very similar perspectives, differ in one important fashion: whether individuals have the moral right to withhold test results from family members. The concerns are with the confidentiality of test results versus the fiduciary claims of others. Although contrasting with the position of the CSHD with respect to the ethical conclusion reached, a common starting point recognizes the context within which predictive testing takes place as a complex system of interrelationships. The divergence appears in the strategy used to address the issue, with the CSHD placing heavy emphasis upon the value of counselling to resolve competing claims but simultaneously reaffirming individual autonomy. The alternative is to place more emphasis upon judicial mediation between conflicting claims. The CSHD may provide a valuable model, stressing as it does an interactive consensus rather than relying on a more legalistic approach to competing rights claims.

The position of Lamport proceeds somewhat further than that of Smurl and Weaver by asserting that high-risk parents have an obligation to have testing because of a responsibility to their future offspring. This more extreme position raises the slippery slope thesis advanced by those who express reservations about the technology. The slippery slope argument is that current legal protection of autonomy, in the form of the right to refuse testing, will be eroded as prenatal diagnostic technology is developed. This issue has also been a concern of the CSHD, which has strongly resisted third-party claims with respect to adult predictive testing.

The two issues raised in this section illustrate the coexistence of competing rights claims (those of individuals at risk for Huntington's disease and those of other individuals or groups) and the ethical requirement of in-depth counselling in light of the complex nature of the technology and the moral issues involved. Perhaps the salient feature is the centrality of the principle of autonomy. Individual autonomy is considered to be the fundamental ethical value, and participants on both sides of debates in this section adopt the fundamental perspective that a discourse of rights is sufficient to address all ethical issues encountered.

Social Contextualization of Issues

Participants in the discourse concerning social contextualization adopt a different perspective, questioning the overall contribution of prenatal diagnosis to the public good. Consequently, a language of rights is not always adequate to address the issues raised. The matter is not necessarily best viewed as a conflict between private and public good, although it is sometimes that. Rather, it appears to be an attempt to analyze complex sets of interrelated social effects that are more difficult to elaborate than the issues of the first section. It appears that the clash of two differing perspectives and the inadequacy of the traditional conceptual tools of medical ethics to address the issues raised at the second level of discourse have in large part determined its character, which has at times been acrimonious.

To begin with, the development of prenatal diagnosis has taken place in a context that has referred to the benefits of this technology as offering increased reproductive autonomy to women by providing more control and choice regarding birth. But those who express concerns about the development of prenatal diagnosis remain unconvinced at this time that, in its current context at least, prenatal diagnosis will in the long term have more positive than negative social effects.

Much of the criticism of the rapid development of prenatal diagnosis takes place in the context of concerns about the Human Genome Project and other reproductive technology. Issues regarding effects of technological development that are somewhat more subtle and long term than those discussed earlier in this report are raised.

Technological Sophistication and Limits to Autonomy

One locus of criticism is the observation that the increasing role of complex technologies in the childbearing process limits the control women exercise over reproduction by investing a large degree of the decision-making process in medical experts. Without a doubt, Canada has witnessed the introduction of technologies that have required a progressively greater educational sophistication to understand fully. It has been argued that, though ostensibly providing expanded choice for women, the technological expansion has created a greater dependency upon the experts who administer it. The argument is, in part, that the routine use of prenatal diagnostic procedures, though providing information of use to a small number of individuals, creates a culture in which the childbearing function becomes less in control of pregnant women and more in control of medical experts. What is somewhat less clear is whether or not this is considered to be adequate reason to limit the development of such technology.

With respect to predictive testing for Huntington's disease, some authors have reported that a high percentage (89 percent) of individuals have difficulty fully understanding the technology (Tyler et al. 1990) because the current process of marker analysis is so complex. Such technology-related difficulty was noticed particularly with respect to exclusion testing. Tyler et al. found that in surveys of attitudes toward predictive testing for Huntington's disease (Kessler et al. 1987; Meissen and Berchek 1987), as the level of understanding of the test decreased, people tended to decide to continue a pregnancy that was identified as at higher risk on exclusion testing.

Such findings illustrate that a commitment to the ethical principle of autonomy, as reflected by fully informed choice, requires a commitment to adequate counselling resources. This principle has been recognized in the CSHD and by others offering the procedure. One conclusion is that "counselling must be regarded as an integral part of the testing procedure, and in its absence testing would fall short of the expected standard of practice" (Harper et al. 1990, 1089).

Recent commentators have focussed upon the necessity for those who develop public policy to be aware that genetic tests must be offered in the context of adequate counselling resources. This is especially true for late-onset disorders, given the special issues involved. Genetic counselling has been an important part of current programs providing predictive testing for Huntington's disease in Canada and elsewhere. But "there are three obstacles to the appropriate proliferation of genetic tests once their validity is demonstrated: (1) an insufficient number of health care professionals ready to use them, (2) inadequate training of those who are likely to provide genetic services as they expand, and (3) gaps in our knowledge of how to communicate probabilistic information and how people make decisions regarding genetic risks" (Holtzman 1988, 627).

The disparity between the increasing sophistication of technologies involved in prenatal diagnosis and the knowledge base of those seeking services has implications. It raises questions about introducing such procedures without developing appropriate approaches in such areas as education. It may be argued that such a disparity has always existed in medicine. However, it may become less acceptable given the recent shift toward greater autonomy for consumers of health care services.

Genetic Counselling and Fully Informed Choice

Quality, in-depth counselling is required to ensure fully informed choice, focussing on the role of the counsellor to provide information about risk factors and explore issues surrounding competing ethical claims (e.g., related to the predictive testing of children for late-onset disorders). Some authors have raised the related issue of a perceived inadequacy of current genetic counselling approaches to provide detailed information about the condition and about options other than termination (Asch 1989; Henifin et al. 1989). In the current Canadian context of predictive testing for Huntington's disease, this is a less pressing issue because individuals who seek the service are often actively involved in care for an affected parent, and are generally well informed. The situation may change if screening for late-onset disorders becomes more widely available.

Genetic counselling should include information about services and support groups for individuals with specific disabilities as well as entitlement to and the availability of financial assistance. Concern has been raised that the current context of genetic counselling itself is biased in favour of termination in cases of prenatally diagnosed disability, a situation that reflects and reinforces negative social attitudes toward disabled persons (Rothman 1986; Clarke 1991). This viewpoint raises questions about the possibility of prenatal screening contributing, if inadvertently, to a long-term decrease in a social willingness to provide support for disabled persons.

In light of the complexity of technical issues involved in the marker analysis for Huntington's disease (and any disorders requiring this technology in the future), the dilemmas associated with the late onset of symptoms, and the more subtle potential for contributing to a negative shift in social attitudes toward disabled persons, reassessment of what is needed in the counselling process is in order. CSHD may serve as a model, with its emphasis on in-depth pre-test exploration of motivation for testing and the ethical issues mentioned above.

Social Attitudes Toward Disabled Persons

Concerns that genetic screening will contribute to a decreasing social tolerance of disability and individual difference have been voiced in the popular media (Canadian Broadcasting Corporation 1991) and in the academic literature (Lippman 1991; Asch 1989; Hubbard 1990; Henifin et al. 1989). One commentator states: "prenatal diagnosis presupposes that certain fetal conditions are intrinsically not bearable. Increasing diagnostic capability means that such conditions, as well as a host of variations that can be detected *in utero*, are proliferating, necessarily broadening the range of what is not 'bearable' and restricting concepts of what is 'normal.' It is, perhaps, not unreasonable to ask if the 'imperfect' will become anything we can diagnose" (Lippman 1991, 25).

Central to such a view is the perception that technology, once developed, creates pressure for its own use. The ability to screen for genetic disability places a pressure upon women to use this technology. Critics argue that this is particularly true in a society in which resources for long-term support of the disabled are limited. Basically, the question being asked is, will one effect of the ability to diagnose disability prenatally be to reduce the willingness of society to provide support for disabled individuals, focussing instead on a strategy of prevention through genetic screening and abortion? Also of concern is whether insurers and employers have the right of access to genetic information. If women's decisions regarding genetic testing are to be made in the context of inadequate support for disabled individuals and systematic discrimination by insurers and employers against individuals at risk for late-onset disorders such as Huntington's disease, can such decisions be construed as fully informed, free choice?

The concern articulated by these observers is that one overall effect of prenatal diagnosis (along with other reproductive technologies) is to attribute the responsibility for disability to individual women, simultaneously minimizing the responsibility of a humane society to care for its disabled members. It has been argued that one element of disability is socially constructed. Whether or not a genetic condition is seen as a disability is determined, in part, by society's response to it. This may seem less obvious in the case of Huntington's disease, with its loss of cognitive and physical control. However, some observers have noted that the degree of anxiety about the future development of a disorder relates to the perceived treatment of the affected parent (Wexler 1979). The related question is whether the perceived degree of social support available to those who do develop symptoms will influence reproductive decisions.

One obvious conclusion is that prenatal predictive testing for late-onset disorders, like prenatal diagnosis generally, takes place within a context of social interrelationship. Attempts to develop ethically defensible policies must take this into account. One of the espoused goals of genetic counselling is to increase reproductive options. Critics would say that, as prenatal diagnosis becomes common, it will not be unrealistic to propose a scenario wherein society does not provide adequate support for disabled persons, looks with disfavour upon someone who knowingly gives birth to a disabled child, discriminates against those at risk for a late-onset disorder with respect to insurance and employment, and yet says, "We'll give you information that your child will be disabled, but it's your free choice what to do." Critics argue that freedom in this context would be illusory.

There would seem to be some validity to these concerns, particularly in light of individuals writing in the area of law and medicine who have argued that there are ethical and legal grounds for mandatory genetic screening and for women to be criminally charged for failing to obtain it if they belong to a designated high-risk group. Arguments have referred both to the welfare of the affected fetus and to the general welfare of society.

Legal Aspects

Some commentators have argued that a woman has a legal and moral duty to bring her child into the world as healthy as is reasonably possible. For example, Robertson thinks prenatal screening to be a moral obligation and suggests it should be demanded by statute, with criminal penalties for women who fail to obtain it (Robertson 1983). This is contrary to the stance of geneticists.

With specific reference to pre-symptomatic testing for Huntington's disease, Margery Shaw says, "Knowingly, capriciously, or negligently transmitting a defective gene that causes pain and suffering and an agonizing death to an offspring is certainly a moral wrong if not a legal harm" (Shaw 1987b, 245). This therefore points out a danger of coercion that must be guarded against.

Legal approaches to this question have generally taken the forms of wrongful birth and wrongful life torts. Wrongful birth refers to actions initiated by parents of a child born with a disability against clinicians who are claimed to have been negligent in providing available prenatal diagnosis to members of an at-risk group. In such actions it is claimed that if prenatal diagnosis had been made available, pregnancy would have been terminated. American courts have found in favour of plaintiffs in a number of cases, usually awarding costs above those of raising a non-disabled child and, in some cases, damages for psychological trauma to parents (*Curlender v. Bio Science Laboratories* 1981; *Naccash v. Burger* 1982; *Karlsons v. Guerinot* 1977).

Wrongful life actions are brought by parents on behalf of their children against physicians for bringing them into the world, thereby causing the suffering related to their disability. Such actions are grounded in the claims that wrongful life is worse than no life at all. To date, courts in the United States have been generally unwilling to make this judgment. The existence of such actions does, however, introduce a troubling conceptual framework.

Although American judicial precedent does not determine Canadian common law judgments, the reasoning of American courts may influence Canadian decisions. As such, the opinion of the court in *Curlender v. Bio Science Laboratories* is of note in that it refers also to possible limitations to parental prerogative in reproductive decision making:

> If a case arose where, despite due care by the medical profession in transmitting the necessary warnings, parents made a conscious choice to proceed with a pregnancy, with full knowledge that a seriously impaired infant would be born ... we see no sound public policy which should protect those parents from being answerable for the pain,

> suffering and misery which they have wrought upon their offspring. (*Curlender v. Bio Science Laboratories* 1981, 488)

Legal arguments made in this case judgment and expressed in the legal journals by individuals such as Shaw and Robertson have referred to the suffering inflicted by parents who pass on a deleterious gene. However, arguments in favour of mandatory genetic screening have also made claims on behalf of the proposed common good. These arguments, though the exception and with little support, are more troubling, having clearly eugenic intent. For example, George P. Smith II in *Genetics, Ethics and the Law* states that:

> Societal problems such as population control, the cost of supporting the handicapped, and the general welfare of the population favor the trend toward mandatory genetic screening ... The state's interest in improving the quality of a population's genetic pool in order to minimize suffering, to reduce the number of economically dependent persons, and possibly, to save mankind from extinction arguably justifies the infringement of individuals' civil liberties. (Smith 1981, 19)

Margery Shaw makes a similar argument with specific reference to Huntington's disease. Leaders of the CSHD have strenuously disagreed with such a position, saying that the major goal of pre-clinical detection of Huntington's disease is to improve the quality of life for at-risk persons (Hayden et al. 1987).

The potential of a eugenic ideology developing should be actively and vigorously resisted, particularly arguments such as Smith's that are based in part upon economic considerations. The best defence against this possibility is an informed and aware public.

To summarize the second level of ethical discourse on prenatal diagnosis and predictive testing: There are concerns that there may be increasing pressure, including economic pressure, to limit reproductive freedom. The overwhelming preponderance of ethicists, geneticists, lawyers, and the public are strongly opposed to such a trend. However, it is important to continue to be aware of and vigilant against this possibility.

Discussion

This report has taken the view that there are essentially two levels of discourse that must be addressed when considering predictive testing for Huntington's disease in the context of current developments in reproductive and genetic technologies. Although this distinction is somewhat arbitrary, as the many dilemmas encountered are multidimensional and call for responses at many different levels, it does facilitate consideration of very complex issues.

The first level of discourse concerns itself with questions related to what might be called the internal structures defining the interactions between the participants in the counselling situation itself. Discourse at this level accepts implicitly that prenatal diagnosis is an appropriate endeavour, and it is addressed to the structuring of relationships within this context. As such, it refers to the traditional principles of medical ethics such as autonomy, beneficence, confidentiality, and justice. Resolution of ethical dilemmas within this framework consists of mediation of conflicting rights claims through a process that attempts to weigh proportionately the relevance of the various ethical principles operant in each individual case.

However, when reference is made to individuals outside the counselling situation itself, such reference also pertains to competing rights claims such as fiduciary or non-fiduciary claims of third parties. Even referral to a proposed common good, such as that of Smith (1981, 19) in support of mandatory screening, conceives of the common good as the collected individual rights claims of other individuals in society. This differs, it would appear, from a classical common good approach in which the structures defining individual interrelationships emerge from an analysis of the cooperative enterprises of the collective. Classically, the responsibilities implied for the individual are correlative to participation in the common good.

In this report, discussion at the first level was focussed upon essentially two issues: (1) prenatal testing for individuals who did not want termination in the case of an increased risk estimate; and (2) claims of third parties to have access to predictive testing results or to determine whether or not testing should be done. The other important issue that underlay these discussions was the ethical imperative to provide in-depth counselling because of complexities in prenatal predictive testing for a late-onset disorder using marker analysis. Certain of the ethical dilemmas reported in the literature were not discussed because they have not been contested in the literature and are not unique to the mandate of the Royal Commission on New Reproductive Technologies; that is, they are common to many medical situations and resolved in an unproblematic fashion through recourse to traditional ethical approaches (see Huggins et al. 1990).

Perceived conflict surrounded the CSHD policy of refusal to perform prenatal predictive testing for individuals for whom termination of the pregnancy was not an option. Central to the debate is the treatment of parents as third parties. The initial reasoning for the position of the CSHD was presented with respect to the testing of minor children, and, by analogy, to the prenatal situation. The competing rights claims in this case were the primacy of the autonomy of children versus parental autonomy and the right of parents to make decisions regarding their minor children. It was proposed that how this should be resolved is still unclear.

Of note in this situation is the resolution of the majority of such situations through counselling (Bloch and Hayden 1990). The counselling alternative, compared to a process of mediating rights claims, clarifies coexisting fundamental values, permitting a resolution that arises out of the experience of the participants in the dialogue rather than being imposed by referral to a third party.

Heavy emphasis in counselling on what might be called value clarification may provide a model for the resolution of related issues in testing for other late-onset disorders. The need for in-depth counselling was also described with respect to fully informed choice. The situation involving exclusion testing raised the issue most explicitly. It was proposed that the difficulties encountered may indicate an increased requirement for counselling resources for disorders assessed by marker analysis.

The final issue in the first level of discourse, that of third-party claims, has been conceived of as a conflict between the principles of autonomy and beneficence. The claims of individuals' rights to autonomy and confidentiality, concretized in the right to refuse testing, are seen to be in conflict with the fiduciary and non-fiduciary claims of third parties for information valuable to themselves.

The CSHD has strongly defended individual autonomy and has been supported by the IHA and WFN. An international survey of geneticists (Wertz and Fletcher 1989) found almost unanimous consensus against third-party (non-fiduciary) access without individuals' consent (100 percent in Canada). Almost half of the geneticists (46 percent) said there should be no third-party access at all. Consensus was not as strong in cases of claims of spouses and relatives.

Wertz and Fletcher suggest that, as institutions have the economic power to force consent, regulations should be introduced to prevent institutional third parties from access to test results, even with consent, unless access would benefit the individual. Even this exception raises the possibility of employers having access to information about individuals' susceptibility to workplace hazards, with subsequent decreased motivation to reduce the hazards themselves. Therefore, the issue of access to genetic information remains one of the major ethical issues to be considered at this time.

The second section of the report was concerned with broader social issues of the relationship of prenatal diagnosis (including prenatal predictive testing for Huntington's disease) to general social reality. Concerns expressed in this area included the long-term effect of the development of the technology on social attitudes toward women, disabled persons, and children, and the effect of reproductive technology on society in general. Although the issue does not specifically relate to prenatal testing for late-onset disorders, the well-articulated and strong concerns of such commentators should be addressed by those developing such programs.

The concerns expressed in the second section appear to represent a radically different conceptual grounding than those in the first section. These concerns are not expressed primarily with reference to conflicting rights claims but rather appear to be grounded in an awareness of the complex system of relationships that characterize any society and the perception that developments in one part of the social system necessarily have an impact on the whole system. As such, the reservations expressed by authors in this section do not have as their object the individual right of access to doable technology. Instead, the object of concern is how the development of reproductive technology may contribute to or detract from the common good.

The different conceptual framework and analytical agenda underlying the concerns of the critics of the technology determine the fundamental unit of inquiry from this perspective as a multiplicity of relationships that cannot be dissociated. One commentator states that the "disjunction" between individual and social agendas "underscores the need to avoid premature closure of discussion and to avoid reducing it to sterile debates between 'pros' and 'cons' ... [since this] ... decontextualizes these technologies, severing their essential relatedness to time and place and isolating them from the broader health and social policy agenda of which they are a part" (Lippman 1991, 48-49).

Also part of the concerns of this constituency is the recognition that previous technological developments in the medical field and elsewhere have had unpredicted and very negative consequences. There is growing recognition that the introduction of new technology results in often radical changes to society by fundamentally changing the structures that define the interrelationships between individuals and between individuals and the technology. In the 1989 Massey Lectures entitled *The Real World of Technology*, Ursula Franklin comments on the unintended consequences of certain recent technological development as follows:

> What turns the promised liberation into enslavement are not the products of technology *per se* ... but the structures and infrastructures that are put in place to facilitate the use of these products and to develop dependency on them.

And further,

> Once a given technology is widely accepted and standardized, the relationship between the products of the technology and the users changes. Users have less scope, they matter less, and their needs are no longer the main concern of the designers. There is, then, a discernable pattern in the social and political growth of a technology that does not depend on the particular technical features of the system in question. (Franklin 1990, 102)

Two perceptions are central to the position of those expressing concern about the development of reproductive technology, including prenatal diagnosis. First, the introduction of new technology has historically had unintended, often negative social effects. Second, adequate analysis of the desirability of developing this particular technology must entail attempts to determine whether its introduction will nurture or erode the previously evolved structures that support health care and other social systems. The recognition that these broader social concerns may at times exist in tension with individual concern is implicit in this position.

What are the implications of the introduction of these concerns into the discussion currently taking place? This latter conceptual framework has affinity to what has been proposed earlier as a classical common good approach, both in the basic perspective it adopts and because it is grounded in discussions of subtle and not easily accessible systems of relationships between different social structures and attempts to determine how developments in one area effect changes to other structures.

Resolution of radically different issues raised by such a position presents serious difficulties. Serious consideration of such a perspective would, in an ideal world, include analysis of existing and potential structures for approaching public consensus on general conceptions of the public good. Minimally, policy decisions relating to the development of technologies such as prenatal diagnosis should be made with adequate public input. One suggestion has been that such discourse may profitably follow models taken from current theory of conflict resolution (Melchin 1993). The issue of public input also raises concrete questions for policy makers. There exists in the literature a radical divergence of opinion regarding who should make which decisions about what technology is researched and developed.

One pole in this discussion is the following:

> In the final analysis, the private researcher charts the course of scientific investigation. He will determine the balance between freedom of scientific inquiry and concepts of what is socially good; he will determine whether his research should be totally utilitarian, providing the greatest good to the greatest number even if it may compromise the rights of some individuals, and how his research should accommodate the competing interests of each subgroup in society. (Smith 1981, 133)

At the opposite pole is the following:

> For science and technology to be useful and responsive to people's needs, scientists, along with everyone else, will have to recognize that science is no more immune from ideological commitments than are other human activities and that we therefore need better and more democratic mechanisms than we now have to decide what science needs to be done and how best to do it. (Hubbard 1990, 211)

One area of future government activity might be development of concrete structures to ensure input into decision making from those that are affected by technological developments.

A second issue that relates to genetic testing generally is the issue of wrongful birth suits. Recognition of such claims would dangerously affect the concept of free choice as expressed through the choice to refuse to be tested. Therefore, this issue is worthy of legislative consideration.

Third, given that technologies are not introduced in a social vacuum, the increasing sophistication of reproductive and genetic technology may necessitate reevaluation of current educational approaches, both for those offering the service and, more generally, in the public education system.

One area of consideration is how the education system might better prepare its consumers to deal with the increasingly demanding ethical and social issues. This could affect the issue of fully informed choice on the individual level and would provide a basis, in the long term, for more creative public input into the decision-making process.

Fourth, any serious consideration of the issue of the effects of reproductive technology on people with disabilities necessarily implies a consideration of resource allocation questions. This is particularly true with respect to prenatal testing for a disorder such as Huntington's disease, which results in significant need for institutional care. The attractiveness of preventing, by selective abortion, disabilities that require long-term care may increase. The possible negative effects of such a development on social attitudes toward persons with disabilities who place a great financial burden on the health care system must be considered in this context, and any decrease in reproductive choice, or coercion in that regard, will need guarding against. It is important that in allocating funding, the needs of affected persons are taken into account, not just the development of diagnostic technologies.

Conclusions

The first level of discourse is concerned with the question, how should we administer this technology? Central to the discussion in this area is the ethical principle of individual autonomy, and approaches have generally attempted to maximize individual autonomy. The second level of discourse centres upon the question, should we be using this technology at all? Discussion at this level is concerned more with long-term social consequences. Therefore, the discussion adopts a different perspective more concerned with questions of the common good.

There exists, given the coexistence of these two perspectives, a tension between individual and public claims. A discourse of rights seems inadequate to resolve this tension and there is, therefore, a need to develop structures that will contribute to consensus regarding the desirability of developing genetic screening programs.

Within the first level of discourse, there exists a need for measures that protect the principle of fully informed free choice. These may include legislative protection from third-party claims, reassessment of genetic counselling approaches, and increased public education regarding the technological developments being introduced and the available reproductive options.

Current ethical imperative, therefore, may include a continual process of reassessment of current services and a structured assessment process (the second level) to be applied to newly developing technologies, a process that includes public input at the decision-making level.

Given the existence of two levels of ethical issues, policy response may need to be made on more than one level. In the context of service delivery, interventions should attempt to ensure that individuals are presented with this service in an environment that fully protects their freedom to choose to use or not use the technology. At the level of social policy, structures should be developed that facilitate public discourse and foster consensus, and that attempt to ensure that further developments in the area of genetic screening contribute in a positive way to the developing social context.

To quote Daniel Callahan,

> Medical technologies should not be publicly or professionally sanctioned unless they can be shown to be significantly efficacious in achieving their intended goals, cost effective in their dissemination, and beneficial in their long-term medical, social, and cultural consequences. (Callahan 1990, 191-92)

Although it may be argued that such a process is impractical and expensive, if we are to continue to be a caring and free society, we cannot afford to neglect this.

Bibliography

Asch, A. 1989. "Reproductive Technology and Disability." In *Reproductive Laws for the 1990s*, ed. S. Cohen and N. Taub. Clifton: Humana Press.

Becker, C. 1988. "Legal Implications of the G-8 Huntington's Disease Genetic Marker." *Case Western Reserve Law Review* 39: 273-305.

Bloch, M., and M.R. Hayden. 1990. "Opinion: Predictive Testing for Huntington Disease in Childhood: Challenges and Implications." *American Journal of Human Genetics* 46: 1-4.

Bowen v. American Hospital Association, 476 U.S. 610 (1986).

Brandt, J., et al. 1989. "Presymptomatic Diagnosis of Delayed-Onset Disease with Linked DNA Markers: The Experience in Huntington's Disease." *JAMA* 261: 3108-14.

Callahan, D. 1990. *What Kind of Life: The Limits of Medical Progress*. New York: Simon and Schuster.

Canadian Broadcasting Corporation. 1991. "CBC Ideas: Technologizing Reproduction." Toronto: CBC.

Clarke, A. 1991. "Is Non-Directive Genetic Counselling Possible?" *Lancet* (19 October): 998-1001.

Cohen, S., and N. Taub, eds. 1989. *Reproductive Laws for the 1990s*. Clifton: Humana Press.

Curlender v. Bio Science Laboratories, App., 165 Cal. Rptr. 477 (1981).

Destro, R.A. 1986. "Quality of Life Ethics and Constitutional Jurisprudence: The Demise of Natural Rights and Equal Protection for the Disabled and Incompetent." *Journal of Contemporary Health Law and Policy* 2: 71-130.

Franklin, U.M. 1990. *The Real World of Technology* (CBC Massey Lecture Series). Toronto: CBC Enterprises.

Gusella, J.F., et al. 1983. "A Polymorphic DNA Marker Genetically Linked to Huntington's Disease." *Nature* 306: 234-38.

Harper, P., M.J. Morris, and A. Tyler. 1990. "Genetic Testing for Huntington's Disease: Internationally Agreed Guidelines Are Being Followed." *British Medical Journal* 300: 1089-90.

Hayden, M., et al. 1987. "Ethical Issues in Preclinical Testing in Huntington Disease: Response to Margery Shaw's Invited Editorial Comment." *American Journal of Medical Genetics* 28: 761-63.

Henifin, M.S., R. Hubbard, and J. Norsigian. 1989. "Position Paper: Prenatal Screening." In *Reproductive Laws for the 1990s*, ed. S. Cohen and N. Taub. Clifton: Humana Press.

Holtzman, N.A. 1988. "Recombinant DNA Technology, Genetic Tests, and Public Policy." *American Journal of Human Genetics* 42: 624-32.

Hubbard, R. 1990. *The Politics of Women's Biology*. New Brunswick: Rutgers University Press.

Huggins, M., et al. 1990. "Ethical and Legal Dilemmas Arising During Predictive Testing for Adult-Onset Disease: The Experience of Huntington Disease." *American Journal of Human Genetics* 47: 4-12.

Karlsons v. Guerinot, 57 AD. 2d 73, 394; N.Y.S. 2d 933 (N.Y. App. Div. 1977).

Kessler, S., et al. 1987. "Attitudes of Persons at Risk for Huntington Disease Toward Predictive Testing." *American Journal of Medical Genetics* 26: 259-70.

Lamport, A.T. 1987. "Presymptomatic Testing for Huntington Chorea: Ethical and Legal Issues." *American Journal of Medical Genetics* 26: 307-14.

Lippman, A. 1991. "Prenatal Testing and Screening: Constructing Needs and Reinforcing Inequities." *American Journal of Law and Medicine* 17: 15-50.

Meissen, G.J., and R.L. Berchek. 1987. "Intended Use of Predictive Testing by Those at Risk for Huntington Disease." *American Journal of Medical Genetics* 26: 283-93.

Melchin, K. 1993. "Pluralism, Conflict and the Structure of the Public Good." In *The Ensuing Conscience: Critical Responses to the Work of Charles Davis*, ed. M. Lalonde. (Unpublished.)

Naccash v. Burger, 223 Va. 406, 290 S.E. 2d 825 (1982).

Pelias, M. 1991. "Duty to Disclose in Medical Genetics: A Legal Perspective." *American Journal of Medical Genetics* 39: 347-54.

Re Infant Doe, No. GU, 8204-00 (Cir. Ct. Monroe County, Ind., Apr. 12, 1982).

Robertson, J.A. 1983. "Procreative Liberty and the Control of Conception, Pregnancy and Childbirth." *Virginia Law Review* 69: 405-64.

Rothman, B.K. 1986. *The Tentative Pregnancy: Prenatal Diagnosis and the Future of Motherhood.* New York: Penguin Books.

Shaw, M. 1987a. "Response to Hayden, Bloch, Fox and Crauford: Presymptomatic and Prenatal Testing in Huntington Disease." *American Journal of Medical Genetics* 28: 765-66.

—. 1987b. "Testing for the Huntington Gene: A Right to Know, a Right Not to Know, or a Duty to Know." *American Journal of Medical Genetics* 26: 243-46.

Smith, G.P., II. 1981. *Genetics, Ethics and the Law.* Gaithersburg: Associated Faculty Press.

Smurl, J.F., and D.D. Weaver. 1987. "Presymptomatic Testing for Huntington Chorea: Guidelines for Moral and Social Accountability." *American Journal of Medical Genetics* 26: 247-57.

Tyler, A., and M. Morris. 1990. "National Symposium on Problems of Presymptomatic Testing for Huntington's Disease, Cardiff." *Journal of Medical Ethics* 16: 41-42.

Tyler, A., et al. 1990. "Exclusion Testing in Pregnancy for Huntington's Disease." *Journal of Medical Genetics* 27: 488-95.

Wasmuth, J.J., et al. 1988. "A Highly Polymorphic Locus Very Tightly Linked to the Huntington's Disease Gene." *Nature* 332: 734-36.

Went, L. 1990. "Ethical Issues Policy Statement on Huntington's Disease Molecular Genetics Predictive Test." *Journal of Medical Genetics* 27: 34-38.

Wertz, D.D., and J.C. Fletcher. 1989. "Ethics and Genetics: An International Survey." *Hastings Center Report* 19 (July-August, Special Suppl.): 20-24.

Wexler, N.S. 1979. "Genetic 'Russian Roulette': The Experience of Being 'At Risk' for Huntington's Disease." In *Genetic Counseling: Psychological Dimensions,* ed. S. Kessler. New York: Academic Press.

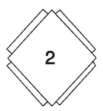

Prenatal Testing
for Huntington Disease:
Psychosocial Aspects

Shelin Adam and Michael R. Hayden

Executive Summary

Adult predictive and prenatal testing programs for Huntington disease have been available in Canada since 1986. However, the extent of the demand for prenatal testing, and the reasons why some people choose not to have the prenatal test for this late-onset disorder, have not been well documented. In addition, the knowledge and attitudes of adult predictive testing candidates and their partners about prenatal testing are not well known, nor are the psychological effects of prenatal testing well understood.

As of September 1991, 425 individuals had entered the Canadian Collaborative Study of Predictive Testing for Huntington Disease and, of these, 47 individuals or their partners had become pregnant. Of this group, 14 couples (30%) requested prenatal testing, 24 couples (51%) did not want prenatal testing, and 9 at-risk individuals (19%) had already received a decreased risk through adult predictive testing and therefore were not eligible for the prenatal test. Of the 14 couples who initially requested prenatal testing, 7 withdrew. Thus, demand for the prenatal test by eligible candidates was 7/38 or 18%, which is much lower than the 32-65% expected on the basis of early survey data.

This paper was completed for the Royal Commission on New Reproductive Technologies in May 1992.

The most frequently cited reason for declining prenatal testing was the hope that a cure would be found in time for their children. While the majority of adult predictive testing candidates (71%) in our study had accurate information about definitive prenatal testing, many (63%) did not have a correct understanding of exclusion prenatal testing. Although no serious adverse events such as suicide planning or psychiatric hospitalization have occurred, a particular need for careful counselling was identified for those at-risk candidates and their partners who have one prenatal test and feel compelled to use the test again in future pregnancies. Even though prenatal testing for Huntington disease is not requested as often as originally expected, it still remains a desired option for some at-risk persons and their partners.

Introduction

The identification of closely linked deoxyribonucleic acid (DNA) restriction fragment-length polymorphisms has made both adult predictive and prenatal testing possible for many adult-onset disorders, including polycystic disease of kidneys (Reeders et al. 1985), familial Alzheimer's disease (Goate et al. 1991), familial Creutzfeldt-Jakob disease, and Huntington disease (Collinge et al. 1991; Gusella et al. 1983; Wasmuth et al. 1988). However, although adult predictive testing for Huntington disease has received international attention in the last few years, little is known about the acceptability and demand for prenatal testing. In addition, the factors influencing the decision to use prenatal testing for this currently incurable, adult-onset disorder are not well understood.

Prenatal testing for Huntington disease can be offered in various ways (Fahy et al. 1989). "Exclusion" prenatal testing is possible when the at-risk parent is at 50% risk for Huntington disease and either does not wish to or is unable to determine his or her personal risk for the disease. Such testing allows the risk of the fetus (25%) to be changed to either very low (i.e., excluded) or approximately 50% (i.e., the same as the at-risk parent), depending on which of the grandparents' chromosomes the fetus has inherited. "Definitive" prenatal testing is available for a parent affected with Huntington disease or identified, through predictive testing, as being at increased risk. Using this approach, the risk of the fetus is altered from approximately 50% to very high (approximately 96%) or very low (2% or 3%). The final option is a stepwise combination of these two approaches, or "exclusion-definitive" testing. The first step of the prenatal test is exclusion testing. If the fetus is found to be at low risk (i.e., excluded), no further testing is necessary. However, if the fetus is found to have a risk similar to that of the at-risk parent (i.e., approximately 50%), the next step is to perform adult predictive testing on the parent to determine the status of that parent and thus the risk of the fetus.

Before predictive or prenatal testing became widely available, four U.S. studies surveyed the attitudes of individuals at 50% risk for Huntington disease (Markel et al. 1987; Meissen and Berchek 1987; Kessler et al. 1987; Mastromauro et al. 1987) toward adult predictive and prenatal testing. Between 32% and 65% of those at risk indicated they would use or would have used prenatal testing if it were or had been available. However, it is difficult to use these studies to judge the demand for prenatal testing, as many of those surveyed were beyond childbearing age or had already completed their families. In each study more people indicated they would use predictive testing than those who said they would use prenatal testing.

Studies of participants in prenatal testing for Huntington disease are few and generally limited to case reports (Hayden et al. 1987; Quarrell et al. 1987; Millan et al. 1989; Spurdle et al. 1991). There have been two reports on the low uptake of this technology. Craufurd et al. (1989) reported that although 81% of their 109 candidates indicated they would request prenatal testing if pregnant, exclusion tests were done for only 3 couples, in contrast to 33 adult predictive tests performed. Unfortunately, the authors did not report how many of the candidates became pregnant and chose not to use prenatal testing. Tyler et al. (1990) offered only exclusion prenatal testing and not adult predictive testing at the outset of their program. Of the 90 couples referred to their centre over three years, 15 participated in prenatal testing. However, from this study the demand for prenatal testing is difficult to estimate because some people who chose prenatal testing might have used adult predictive testing first (if it had been available) to determine whether prenatal testing was necessary. A low-risk adult predictive testing result would have obviated the need for prenatal testing.

In this study, we report on our experience with prenatal testing in the Canadian Collaborative Study of Predictive Testing for Huntington Disease. This study is particularly suited to look at the demand for prenatal testing, because of its large size and because, unlike some other centres, both prenatal and predictive testing for Huntington disease were offered from the outset of the program. The purpose of this study was to assess the demand for prenatal testing for Huntington disease in Canada and to learn some of the reasons why at-risk individuals chose to use prenatal testing or not. As of September 1991, 425 people had entered the program (Figure 1). Forty-seven of these individuals or their partners had become pregnant. Nine of them had previously received a decreased risk assessment through adult predictive testing and thus were ineligible for prenatal testing. Of the remaining 38 couples, 14 (37%) requested prenatal testing; 24 (63%) declined.

The results of psychosocial assessment for participants in prenatal testing are provided in this study. Prenatal testing has not led to any serious adverse outcomes, and the indices of psychological functioning throughout the follow-up period have been similar to those at baseline. To learn more about the factors distinguishing those who chose to use prenatal testing from those who did not, we assessed the two groups using questionnaires and personal interviews.

Methods

Patients and Questionnaires

Predictive and prenatal testing for Huntington disease began in British Columbia in 1986 and became available across Canada in 1988. At-risk individuals were notified about the program through the Huntington Society of Canada newsletter, various media sources such as television and newspapers, and letters sent to at-risk people known to the local genetics centre.

At the first session, all candidates requesting adult predictive testing completed a questionnaire assessing their attitudes toward predictive and prenatal testing. Knowledge of prenatal testing was assessed by five true or false questions (Table 1a-e). Attitudes of predictive testing candidates toward prenatal testing were assessed by asking: "If you or your spouse were pregnant, would you use prenatal testing?" The options for response were "yes," "no," and "uncertain" (Table 2). A second question asked if the results of the prenatal test showed that the fetus probably had the gene for Huntington disease, would the reader complete the pregnancy, would she terminate it, or was she uncertain as to what she would do (Table 3). Responses to these questions were subdivided into three age categories — less than 30 years of age, between 30 and 40 years, and greater than 40 years. Differences in responses between the two sexes were also analyzed.

A separate questionnaire was later developed and sent by mail to the 24 people who were eligible for, but chose not to have, a prenatal test. This questionnaire addressed issues such as the number and outcome of pregnancies they had had while participating in the program, their current risk status, and their attitudes toward pregnancy termination. Candidates were asked to select up to five reasons for not choosing prenatal testing (Table 9). A similar questionnaire was sent to the partners of the at-risk candidates.

Psychosocial Assessment

All candidates for predictive and prenatal testing participated in a protocol of psychosocial assessment and pre- and post-test counselling. The assessment consisted of an extensive battery of demographic and psychosocial questionnaires used to assess current psychological status. Two instruments were selected for measurement purposes. The General Severity Index (GSI) of the Symptom Checklist 90-R (SCL 90(R)) measures the general level of psychiatric distress (Derogatis 1977). This test has been standardized on a general adult population and has a mean of 50 and a standard deviation of 10. A second instrument, the Beck Depression Inventory, measures depression (Beck et al. 1961). A score above 10 on this scale is considered to be indicative of a clinical depression.

Statistical Analysis

Chi-squared analyses (for categorial variables) and t-tests (for continuous variables) were used to determine whether there were any differences on baseline demographic variables between the groups requesting and not requesting prenatal testing. Chi-squared tests were also used to determine whether predictive testing participants responded differently according to their age and sex about their attitudes toward prenatal testing and termination of pregnancy. One-way analysis of variance (ANOVA) or a non-parametric equivalent (Kruskall-Wallis test) and t-tests were used to test for differences in psychological distress and depression at baseline and follow-up points between participants who received a modification of risk (increased or decreased) in adult predictive testing, and those who received prenatal testing results. Difference scores (i.e., follow-up score minus baseline score) were used in the analysis of follow-up data. For all analyses, 0.05 was set as the criterion for statistical significance.

DNA Analysis

Blood samples were taken from each couple and other available relatives. DNA was extracted and digested with appropriate restriction enzymes. A maximum of 13 restriction fragment-length polymorphisms was used to determine the informativeness of the test. Where possible, the analysis was done before the pregnancy occurred.

Prenatal Procedures

When a prenatal test was requested, transcervical chorion villus biopsy was used to obtain fetal DNA samples at 9 to 11 weeks of gestation. If termination of the pregnancy was indicated and requested, the pregnancy termination was done by curettage as soon as possible.

Results

Knowledge of Participants About and Attitudes Toward Prenatal Testing

The knowledge of the large group in the program regarding general aspects of prenatal testing when they entered the program was assessed as good (Table 1). Of the 400 who responded, 285 (71%) understood how definitive testing was performed and 315 (79%) were aware that exclusion testing was available. However, only 149 of 400 (37%) understood that it was not necessary to determine the risk of the parent to do exclusion testing for the fetus. Little difference was found between the two sexes or the three age groups with respect to these questions. However, only 18 of 75 (24%) women more than 40 years of age understood exclusion testing, while 16 of 45 (36%) men in the same age group and 38 of 74 (51%) women younger than age 30 answered this question correctly.

Regarding attitude, 169 of the 390 (43%) respondents to the questionnaire in the first session indicated that they would use prenatal testing if they or their spouse were pregnant (Table 2). There was a significant difference in the response to this question depending on the age of the participant (p = 0.002). This was primarily due to different attitudes expressed by women over 40 years of age, who were more likely to choose prenatal testing than younger women. No significant differences were seen in men of different ages.

Sixty-seven (40%) of 167 respondents who said they would use prenatal testing said they would definitely terminate the pregnancy if the test showed an increased risk for the fetus. Forty-one of 167 (25%) said they would complete the pregnancy and 50 of 167 (35%) were uncertain (Table 3). These responses were significantly different depending on the age of the participant (p = 0.002). Only 6 (16%) participants under the age of 30 said they would terminate a fetus at increased risk, while a much larger proportion of persons over age 30 would choose to terminate the pregnancy. There were no differences based on the sex of the participant. Most of the participants over 40 years of age who stated they were likely to use prenatal testing already had two or more children (Table 4).

Number and Outcome of Pregnancies

In all, 18 prenatal tests were requested by the 14 participants in the prenatal testing program; one person requested three prenatal tests in successive pregnancies and two people requested two prenatal tests each. However, 11 prenatal tests were actually performed for seven couples. Four definitive prenatal tests were performed in which the parent was affected, and one was performed in which the parent was at an increased risk for Huntington disease. Six exclusion tests were performed where the at-risk parent was at 50% risk. The results of these prenatal tests are shown in Table 5. The reasons why the seven other prenatal tests were not done included miscarriage in three pregnancies, termination of pregnancy not accepted as an option in three pregnancies, and one termination for personal reasons irrespective of the prenatal result.

Six out of the seven increased risk pregnancies were terminated. Three couples had had prenatal testing on more than one occasion. One person was affected and requested definitive testing. She had received an increased risk result in the first pregnancy and had terminated that pregnancy. A decreased risk result was given in the second pregnancy but the pregnancy was miscarried. In her third pregnancy a decreased risk result was given and the pregnancy was continued. Another two couples had had two previous pregnancies, both of which had shown an increased risk from an exclusion test and had been terminated. Both couples had a third pregnancy during which neither chose to use prenatal testing.

Psychosocial Assessment for Participants in Prenatal Testing

Psychosocial assessment was available for six of the seven participants in prenatal testing; one refused the follow-up. Their mean scores on the GSI are shown in Table 6. Figure 2 illustrates the comparison of the mean change from the baseline score at each of the follow-up points. All scores are within the normal range, indicating that the group has coped well with prenatal testing regardless of whether the results have shown increased or decreased risk. Comparison of these scores with the mean scores of the participants in adult predictive testing has not revealed any significant differences. However, although the prenatal group shows an increase in psychological distress as measured by the SCL 90(R) from the two-month follow-up to the six-month follow-up, the adult predictive testing group does not exhibit a comparable increase (Figure 2). Similar results are seen using the Beck Depression Inventory and comparing these scores with those of adults who have participated in predictive testing (Table 7). These comparisons are limited due to the small number of individuals in the prenatal testing group.

Individuals Not Eligible for Prenatal Testing

Nine of the 47 participants who became pregnant while in the predictive testing program had received a decreased risk, and therefore prenatal testing was not necessary. When asked about reproductive plans in a questionnaire at the first session, five of the nine indicated that they would not have had (more) children if their risk was increased or if the testing was uninformative, and three indicated that they wanted (more) children regardless of the results of the predictive test. One person did not respond to the question.

Comparison of Attitudes and Sociodemographic Variables of Participants Who Chose Prenatal Testing or Not

Twenty-four participants in the adult predictive testing program who knew about the availability of prenatal testing became pregnant and chose not to use the option. Sociodemographic variables of these individuals were compared with those of the 14 who requested prenatal testing (Table 8). No significant differences were found between the two groups in terms of sex ratio, age, and education level. However, the mean number of children was significantly different (p = 0.02). More individuals who had chosen not to have prenatal testing already had children. The religious practices of the

Figure 1. Demand for Predictive Testing in the Canadian Collaborative Study of Predictive Testing for Huntington Disease

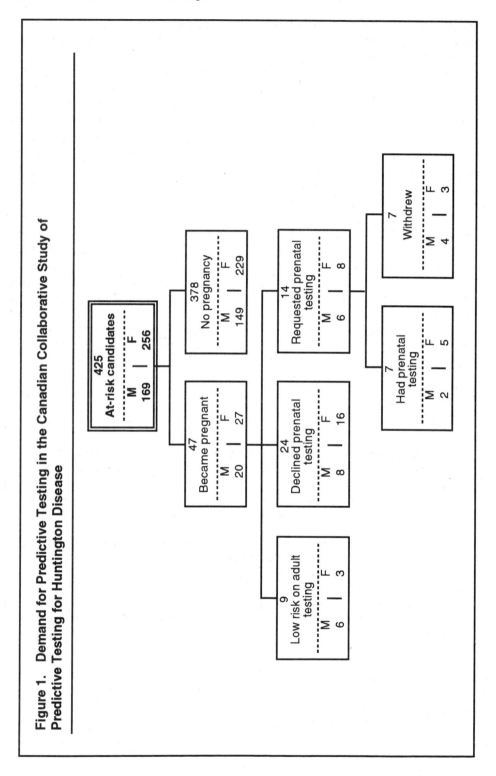

two groups also differed significantly (p = 0.05). More individuals in the group that did not choose prenatal testing indicated that they were practising members of a religious organization.

The 24 candidates were asked to complete a separate questionnaire; their spouses received a similar questionnaire. Seventeen (71%) of the candidate questionnaires and 16 (67%) of the spousal questionnaires were returned. The respondents were representative of the original group of 24 in terms of sex ratio and age. Regarding termination of pregnancy, 3 of 17 respondents answered that termination should not be available under any circumstances; 10 thought that termination should be available only under certain circumstances; and 3 individuals thought that it should be available on demand. One person did not respond.

In indicating their most important reasons for not having prenatal testing, 14 of 17 (82%) candidates stated that they did not have the test because they believed that a cure will be found before their children develop Huntington disease (Table 9). The desire to have a child was greater for 12 of 17 (71%) than the distant threat that the child could someday develop Huntington disease. Seven (41%) had serious concerns about the safety of the prenatal procedure, and the same number also indicated that they wanted to determine their own status before making any decisions about prenatal testing or that they did not consider termination to be an option. Their spouses' reasons for not wanting prenatal testing were similar to those of the at-risk partners; however, in five cases the partner's opposition to prenatal testing was given by the candidate as one of the reasons against prenatal testing.

Table 1a. Responses of Adult Predictive Testing Candidates to Question 1 of Knowledge and Attitudes Questionnaire, by Sex and Age (n = 400)

"If the parents decide that they want to know definitively whether or not the fetus carries the gene for Huntington disease, this means that the at-risk parent must also know his/her status."

| | Age categories | | | | | | |
| | < 30 | | 30-40 | | > 40 | | |
Response	M	F	M	F	M	F	Total
Correct	28	43	50	72	37	55	285
(%)	(71.8)	(58.1)	(69.4)	(75.8)	(82.2)	(72.4)	(71.2)
Incorrect	11	31	22	23	8	20	115
(%)	(28.2)	(41.9)	(30.6)	(24.2)	(17.8)	(27.6)	(28.8)
Total	39	74	72	95	45	76	400
(%)	(100.0)	(100.0)	(100.0)	(100.0)	(100.0)	(100.0)	(100.0)

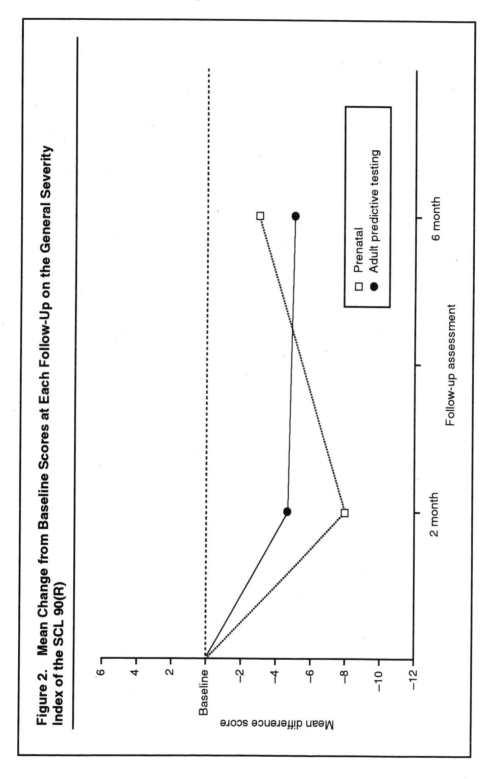

Figure 2. Mean Change from Baseline Scores at Each Follow-Up on the General Severity
Index of the SCL 90(R)

Table 1b. Responses of Adult Predictive Testing Candidates to Question 2 of Knowledge and Attitudes Questionnaire, by Sex and Age (n = 400)

"It is possible to provide information that the fetus is either at a very low risk of having the gene for Huntington disease or at a risk that is approximately the same as that of the at-risk parent."

| | Age categories | | | | | | |
| | < 30 | | 30-40 | | > 40 | | |
Response	M	F	M	F	M	F	Total
Correct	29	58	54	80	35	59	315
(%)	(74.4)	(78.4)	(75.0)	(84.2)	(77.8)	(78.7)	(78.8)
Incorrect	10	31	18	15	10	16	85
(%)	(25.6)	(21.6)	(25.0)	(15.8)	(22.2)	(21.3)	(21.2)
Total	39	74	72	95	45	75	400
(%)	(100.0)	(100.0)	(100.0)	(100.0)	(100.0)	(100.0)	(100.0)

Table 1c. Responses of Adult Predictive Testing Candidates to Question 3 of Knowledge and Attitudes Questionnaire, by Sex and Age (n = 400)

"It is not necessary to establish the Huntington disease status of the at-risk parent to perform exclusion testing."

| | Age categories | | | | | | |
| | < 30 | | 30-40 | | > 40 | | |
Response	M	F	M	F	M	F	Total
Correct	16	38	25	36	16	18	149
(%)	(41.0)	(51.4)	(34.7)	(37.9)	(35.6)	(24.0)	(37.3)
Incorrect	23	36	47	59	29	57	251
(%)	(59.0)	(48.6)	(65.3)	(62.1)	(64.4)	(76.0)	(62.7)
Total	39	74	72	95	45	75	400
(%)	(100.0)	(100.0)	(100.0)	(100.0)	(100.0)	(100.0)	(100.0)

Table 1d. Responses of Adult Predictive Testing Candidates to Question 4 of Knowledge and Attitudes Questionnaire, by Sex and Age (n = 400)

"The results cannot indicate that the fetus has a high risk of inheriting the gene for Huntington disease while the at-risk parent has a low risk."

Response	Age categories						
	< 30		30-40		> 40		
	M	F	M	F	M	F	Total
Correct	34	62	57	85	35	66	339
(%)	(87.2)	(83.8)	(79.2)	(89.5)	(77.8)	(88.0)	(84.8)
Incorrect	5	12	15	10	10	9	61
(%)	(12.8)	(16.2)	(20.8)	(10.5)	(22.2)	(12.0)	(15.2)
Total	39	74	72	95	45	75	400
(%)	(100.0)	(100.0)	(100.0)	(100.0)	(100.0)	(100.0)	(100.0)

Table 1e. Responses of Adult Predictive Testing Candidates to Question 5 of Knowledge and Attitudes Questionnaire, by Sex and Age (n = 400)

"You do not *have* to terminate the pregnancy, if the test results indicate that the fetus probably does have the gene for Huntington disease."

Response	Age categories						
	< 30		30-40		> 40		
	M	F	M	F	M	F	Total
Correct	36	69	70	91	42	66	374
(%)	(92.3)	(93.2)	(97.2)	(95.8)	(93.3)	(88.0)	(93.5)
Incorrect	3	5	2	4	3	9	6
(%)	(7.7)	(6.8)	(2.8)	(4.2)	(6.7)	(12.0)	(6.5)
Total	39	74	72	95	45	75	400
(%)	(100.0)	(100.0)	(100.0)	(100.0)	(100.0)	(100.0)	(100.0)

Table 2. Responses by Age and Sex of Predictive Testing Candidates to the Question "If You or Your Spouse Were Pregnant, Would You Use Prenatal Testing?" (n = 390)

	Age categories			
	< 30	30-40	> 40	Total
All candidates (%)				
Yes	37 (33.6)	73 (44.0)	59 (51.8)	169 (43.3)
No	25 (22.8)	48 (28.9)	15 (13.1)	88 (22.6)
Uncertain	48 (43.6)	45 (27.1)	40 (35.1)	133 (34.1)
Total	110 (100.0)	166 (100.0)	114 (100.0)	390 (100.0)
				p = 0.002
Female candidates (%)				
Yes	24 (33.3)	43 (45.7)	39 (56.5)	106 (45.1)
No	19 (26.4)	28 (29.8)	8 (11.6)	55 (23.4)
Uncertain	29 (40.3)	23 (24.6)	22 (31.9)	74 (31.5)
Total	72 (100.0)	94 (100.0)	69 (100.0)	235 (100.0)
				p = 0.002
Male candidates (%)				
Yes	13 (34.2)	30 (41.7)	20 (44.4)	63 (40.6)
No	6 (15.8)	20 (27.8)	7 (15.6)	33 (21.3)
Uncertain	19 (50.0)	22 (30.6)	18 (40.0)	59 (38.1)
Total	38 (100.0)	72 (100.0)	45 (100.0)	155 (100.0)
				p = 0.218

Table 3. Responses of Individuals Who Said They Would Use Prenatal Testing to the Question "If the Fetus Was Shown to Have an Increased Risk, What Would You Do?" (n = 167)

	Age categories			
	< 30	30-40	> 40	Total
Complete (%)	11 (29.7)	12 (16.6)	18 (31.0)	41 (24.6)
Terminate (%)	6 (16.2)	39 (54.2)	22 (38.0)	67 (40.1)
Uncertain (%)	20 (54.1)	21 (29.2)	18 (31.0)	59 (35.3)
Total (%)	37 (100.0)	72 (100.0)	58 (100.0)	167 (100.0)
				p = 0.002

Table 4. Number of Children per Family, by Age

No. of children (%)	< 30		30-40		> 40	
0	87	(76.3)	62	(36.9)	12	(10.0)
1	14	(12.3)	35	(20.8)	14	(11.7)
2 or more	13	(11.4)	71	(42.3)	94	(78.3)
Total	45	(100.0)	220	(100.0)	269	(100.0)

Table 5. Results of Testing Performed During Eleven Pregnancies for Seven Couples

	Definitive tests (3 couples)		Exclusion tests (4 couples)
	Affected	Increased risk	
Increased risk	1	1	5
Decreased risk	3	0	1
Total	4	1	6

Table 6. Comparison of Mean Scores on GSI of SCL 90(R) at Baseline, and at Two- and Six-Month Follow-Ups

Groups	Baseline		2 months		6 months	
	n	mean ± SD	n	mean ± SD	n	mean ± SD
Prenatal testing	7	48.0 ± 11.0	6	−8.0 ± 10.5	6	−3.7 ± 9.8
Predictive testing	95	51.6 ± 10.8	92	−5.02 ± 9.3	92	−5.5 ± 10.0
p value		0.39		0.45		0.67

Table 7. Comparison of Median Scores on Beck Depression Inventory at Baseline, and at Two- and Six-Month Follow-Ups

Groups	n	Baseline median (min-max)	n	2 months median (min-max)	n	6 months median (min-max)
Prenatal testing	7	4.0 (0.0-8.0)	6	-0.5 (-4.0-0.0)	6	0.0 (-4.0-3.0)
Predictive testing	95	3.0 (0.0-9.0)	86	-1.0 (-6.0-8.0)	89	-1.0 (-7.0-8.0)
p value		0.88		0.99		0.71

Table 8. Sociodemographic Comparison of Groups Choosing or Not Choosing Prenatal Testing

Variable	Group membership Prenatal test (n = 14)	No prenatal test (n = 24)	p value
Mean age (min-max)	26.8 (17-36)	30.1 (21-41)	n.s.
Sex			
Men	5 (36%)	8 (33%)	n.s.
Women	9 (64%)	16 (67%)	
Mean number of children (min-max)	0.21 (0.0-2.0)	0.96 (0.0-4.0)	0.02
Education			
<High school	2	4	n.s.
>High school	11	19	
Religious practices			
Religious group member	3	12	
Non-religious/ non-practising	10	9	0.05

n.s. = not significant.

Table 9. Reasons Given by Questionnaire Respondents for Choosing Not to Have Prenatal Testing (Up to Five Reasons Were Allowed)

	No. of times given as a reason	
Reasons	**At-risk persons (n = 17)**	**Spouses (n = 16)**
Candidate believed that a cure would be found in time for his or her children.	14	11
Candidate's desire for a child outweighed the possibility that the child may someday develop Huntington disease.	12	10
Candidate could not handle the emotional and psychological consequences of an elective termination of a pregnancy.	7	8
Candidate had serious concerns regarding the safety of the prenatal test.	7	7
Candidate wanted to determine his or her status before making a decision about prenatal testing.	7	n.a.
Candidate did not believe prenatal genetic testing was ethically, morally, or religiously justifiable.	6	5
Candidate's partner was opposed to prenatal testing.	5	7
Candidate felt that the prenatal test was too inaccurate to risk the termination of a potentially healthy child.	5	6
Candidate felt the child should make his or her own decision about predictive testing.	2	0
Candidate felt that to test the current pregnancy would be unfair to previous children who were not tested.	2	1
Prenatal testing was not possible in candidate's family.	2	2
Candidate was unaware that prenatal testing was possible or available.	1	2

Discussion

Prenatal testing for Huntington disease has now been offered in Canada for about five years. This ongoing national program has provided the opportunity to study the knowledge and attitudes of people at risk who choose or decline prenatal testing. During this period, over 425 people have participated in predictive testing. Of the 38 who became pregnant and were eligible for prenatal testing, 14 (37%) have entered the prenatal testing program. Of the 14, only 7 actually took the prenatal test. The other 7 withdrew, primarily due to miscarriage or not wanting to consider termination of pregnancy as an option. Clearly, the demand for prenatal testing for this late-onset, autosomal dominant disorder is lower than the expected demand suggested by the four U.S. studies that had been conducted before the development of these programs (Markel et al. 1987; Meissen and Berchek 1987; Kessler et al. 1987; Mastromauro et al. 1987).

Two variables appeared to influence the choice to participate in prenatal testing. The first factor was the number of existing children in the family. Most people requesting prenatal testing were childless. In contrast, most of those who became pregnant during this study but who chose not to participate in prenatal testing had at least one child. A reason why people who already have children are less willing to participate in prenatal testing could be that they do not want some of their children to be aware of their risks for Huntington disease while their other children do not know.

The analysis of the responses of all at-risk candidates to the question of whether they or their spouse would consider prenatal testing revealed that most people who responded that prenatal testing was acceptable were over 40 years of age. However, no pregnancies were in this age category, and though the procedure might have been acceptable, it was not undertaken for this group. People under 30 years of age were less likely to consider prenatal testing, and only a small proportion (16%) of these said they would terminate a pregnancy if the fetus were shown to have an increased risk. Rejection of termination as an option was a major reason for the withdrawal of 4 of the 14 individuals who initially requested prenatal testing. In addition, 7 of 17 (41%) individuals who became pregnant but did not choose prenatal testing indicated that it was because they did not consider termination to be an option. Those who rejected termination as an option may have been influenced by religious conviction. Our study revealed that those who chose prenatal testing were less likely to be affiliated with a particular religion than those who did not.

The most common reason for refusing prenatal testing was the belief that a cure for Huntington disease would be found. They felt prenatal testing was not necessary because even if Huntington disease were to develop, appropriate therapy would be available that would either cure or halt the progression of the illness. Recent publicity concerning genetic discoveries has clearly raised the expectations of people at risk for

Huntington disease that the eventual cloning of the gene will result in effective therapy. Although this is a possibility, it is not a certainty; to believe so may create unrealistic expectations for the at-risk population.

Most people who entered the predictive testing program already had significant information concerning many aspects of prenatal testing before they were counselled. Exclusion testing was understood the least, and women over 40 years of age rated most poorly on this question. The issue most commonly confused was that it is possible to alter the risk status of the fetus without establishing the status of the at-risk parent. This finding is similar to that previously described by Tyler et al. (1990), who also found that nearly 90% of their cohort was confused by certain aspects of exclusion testing.

Lack of knowledge of prenatal testing does not appear to be a factor in the low use of this testing, as only one person in this study was unaware of the availability of testing.

One of the major concerns about prenatal and adult predictive testing has been the impact of these new technologies on the participants' quality of life. We have shown previously that adult predictive testing for Huntington disease has led to some improvement in the quality of life for those who have received either a decreased or an increased risk result (Huggins et al. 1992; Bloch et al. 1992). The results of the psychosocial assessment in the prenatal testing group, including the SCL 90(R) and Beck Depression Inventory, show that these individuals are similar to other predictive testing candidates at baseline. After receiving results, participants undergoing prenatal testing had a reduction in their scores at two months, which may indicate a reduction in psychological distress; however, at six months they may be returning closer to the baseline levels. This curve is somewhat different from that of the adult predictive testing cohort, who also had a reduction in their indices of distress, with improved well-being after receiving results, but who have maintained the level after six months and one year. Of the six participants in the prenatal group who were followed for six months, four (all of whom received an increased-risk prenatal result) have become pregnant again and thus were not available for longitudinal follow-up. Overall, no serious adverse responses to prenatal testing for Huntington disease have been revealed.

Some couples participating in prenatal testing found the availability of the test impelled them to use it in the first pregnancy, and they could justify the initial use of prenatal testing only if they continued to use the same technology in future pregnancies. Several couples have requested prenatal tests for each pregnancy, including two individuals who each had two prenatal tests and one individual who had three successive prenatal tests for three successive pregnancies. Careful in-depth counselling is needed to free couples from feeling they must necessarily repeat the prenatal test for every pregnancy. We have explained to couples in this situation that their circumstances may be different from what they were before the previous test and that they need to consider carefully whether the risks and benefits still warrant a prenatal test. The psychological distress that could result from the loss of repeated pregnancies has to be balanced against the possible relief from knowing that the current pregnancy is at low risk for having inherited the gene for Huntington disease. Freeing patients from the technological imperative and allowing them to make an independent choice in every pregnancy are an important part of pre-test counselling.

Of the 47 participants who became pregnant, nine had previously received a decreased risk result and did not need prenatal testing. Predictive testing has given them the knowledge that they can have children who are at low risk for Huntington disease. Five of these participants had indicated they would not have more children without having a predictive test and learning that the risk was reduced.

Six of the seven individuals who received an increased risk result on prenatal testing chose to terminate the pregnancy. The abortions were performed shortly after receiving the results, and the counsellors played an important role in making the arrangements with as little stress and delay as possible. On the basis of this experience and the experience in Wales (Tyler et al. 1990), most high risk pregnancies are likely to be terminated. Most people who would not consider termination of pregnancy will choose not to participate in prenatal testing.

Parents who do not accept termination of pregnancy as an option have to balance the complexities and difficulties associated with having a child at increased risk with the possibility of obtaining information that the fetus could be at low risk for Huntington disease. With counselling, patients understand that there is no difference in performing predictive testing before birth or during childhood; the testing is justified in childhood only if an advantage can clearly be demonstrated for the child (Bloch and Hayden 1990). No treatment has yet been discovered or developed that might prevent or delay the onset of Huntington disease, and predictive testing in childhood could be disadvantageous to the child because of possible distortions of parent-child or sibling relationships. The knowledge of being at risk could also result in significant diminishing of self-esteem and sense of worth for a developing child.

For exclusion testing, there is the added dimension that if the fetus has an increased risk close to 50%, the risk is similar to that of the at-risk parent. The onset of symptoms in a parent would be equivalent to a definitive predictive test in the child, as each would probably have inherited the same chromosome 4 from the affected grandparent. When the implications of prenatal testing of Huntington disease are explained to parents who do not consider termination of pregnancy to be an option, most parents do not want the testing. Ongoing education and in-depth counselling are needed to explain the intricacies and complexities of prenatal testing to every prospective couple.

Because of the complexity of counselling for prenatal definitive and prenatal exclusion testing, beginning the DNA testing for prenatal testing before becoming pregnant is preferable so that sufficient time is allowed to assimilate all of the complex information about prenatal testing. In our study, three of the seven couples requested information about prenatal testing before a pregnancy occurred. However, many people who enter a prenatal testing program may already be pregnant, which places them and the counsellors under time constraints. It is important, therefore, to educate the at-risk population about prenatal testing before pregnancy occurs.

The cloning of the gene for Huntington disease will have an impact on the demand for and attitudes of at-risk individuals toward prenatal testing. If Huntington disease were due to a single mutation or a few mutations, an opportunity would exist for definitive testing for patients who were previously unable to choose this option. Three out of four people who chose exclusion testing in our study did not have the option of definitive testing because they had too few family members. If the chances for definitive testing were improved, the number of requests for exclusion testing might decrease. Of the 17 individuals in our study who chose not to use prenatal testing, five believed the prenatal test was too inaccurate to risk termination of a potentially healthy child. The finding of a specific mutation causing Huntington disease will obviously improve the accuracy and may make prenatal testing more acceptable for some people.

Increased requests for prenatal testing due to possible improvement in the accuracy of the test are likely to be offset by other factors. Optimism about a cure was the predominant reason for not considering prenatal testing. The possibility of effective therapy that may arise as a result of understanding gained after cloning of the gene for Huntington disease is likely to reduce the demand for prenatal testing further because termination of a pregnancy for a curable adult-onset illness will likely be even less acceptable. For other late-onset autosomal dominant disorders, such as polycystic disease of kidneys, for which some effective therapies may retard progression, prenatal testing is considered to be an unpopular option with exceedingly low demand (Kerzin-Storrar et al. 1991). As further treatments are developed, or where the patient population believes that effective therapy is imminent, prenatal testing for late-onset genetic disorders is likely to be seen as desirable by only a minority.

Despite the complexity of prenatal testing for Huntington disease and the need for in-depth counselling and support, prenatal testing for Huntington disease should still remain a valid option for the small number of individuals who wish to have it. Although our sample size is limited and the long-term follow-up of the group is confounded by additional pregnancies, our study indicates that with continued availability of support, prenatal testing is safe. Careful, long-term assessment and documentation of the impact of prenatal testing are needed before reaching final conclusions about the impact of prenatal testing on the psychosocial well-being of people at risk for Huntington disease.

Acknowledgments

We thank our colleagues Patti Whyte, Maurice Bloch, Marlene Huggins, and Jane Theilmann in Vancouver; and Dr. M.H.K. Shokeir, Alice Gibson, Dr. H. Soltan, Jo-Anne Kane, Dr. W. Meschino, Dr. A. Summers, Dr. O. Suchowersky, Marylou Klimek, Dr. J.P. Welch, Anne Fuller, and all the other investigators in the Canadian Collaborative Study of Predictive Testing for Huntington Disease. The information in this study has formed part of a separate submission to the *Journal of Medical Genetics*.

Bibliography

Beck, A.T., et al. 1961. "An Inventory for Measuring Depression." *Archives of General Psychiatry* 4: 561-71.

Bloch, M., and M.R. Hayden. 1990. "Opinion: Predictive Testing for Huntington Disease in Childhood: Challenges and Implications." *American Journal of Human Genetics* 46: 1-4.

Bloch, M., et al. 1992. "Predictive Testing for Huntington Disease in Canada: The Experience of Those Receiving an Increased Risk." *American Journal of Medical Genetics* 42: 499-507.

Collinge, J., et al. 1991. "Presymptomatic Detection or Exclusion of Prion Protein Gene Defects in Families with Inherited Prion Diseases." *American Journal of Human Genetics* 49: 1351-54.

Craufurd, D., et al. 1989. "Uptake of Presymptomatic Predictive Testing for Huntington's Disease." *Lancet* (9 September): 603-605.

Derogatis, L.R. 1977. *SCL-90: Administration, Scoring & Procedures Manual for the R(evised) Version and Other Instruments of the Psychopathology Rating Scale Series*. Baltimore: Johns Hopkins School of Medicine, Clinical Psychometric Research.

Fahy, M., et al. 1989. "Different Options for Prenatal Testing for Huntington's Disease Using DNA Probes." *Journal of Medical Genetics* 26: 353-57.

Goate, A., et al. 1991. "Segregation of a Missense Mutation in the Amyloid Precursor Protein Gene with Familial Alzheimer's Disease." *Nature* 349: 704-706.

Gusella, J.F., et al. 1983. "A Polymorphic DNA Marker Genetically Linked to Huntington's Disease." *Nature* 306: 234-38.

Hayden, M.R., et al. 1987. "First-Trimester Prenatal Diagnosis for Huntington's Disease with DNA Probes." *Lancet* (6 June): 1284-85.

—. 1988. "Improved Predictive Testing for Huntington's Disease by Using Three Linked DNA Markers." *American Journal of Human Genetics* 43: 689-94.

Huggins, M., et al. 1992. "Predictive Testing for Huntington Disease in Canada: Adverse Effects and Unexpected Results in Those Receiving a Decreased Risk." *American Journal of Medical Genetics* 42: 508-15.

Kerzin-Storrar, L., et al. 1991. "A Regional Genetic Family Register: Opportunity for Active — Rather than Reactive — Genetic Counselling." *American Journal of Human Genetics* 49 (Suppl.): 42, Abstract No. 208.

Kessler, S., et al. 1987. "Attitudes of Persons at Risk for Huntington Disease Toward Predictive Testing." *American Journal of Medical Genetics* 26: 259-70.

Markel, D.S., A.B. Young, and J.B. Penney. 1987. "At-Risk Persons' Attitudes Toward Presymptomatic and Prenatal Testing of Huntington Disease in Michigan." *American Journal of Medical Genetics* 26: 295-305.

Mastromauro, C., R.H. Myers, and B. Berkman. 1987. "Attitudes Toward Presymptomatic Testing in Huntington Disease." *American Journal of Medical Genetics* 26: 271-82.

Meissen, G.J., and R.L. Berchek. 1987. "Intended Use of Predictive Testing by Those at Risk for Huntington Disease." *American Journal of Medical Genetics* 26: 283-93.

Millan, F.A., et al. 1989. "Prenatal Exclusion Testing for Huntington's Disease: A Problem of Too Much Information." *Journal of Medical Genetics* 26: 83-85.

Quarrell, O.W.J., et al. 1987. "Exclusion Testing for Huntington's Disease in Pregnancy with a Closely Linked DNA Marker." *Lancet* (6 June): 1281-83.

Reeders, S.T., et al. 1985. "A Highly Polymorphic DNA Marker Linked to Adult Polycystic Kidney Disease on Chromosome 16." *Nature* 317: 542-44.

Spurdle, A., et al. 1991. "Prenatal Diagnosis for Huntington's Disease: A Molecular and Psychological Study." *Prenatal Diagnosis* 11: 177-85.

Tyler, A., et al. 1990. "Exclusion Testing in Pregnancy for Huntington's Disease." *Journal of Medical Genetics* 27: 488-95.

Wasmuth, J.J., et al. 1988. "A Highly Polymorphic Locus Very Tightly Linked to the Huntington's Disease Gene." *Nature* 332: 734-36.

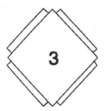

3

Screening for Genetic Susceptibilities
to Common Diseases

Lynn Prior

Executive Summary

Screening programs for genetic susceptibilities to common diseases could have benefits, including allowing individuals to take preventive measures or to otherwise benefit from early diagnosis; they could also have disadvantages, such as discrimination against carriers by employers, insurance companies, or peers; harm to self-image and happiness; damage to parent-child interactions; and societal stigmatization.

Three criteria would have to be met before a screening program should be established: (1) the disease would have to pose a serious health risk to the population, both by its high prevalence and by its seriousness; (2) safe, accurate tests would have to be available, without too many false-positives, which would create undue anxiety, or false-negatives, which would give a false sense of security, and would have to be valid (as shown through testing and following of outcomes over several years); and (3) some intervention would have to be available to decrease the burden of disease, either through preventive measures or through increased ability to offer treatment due to early diagnosis. Such interventions include counselling on reducing exposure to environmental risks and monitoring to detect disease onset at the earliest possible

This paper was completed for the Royal Commission on New Reproductive Technologies in February 1992.

moment; in the distant future, gene therapy may be another possible intervention.

None of the susceptibility genes identified to date fulfil these criteria, and the Human Genome Project is unlikely to identify any genes more eligible than those already known. But the potential for profit, for instance by pharmaceutical companies, which may develop therapeutic agents through a better understanding of the disease process, may result in pressures for screening. It is, therefore, important that guidelines be put in place and criteria specified now.

Screening for susceptibility genes raises serious issues. One is the possibility of discrimination. This must be discussed and recommendations made about what social measures can and should be taken to protect carriers of genes causing disorders against discrimination. Another is the use of prenatal diagnosis for screening for susceptibility genes. There is significant concern about the morality and legality of performing prenatal diagnosis for a gene that may or may not result in a disease that will appear only in later life; this may result in the termination of a fetus that, if it had survived, might never have developed the disorder. There is a consensus that this use of prenatal diagnosis is not justified and should not occur.

Introduction

A variety of common diseases in our society today, such as many types of cancer, cardiovascular disease, and mental illness, are multifactorial disorders. Multifactorial disorders are caused by more than one genetic factor, more than one environmental factor, or, in the conventional view, several of both. When an interaction between genes and environmental factors is needed to cause the disorder, the genetic factors predisposing to the disorders are called susceptibility genes.

Family, adoption, and twin studies suggest that there are susceptibility genes for most common familial disorders. Recent advances in molecular biology provide the means for identifying these genes more precisely by mapping their locations on the chromosomes. Certain differences within these genes have been identified to increase the risk that external influences will cause illness. With the advent of the Human Genome Project, in which scientists are attempting to analyze each of the human being's estimated 100 000 genes, some new susceptibility genes will be detected. Identification of these susceptibility genes has raised the issue of genetic screening for them. Genetic screening is the search in a population of apparently healthy individuals for those with genotypes that place them or their offspring at increased risk for having a particular disease. Screening programs could be used to determine which individuals possess susceptibility genes that increase the risk of a disorder. Such programs might have benefits. Individuals found to be susceptible could take preventive measures or benefit from earlier diagnosis. There could also be disadvantages, such as discrimination against carriers of susceptibility genes by employers, insurance companies, or peers, or there could be harm done to those individuals' self-image and happiness by having this knowledge about their genetic make-up, as well as damage to parent-child interactions, societal stigmatization, and other, more subtle effects (Holtzman 1989).

The objectives of this paper are to discuss methods of screening for susceptibility genes, to review the susceptibility genes that have already been detected, and to consider the feasibility and practicality of screening programs for these genes. In particular this paper will assess their potential application to prenatal diagnosis, a field within the mandate of the Royal Commission on New Reproductive Technologies. It will also consider what criteria characterize a susceptibility gene as being suitable for a screening program in the general population.

Techniques

Deoxyribonucleic acid (DNA) tests can be performed on an individual at any time after conception. Sufficient DNA can be obtained from the chorionic villi in the ninth week of gestation, from the amniotic fluid cells from the fifteenth week (or earlier if early amniocentesis proves acceptable), or from white blood cells and other tissues after birth.

Linkage Studies

Polymorphic variations in DNA sequences are found among individuals both within genes and in the intervening DNA sequences between genes. Polymorphisms are genetic differences, usually harmless, that are common enough to be useful as genetic markers. If they are very close to genes causing disorders, they can be used to track these genes through families and establish their locations on chromosomes (mapping). These differences in DNA sequences can be used as markers to follow the inheritance of genes. They were discovered by the use of the restriction enzymes that are the basis for recombinant DNA technology (genetic engineering). Restriction enzymes recognize specific short DNA sequences and cut the DNA wherever they occur. At sites that show polymorphic variation, the enzyme will recognize and cut the DNA at a particular place when one, but not another, variant is present. Thus, the length of DNA fragments resulting from the cuts by the restriction enzymes will differ in the two polymorphic forms. These differences in fragment length are called restriction fragment length polymorphisms (RFLPs). A RFLP may be located so close to a gene of interest that it is nearly always inherited with (linked to) the gene. Thus, the RFLPs can be used to follow the inheritance of particular disease-causing gene regions. The RFLP is not itself the cause of disease but is a genetic marker for the presence of the specific gene disease.

Demonstrating that a RFLP (or other marker) is closely linked to the gene for a genetic disorder requires study of large families with many affected members. It is a tedious and laborious process. Such markers are not suitable for population screening, since the carrier of the gene for the disorder cannot be identified directly, but only by linkage studies of the family. There are also other types of polymorphic markers. Particularly important is the major histocompatibility complex (MHC) that determines antigenic specificity. There is a high degree of genetic polymorphism in the MHC region, especially in the region coding for the human leukocyte antigens (HLA).   Genetic susceptibility to several diseases, including diabetes and rheumatoid arthritis, has been linked to specific HLA patterns.

Direct Analysis of Mutant Genes

In some cases the gene for a disorder can be identified by the specific DNA alteration that changes its function. Nevertheless, locating the gene's position in the genome (mapping) still requires study of many large families.

Once a mutant gene is identified by its DNA pattern as causing or increasing the risk of disease, the presence of the mutation can be screened for in the population. If the mutation disrupts a restriction enzyme site within the mutant gene, it can be detected directly by analysis of RFLPs. An alternative direct screening method involves specific probes, which are synthesized to recognize either the normal or mutant DNA sequence. This technique has been used to screen for such single-gene disorders as alpha$_1$-antitrypsin (α_1-antitrypsin) deficiency, which predisposes the individual to emphysema.

Limitations of the Techniques

Linkage studies are useful for following the inheritance of a disease-causing gene within a family where the precise mutation is unknown but where the mutation is linked to a RFLP marker. However, use of the technique is limited to families in which at least one (and preferably more than one) member is affected.   Thus, although linkage studies are important in the discovery of susceptibility genes and could be used for predictive testing in particular families, they are not appropriate for screening the general population.

Direct analysis of mutant genes is a more useful technique for screening the population for susceptibility genes since family study is not required.   However, it is possible only after the disease-causing or susceptibility gene is identified and mapped. Also, use of this method can be limited by such complications as variable expressivity, incomplete penetrance, and genetic heterogeneity.

Variable expressivity involves phenotypic variation: in a group of individuals having the same genetic mutation, some may be more severely affected than others. Thus, when screening for a disease that has variable expressivity, it is not possible to inform a person with a positive test result as to the extent that the disorder will be manifested.

Penetrance is the frequency with which a heritable trait is manifested by those carrying a gene coding for it. For a disease with incomplete penetrance, not everyone having the mutant genotype will develop the disease; this also introduces uncertainty into the interpretation of a positive test. In screening for susceptibility genes, the direct analysis of mutant genes determines only if a specific gene mutation is present, not that the disease will or will not result. The disease will not appear in all people with the susceptibility gene. Environmental factors are also involved and are not measured by the DNA tests. The susceptibility gene is only a marker whose predictive value depends on the frequency with which gene-affected individuals actually develop the disease in question.

Genetic heterogeneity means that different gene mutations may cause the same susceptibility or disease. In a screening program, if genetic heterogeneity is present, the fact that a person is found not to have a specific gene mutation does not mean that the person is not susceptible to the disease because they may carry a different gene mutation. Thus, DNA tests may cause a false sense of security when a test is negative.

Criteria for Establishing Screening Programs

Before a screening program is established, criteria such as the frequency and severity of the disease, the availability of safe and accurate tests, and the ability to intervene successfully in preventing or ameliorating the disease should be considered.

Frequency and Severity of the Disease

To be suitable for mass population screening of a gene that increases susceptibility to a specific disease, the condition must imply a serious health risk to the general population. The disease must have a sufficiently high prevalence in the population to justify the expense of screening. It has been recommended that the frequency of the susceptibility gene must be at least 5 percent (Omenn 1982). Also, to be a candidate for screening programs, not only must the disease be prevalent in the population but it must be serious. For example, lung cancer and obstructive pulmonary disease are such general health hazards that the recognition of potential high-risk individuals merits assessment.

The relative risk of illness in genetically susceptible persons from susceptibility genes should be at least 3:1 and preferably 10:1 or greater, compared to the unaffected population, before screening programs are considered (Murray 1986).

Availability of Safe, Accurate Tests

A screening program for a particular trait should not be implemented unless the benefits of the program outweigh the risks. The possible risks include unnecessary treatment, a false sense of security for those with negative test results, anxiety and an increased sense of vulnerability induced by a positive test in people who might prefer not to know, prejudice against those with certain genetic differences, and the possible abuse of test results by employers or insurance companies. Such risks should be compared to the benefits gained by the program.   Furthermore, the predictive value of the test must be known to determine the benefits of a screening program.

Tests must be valid and reliable to be of predictive value. Before screening the population for the presence of a certain trait, the validity of the test to be used should be determined in a large test population of individuals with and without the trait. Those people tested should be monitored to determine how many with negative results remain free of disease and how many with positive results develop the disease. This process may take many years, as many multifactorial disorders have their onset over a wide age range. Validity is the probability that the test will correctly distinguish between those with the trait and those without. The parameters of sensitivity and specificity are used to determine validity.

Sensitivity is the frequency with which a test will be positive when the genotype in question is present — the degree to which a test can identify all subjects who exhibit a particular trait. Overly sensitive tests tend to be over-inclusive, resulting in false positives so that subjects who do not have a specific trait test positively.   Genetic heterogeneity can decrease sensitivity. If a mutation at one site in a gene is being screened for, and the test is negative, it does not exclude the possibility that the person has mutations in other regions of the same gene or in different genes that could cause the same susceptibility.   Thus, in the presence of genetic heterogeneity, people having a negative test result can still have a susceptibility to a given disease, and may show up a "false negative," in that they develop the disease.

Specificity refers to the frequency with which a test will be negative when the genotype in question is absent — the identification of only those subjects who have the trait being tested for. Overly specific tests tend to be under-inclusive, resulting in many false negatives so that subjects who have the trait in question are not identified as having it.   Reduced penetrance can decrease the specificity of a given test. A person may have a mutation in the gene being screened, but this mutation could have reduced penetrance; thus, the susceptibility due to the gene may never manifest itself, despite the positive test result. This problem seldom arises with severe disorders with simple Mendelian inheritance, but it is pervasive in the case of susceptibility genes for common complex disorders.

The use of an overly sensitive test would result in the misclassification of non-susceptible people as susceptible, which would cause them unneeded concern. Similarly, if a test were overly specific, susceptible people might not be detected, which might expose them to risk factors that might otherwise have been avoided. Sensitivity and specificity are inversely related, and a balance between the two is needed to have a valid test result.

Reliability is the degree to which a given test consistently shows the same result when repeated on the same specimen. The reliability of genetic testing varies by the type of test. Sometimes a subjective element in the interpretation of results is involved in DNA tests, such as deciding when the restriction fragment patterns in a gel form separate bands. This element of subjectivity decreases reliability. In addition, DNA tests are subject to error due to technical difficulties such as the incomplete cutting of DNA by restriction enzymes or the contamination of test samples. Technical problems also reduce the reliability of test results. Good quality control of tests is required.

The validity and reliability of a given test must be known to determine the predictive value — the risk that a person with a positive test result will develop the disease — of a positive test result.

Therapy or Other Meaningful Intervention

Performing genetic tests to determine affected or at-risk individuals incurs all the risks without benefits unless some type of intervention is available that will decrease the burden of disease. Therefore, a screening program should not be undertaken in the general population unless it can be coupled with preventive measures. The same benefit may be gained from treatment after the appearance of symptoms and a clinical diagnosis. Screening uses resources, has the potential to cause harm, and is meaningless, with the possible exception of counselling high-risk couples about reproductive options. It would not be worth the cost of the screening program, or the unnecessary risk of treating people with false-positive results, if no avoidance or amelioration of disease can be expected. However, if irreversible damage has occurred by the time symptoms of the disease appear, and an intervention is known by which disease progression can be slowed or halted, a benefit could be gained by early detection of susceptibilities.

Once at-risk individuals are identified, several possible risk-reducing interventions may be available, depending on the disease in question. If a susceptibility gene that is triggered by known environmental factors is identified, then those factors may be avoided (e.g., the effect of cigarette smoke on people susceptible to lung cancer). Counselling would be important to help those at risk understand their particular risk and recognize ways to avoid triggering the onset of the disease.

Once identified, people at risk could be monitored to detect onset of the disease at the earliest possible moment, which might make a significant difference in the prognosis of treatment. This is especially important for cancers.

Another possibility for risk-reducing intervention that may be available in the more distant future is gene therapy. If a person has a particular gene causing susceptibility to a severe disease, it may be possible to replace this gene by gene therapy. However, the techniques involved are well in the future, and environmental manipulation seems a much more rewarding approach.

Even if no intervention is available to avoid the onset of disease in high-risk people, some writers have suggested that screening for susceptibility genes may be justified since it would allow identified individuals to prepare for the possible onset of disease with the aid of genetic counselling or to make informed reproductive choices. However, it is felt that the expense involved and the potential risks incurred make this option one of low priority in resource allocation.

A problem with genetic screening for susceptibility genes will be to ensure adequate counselling so that people understand their particular risk and the need to take recommended steps to reduce the risk of disease. If people do not use regimes recommended to reduce risks, screening will not be beneficial but will simply mean the individuals are exposed to potential harms. The question arises — would carriers be expected to prevent or avoid the disease, and would society discriminate against those that did not? Also, unless genetic information is protected, employers or insurance companies could discriminate against carriers if they did not comply with the preventive measures.

Susceptibility Genes

Specific genes that confer susceptibility to common diseases, such as certain types of cancer, heart disease, or mental illness, have been identified. Some of these susceptibilities will be discussed. It should be noted that for most of those that are even possible, practical screening applications of this knowledge will not be available for years.

Cancers

Many cancers are due to genetic-environmental interactions. Persons with a genetic predisposition may develop cancer if exposed to viruses or carcinogenic agents that can trigger the disease. Two types of genes play a role in the development of cancer: oncogenes and anti-oncogenes. Oncogenes are those involved in the development of cancer. Normal genes in the body can be transformed into oncogenes by point mutations or deletions in their DNA sequences that can result in unregulated cell growth and, eventually, cancer. Anti-oncogenes work to restrain this unregulated cell growth, but mutations in them can result in the loss of their protective function. Since there are two copies of each autosomal gene, having one copy of a mutant anti-oncogene will not have any immediate effect, but could lead to cancer if the normal gene is lost or mutates to the inactive form. The genetic changes resulting in the transformation of a cell from normal to cancerous (neoplastic) growth are rapidly being deciphered. It seems that the final neoplastic change is the last of several step-wise genetic changes (mutations or deletions of the genetic material) involving oncogenes and anti-oncogenes and may also involve interaction with environmental factors (carcinogens).

Lung Cancer

Lung cancer is the leading cause of death from cancer in men and the second leading cause in women (Silverberg and Lubera 1987). Not all cigarette smokers develop lung cancer, which suggests that some individuals are more susceptible than others. This susceptibility has been shown to have a genetic component. Deletions of regions of DNA in chromosomes 3, 13, and 17 have been associated with lung cancer. For example, one study has linked deletions of the short arm of chromosome 3 to lung cancer (Kok et al. 1987). In the cancerous cells, mutations were found in a specific region of both copies of chromosome 3 in all types of lung cancer studied. It was suggested that in the familial cases the mutant inactive form of the gene was inherited from a parent, and that once the normal form of the gene was lost in a lung cell, cancer would develop. Conversely, in the non-familial sporadic cases, both copies of the gene had to mutate for the cancer to appear. The precise function of the gene involved has not yet been determined. In a more recent study, a search for anti-oncogenes in chromosome 17 was undertaken in the region of the gene for protein 53, a transformation-associated protein (Takahashi et al. 1989), which had previously been implicated as an anti-oncogene (Mowat et al. 1985). The gene coding for p53 was found to be frequently mutated or inactivated by deletions or point mutations. Thus, the disruption of p53 is probably involved in the pathogenesis of lung cancer. However, mutations of the p53 gene are found only in the lung cancer cells; thus, screening for mutations in this gene conferring susceptibility to lung cancer could not be performed.

In other studies, the cytochrome P-450 enzymes have been associated with lung cancer (Marx 1985). Cytochrome P-450 enzymes are involved in the metabolism of toxic chemicals by the addition of oxygen to a wide range of chemical components. These enzymes are important in defending the body against foreign chemicals, but they may also convert some chemicals to active carcinogens. Thus, genetically determined differences in the production or activity of P-450 enzymes can influence susceptibility to cancer. One example is the P-450 enzyme aryl hydrocarbon hydroxylase (AHH). The speed at which the enzyme is induced after exposure to inducing chemicals is genetically determined. People who produce large amounts of AHH are at an increased risk of developing lung cancer, especially if they smoke. A chemical in the cigarette smoke is converted by AHH to an active carcinogen. Variations in the inducibility of AHH may be due to alterations in the AHH gene or in genes that regulate its production.

A second example of a P-450 enzyme affecting susceptibility to lung cancer has been demonstrated (Ayesh et al. 1984). People who possess a polymorphism for the enzyme debrisoquine 4-hydroxylase (D4H), whereby they rapidly metabolize chemicals, are at an increased risk for lung cancer. Further research is required to determine the size of increase in risk. Identification of rapid metabolizers requires urine examination following a test dose of the drug, and would not be suitable for mass screening.

Once the P-450 genes responsible for conferring susceptibility to lung cancer are isolated, it may become technically possible to screen for them at the DNA level. As noted previously, studies of the validity and predictive value of any tests should be done prior to their being undertaken in the general population.

Colon Cancer

Colorectal cancer is the second most common cause of cancer death in the United States. In some single-gene conditions, the susceptibility to colon cancer is inherited dominantly with a high degree of penetrance. These single-gene disorders, several of which are characterized by the appearance of intestinal polyps, account for fewer than 5 percent of all cases of colon cancer.

In addition to the clearly dominant genes that cause colon cancer, genes are now being identified that predispose individuals to colon cancer. Point mutations in the ras proto-oncogenes have been reported in almost 50 percent of colorectal tumours (Forrester et al. 1987; Bos et al. 1987). These mutations convert proto-oncogenes to oncogenes that participate in neoplastic transformation.

Other mutations involved in a susceptibility to colon cancer involve deletions on several different chromosomes. The deleted sequences probably include tumour-suppressor genes whose products would normally control cell growth. In 75 percent of carcinomas, such deletions are found on the short arm of chromosome 17 and on the long arm of chromosome 18. The deleted chromosome 17 region contains the gene for p53, a transformation-associated protein. Protein 53 may suppress neoplastic growth of colorectal epithelium (Baker et al. 1989). A gene from the deleted chromosome 18 region encodes a cell surface protein whose expression is decreased in most colorectal carcinomas (Fearon et al. 1990). As well, some single-gene disorders involving polyps have been mapped to a region on the long arm of chromosome 5 by linkage analysis (Leppert et al. 1987). This region is deleted in approximately 35 percent of sporadic colorectal carcinomas (Bodmer et al. 1987). Recently, a specific mutation for familial polyposis (APC at region q21 of chromosome 5) has been identified in affected members who develop colon cancers, and also in some people with ordinary colon cancers. For the time being, testing for the mutant gene will be limited to relatives of patients with the familial type (Marx 1991). Screening on a population basis is not practical because of the genetic heterogeneity of colon cancer.

Renal Cancer

Renal cancer develops in about 1 individual per 1 000 in the general population. An inherited chromosomal aberration has been shown to impose a high risk of renal cancer (Cohen et al. 1979). In a family with 22 members, 10 were shown to have a transfer of DNA (translocation) between chromosomes 3 and 8. This translocation was found in 8 patients with renal cancer — no family member with normal genes had cancer. Individuals with the translocation had a risk of 87 percent of having developed renal cancer by the age of 59 (Knudson 1979). A small deletion or point mutation in genes in chromosome 3 or 8 or both, at the sites of rearrangement, may be responsible for the susceptibility to cancer. Screening studies performed in the asymptomatic family members identified 3 having the translocation, which allowed for their early diagnosis and treatment. It seems unlikely that this translocation also increases susceptibility to renal cancer in the general population but, if it did, a screening program could be considered.

Bladder Cancer

Deletions appear to be quite frequent in bladder carcinomas. Reports have identified deletions associated with bladder cancer in chromosome 5 (Atkin and Fox 1990), in chromosome 10 (Berger et al. 1986), in chromosome 21 (Babu et al. 1989), and in chromosomes 9, 11, and 17 (Tsai et al. 1990). Since deletions of chromosome 17 have been reported in lung and colorectal cancers, a common mechanism possibly may be involved through the loss of a tumour suppressor gene.

These deletions occur only in the tumour cells of the bladder. Thus, it would not be possible to screen for these deletions in the general population.

Neuropsychiatric Disorders

Applying molecular genetics to ascertain susceptibility genes involved in neuropsychiatric disorders is difficult. The analysis is complex because such disorders are heterogeneous and their genetic components are probably polygenic. Also, the genes involved display low penetrance. There may also be phenocopies of the disorder; that is, a non-genetic type of the disorder that clinically cannot be distinguished from genetically influenced variants.

Schizophrenia

Schizophrenia affects approximately 1 percent of the population. It is generally accepted that genetic factors play an important role in schizophrenia, along with largely unidentified environmental factors. However, these factors are heterogeneous, probably involving mutations at different chromosomal sites. The results of one study revealed a particular region on chromosome 5 to confer a predisposition to schizophrenia in several Icelandic and English families (Sherrington et al. 1988). However, the same region of chromosome 5 was found to be unrelated to the occurrence of schizophrenia in a large Swedish family (Kennedy et al. 1988). There have been other negative reports regarding schizophrenia and chromosome 5 markers (Detera-Wadleigh et al. 1989), and no other positive reports. Subsequent studies involving a third chromosome 5 marker located between the initial two have shown less evidence of linkage to schizophrenia. It has been argued that genetic heterogeneity may explain the absence of chromosome 5 linkage with schizophrenia outside the single study. A suggestion has also been made that the appearance of genetic linkage between chromosome 5 and schizophrenia in the original Icelandic and English sample could have been due to chance (Robertson 1989).

Any susceptibility genes eventually identified to be involved in a predisposition to schizophrenia may represent only minor contributing factors. A 50 percent discordance rate among identical twins (a 50 percent chance that the disease will not be expressed in the genetically identical co-twin of an affected twin) suggests that powerful non-genetic factors are also involved. The penetrance and expression of any schizophrenia susceptibility gene are likely to be influenced greatly by environmental factors. It will be some time, if ever, before any of the genes for schizophrenia are mapped, and it is doubtful that any such genes, if identified, would be useful for screening.

Bipolar Affective Disorder

Bipolar affective disorder has a variable age of onset and affects 0.5 to 1.0 percent of the population.

The first linkage study reported between DNA markers and bipolar affective disorder involved two markers on chromosome 11 in a single large Amish family (Egeland et al. 1987). However, all subsequent studies in other populations have failed to replicate the linkage. A re-evaluation of the Amish study led to the conclusion that the evidence for linkage to chromosome 11 markers was substantially reduced (Kelsoe et al. 1989).

Bipolar affective disorder has also been linked to markers on the X chromosome (Baron et al. 1987). It was estimated that the genes linked to colour-blindness and glucose-6-phosphate dehydrogenase deficiency markers on the X chromosome are carried by one-third of those who have bipolar affective disorder. These linkage studies were confirmed by a second group (Mendlewicz et al. 1987). This strongly supports an X-linked transmission in a subset of bipolar affective disorder. However, data have also been reported that do not support this linkage, such as father-to-son transmission of the illness. This could be accounted for by genetic heterogeneity.

This gene may be mapped, but, because of the genetic heterogeneity of the disorder and its low frequency, it too would seem to be a poor candidate for screening.

Substance Use Disorders

Addiction refers to an overwhelming involvement in seeking and using drugs or alcohol and a high tendency to relapse after withdrawal. Research has shown that alcoholism is determined by genetic and environmental factors. Alcoholism involves different clinical subgroups (Cloninger 1987); thus, it is unlikely that a single marker will confer vulnerability in all families.

A predisposition to alcoholism has been linked to chromosomes 4, 6, and 11 by different research groups. One group has linked alcoholism to a polymorphism in the gene coding for the receptor for dopamine, a neurotransmitter (Blum et al. 1990). The polymorphism was associated with 69 percent of people who were alcoholics. This suggests that other genes or environmental factors are also responsible for the disorder, and that even if one or more of the genes were mapped, mass screening for them would not be appropriate. It is also very likely that programs designed to ameliorate social and environmental factors important in substance abuse constitute a higher priority for resource allocation by society.

Diabetes Mellitus

There are two major forms of diabetes mellitus: insulin-dependent diabetes mellitus (IDDM) and non-insulin dependent diabetes mellitus (NIDDM).

IDDM

IDDM results from a prolonged, selective, and irreversible destruction of insulin-producing pancreatic cells. IDDM affects about 0.3 percent of Caucasian populations (Todd 1990). Development of the disease phenotype is dependent on environmental factors and on the action of several genes, either in concert or in independent groups. Recent studies have shown that the MHC region on chromosome 6 encodes genes that affect susceptibility to IDDM. This area codes for HLA class II antigens: proteins normally expressed on the surface of cells of the immune system. One specific region, the HLA-D region, may provide 60 percent of the genetic contribution to IDDM susceptibility (Rotter and Landaw 1984). Both major and minor susceptibility genes that contribute to the development of IDDM have been identified from this region.

An increased frequency of HLA types DR3 and DR4 has been found among Caucasian IDDM patients. About 95 percent of all patients with

IDDM have HLA-DR3 or DR4 types, or both. Since the risk for IDDM is greater for those having both types, more than one gene likely predisposes a person to IDDM. In addition, because 50 percent of non-diabetics also carry the DR3 or DR4 types, these HLA types are not alone responsible for the onset of IDDM. The different HLA types are defined by variation in both DR and DQ regions. There is evidence that variation in the DQ region may be more strongly associated with risk for IDDM than variation in the DR region. One polymorphism in the HLA-DQ region protects people from developing IDDM while a second is responsible for a dominant pattern of susceptibility to IDDM in the patients studied (only one copy of the gene is needed to promote disease susceptibility) (Baisch et al. 1990). The protective value of the former overrides the susceptibility effect of the latter. A three-gene heterogeneity model of inheritance has been proposed. This model includes two separate diabetes high-risk genes and one low-risk gene, and is similar to a mouse model of IDDM, in which three recessive genes are required to cause diabetes (Prochazka et al. 1987). Other genes outside the MHC region, such as the insulin and immunoglobulin genes, appear to have a minor influence on susceptibility to IDDM (Todd 1990).

A concordance rate of 30 to 40 percent for IDDM in monozygotic twins suggests that environmental factors also play an important role in the etiology of IDDM. There is increasing evidence that the disease may be initiated by a virus that acts on a genetically susceptible host (Vogel and Motulsky 1986). Several chemical agents have also been shown to cause IDDM in animals (Vadheim et al. 1990).

Although HLA types have been associated with IDDM susceptibility, the specific genes involved have not yet been identified. Because 60 percent of the genetic susceptibility to IDDM is contributed by HLA genes, a marker for HLA-linked genetic susceptibility would allow for identification of those at an increased risk for IDDM. However, a person with either the HLA-DR3 or DR4 type has only a 1/150 chance of becoming diabetic (Vadheim et al. 1990) so that the great majority of people with either HLA-DR3 or DR4 will never develop IDDM. Similarly, the HLA-DQ variants associated with IDDM susceptibility occur in 60 to 75 percent of DR4-carrying non-diabetics. Thus, population screening for these HLA genes would produce many more false positives than true positives. The specificity would be insufficient to justify establishing a screening program. Even testing siblings of patients to detect susceptibility is not commonly done because no effective preventive measures are available.

NIDDM

NIDDM is a much milder form of diabetes, and onset occurs later (usually after 40 years of age compared to before 30 years of age) than in IDDM. NIDDM affects about 3 percent of the population and makes up about 90 percent of all diabetes cases (Vogel and Motulsky 1986). Genetic factors play an important role, as shown by a high identical twin concordance rate, but specific genes have not yet been identified. Insulin resistance contributes greatly to the pathogenesis of NIDDM. An insulin response requires the function of many proteins encoded by many genes, and a mutation in any of these genes could possibly contribute to causing NIDDM. Mutations in the insulin gene (Steiner et al. 1990) and insulin receptor gene (Taylor et al. 1990) have been reported in NIDDM patients and appear to increase the risk of developing NIDDM. However, the presence of abnormal insulin is not always associated with NIDDM, and disease phenotypes may vary among family members having the same insulin gene mutation. Possible contributions of genetic variation in the insulin receptor to the development of NIDDM are an unknown quantity, and environmental factors are involved. Even if the gene, when mapped, is suitable for screening, the late onset of the disorder and its good response to treatment would make it a poor candidate for a screening program in the general population. In addition, factors such as weight control, balanced diet, and regular exercise, which are available as interventions to decrease the likelihood of becoming diabetic, make screening correspondingly less profitable.

Lipoprotein Disorders

Lipoproteins are complexes of lipids and proteins whose function is to carry cholesterol in the bloodstream to cells where it is metabolized. Lipoprotein levels are determined by genes that code for proteins whose functions are to control the synthesis, processing, binding, and breakdown of lipoproteins. These include the apolipoproteins and receptors. Mutations in these genes may be responsible for a whole range of lipoprotein disorders that can result in coronary artery disease.

Extensive epidemiologic work has identified a variety of risk factors for coronary atherosclerosis. The major ones include hypertension, hypercholesterolemia, low levels of high-density lipoprotein (HDL), high levels of low-density lipoprotein (LDL), age, male sex, diet, and diabetes. Other risk factors include hypertriglyceridemia, high levels of apolipoprotein B (apo B), and low levels of apolipoprotein A-I (apo A-I). There is increasing evidence that genetic predisposition is an important risk factor in coronary artery disease, with a multifactorial and heterogeneous basis.

As mentioned earlier, increased cholesterol levels in the blood are associated with heart disease. Cholesterol is carried in the bloodstream by lipoproteins. Among the four types of lipoproteins are the LDLs and the HDLs. LDL and HDL function in the transport of endogenous cholesterol to body cells. About 70 percent of the total plasma cholesterol level is contained in LDL (Robbins et al. 1984). Thus, the extent to which genetic factors alter the LDL concentrations will affect susceptibility to heart disease.

Apo B is the major protein of LDL. There are two different forms of apo B: B-100 and B-48. B-100 is the part of the LDL molecule that is recognized by the LDL receptor. Polymorphisms in the apo B gene on chromosome 2 have been associated with atherosclerosis susceptibility (Gavish et al. 1989) and myocardial infarction (Hegele et al. 1986). However, how common these polymorphisms are in the general population is undetermined. Several different variations at some of the loci within the apo B gene are likely associated with the development of heart disease, thus making genetic screening impractical.

Binding of LDL to the LDL receptor on the cell surface regulates cholesterol metabolism by suppressing cholesterol synthesis and increasing LDL degradation. Familial hypercholesterolemia is a common autosomal dominant disorder caused by defects in the LDL receptor, disrupting cholesterol metabolism (Leppert et al. 1986). One in 500 people is heterozygous for familial hypercholesterolemia and has elevated LDL cholesterol levels. Fifty percent of affected males have some manifestation of coronary artery disease by the age of 50. Clinical manifestations in females occur 10 to 15 years later (Vogel and Motulsky 1986). The homozygote state is extremely rare, affecting one in one million children. Atherosclerosis results in death from myocardial infarction in the affected homozygotes, usually before 30 years of age. One group identified six different mutations in the LDL receptor gene from 234 unrelated heterozygotes for familial hypercholesterolemia (Langlois et al. 1988). It was concluded that major structural rearrangements account for 2 to 6 percent of mutations causing the disorder, of which deletions are the most common. The high frequency of familial hypercholesterolemia in the general population may partially result from a high mutation rate in the LDL receptor gene, due to its high frequency of repetitive elements. Over 20 different defects in the LDL receptor have been identified (Utermann 1990).

Familial hypercholesterolemia is one of the few disorders that has been considered a candidate for genetic screening, as there are interventions (diet, drugs) that lower the cholesterol and decrease disease progression, even though its frequency is far below the recommended 5 percent. It is a monogenic disorder; thus, the LDL receptor gene could be screened for mutations. However, since more than 20 mutations have been identified, no single test could identify all possible mutations in the LDL receptor gene. Each specimen would have to be tested with several probes, which would be too costly for mass screening.

Apo A-I is the principal protein in HDL, which promotes the removal of cholesterol from arterial walls. Decreased plasma concentrations of HDL and apo A-I have been associated with premature coronary artery disease; low HDL levels have been observed in approximately 58 percent of patients with coronary artery disease (Ordovas et al. 1986). Familial hypoalphalipoproteinemia, characterized by low HDL levels, is an autosomal dominant disorder that causes susceptibility to premature coronary artery disease. A RFLP has been identified that is linked to the apo A-I gene. This polymorphism is associated with familial hypoalphalipoproteinemia and premature coronary artery disease (ibid.). The precise relationship between plasma HDL concentrations and the RFLP is not yet defined.

Genetic abnormalities in LDL metabolism can also result from the attachment of a large glycoprotein (apo(a)) to the apo B-100 moiety of LDL. This complex, Lp(a), reacts poorly with LDL receptors on cell surfaces and thus causes increased cholesterol levels in the blood. The seven forms of apo(a) are inherited and affect Lp(a) levels. Certain individuals with high Lp(a) concentrations are at an increased risk for coronary heart disease (Breckenridge 1990). Again, even if any of the contributing genes could be identified directly, genetic heterogeneity and the complexity of the system make it unsuitable for population-wide screening.

Environmental factors are also involved in coronary arterial disease. Studies have shown that smoking is an important determinant in the development of coronary arterial disease. Compared with non-smokers, smokers have more than twice the risk of developing coronary heart disease (Pathobiological Determinants of Atherosclerosis in Youth Research Group 1990). Insurance companies have already responded by adjusting their premiums to this environmental contribution to susceptibility.

Rheumatic Diseases

One subgroup of the disorders that affect structures of the musculoskeletal system is the inflammatory articular multisystemic diseases that are caused by aberrant immunologic mechanisms. They include rheumatoid arthritis, spondyloarthropathies, and several connective tissue diseases such as systemic lupus erythematosus. These disorders are multifactorial, being influenced by both genetic and environmental factors.

The MHC is a genetically determined regulator of immune responses. The MHC codes for both class I antigens (HLA-A, -B, and -C) involved in cytotoxic T-cell responses and class II antigens (HLA-D) involved in antibody responses. Spondyloarthropathies are associated with class I HLA antigens. Autoimmune diseases such as rheumatoid arthritis and lupus are associated with class II antigens.

Spondyloarthropathies

Spondyloarthropathies generally involve the central part of the skeletal system, particularly the joints of the lower spine. Two subgroups of spondyloarthropathies include ankylosing spondylitis and Reiter's syndrome.

Ankylosing spondylitis is a chronic disease of young adults characterized by inflammatory lesions of the central skeleton. The expression of this disease is dominated by back pain and limited spinal mobility. More than 90 percent of patients with ankylosing spondylitis carry the HLA-B27 type (Arnett 1986). However, since only 20 percent of HLA-B27-positive individuals have the disease, the specificity of a test to identify HLA-B27-positive people would be insufficient to justify a screening program. An infectious agent likely is involved in the pathogenesis, and the class I B27 antigen likely promotes a cell-mediated attack on the selected tissues.

In Reiter's syndrome, there are skin, mucous, and eye lesions as well as musculoskeletal involvement. Reiter's syndrome is also associated with HLA-B27 in 75 percent of cases. It is triggered by several infectious agents, such as *Salmonella, Yersinia,* and *Campylobacter enteritis.* The role of HLA-B27 is unclear.

Rheumatoid Arthritis

Rheumatoid arthritis is a chronic inflammatory disorder involving many symmetrical joints and subcutaneous nodules, eyes, heart, lungs, and nerves. Genetic disposition to rheumatoid arthritis is associated with particular genotypes of the HLA-D region of the MHC. HLA-DR4 is present in 70 percent of affected and in 28 percent of unaffected whites. Other HLA regions are also strongly associated with rheumatoid arthritis. Carrying these specific HLA types increases a person's risk by about 5 percent.

Systemic Lupus Erythematosus

Systemic lupus erythematosus is a multisystem inflammatory disease characterized by numerous autoantibodies directed against cellular and serum constituents. The class II antigen HLA-DR3 shows a strong association with lupus, occurring in 50 percent of patients and in 25 percent of unaffected people.

HLA-linked genes alone do not explain rheumatic diseases. A combination of HLA and non-HLA genetic effects plus environmental factors is required. Tests to identify those susceptible to these diseases on the basis of their HLA types would not have adequate specificity or sensitivity.

Chronic Obstructive Pulmonary Disease

Chronic obstructive pulmonary disease (COPD) is a common disorder, usually characterized by progressive obstruction of airflow and a history of inhalation of irritants such as tobacco. COPD may be divided into two entities: chronic bronchitis and emphysema. Chronic bronchitis is defined by its clinical symptoms, such as excessive mucus secretion in the bronchial tree, leading to a productive cough for at least three months during each of two successive years. Emphysema is described by its pathologic anatomy involving destruction of alveolar walls and abnormal enlargement of airspaces at the end of the bronchioles. An affected COPD individual will have a combination of the two entities.

$Alpha_1$-antitrypsin is a plasma protease inhibitor that protects surrounding tissues from proteolytic enzymes produced by inflamed tissues. There are many alleles, several of which produce an enzyme with reduced activity; heterozygotes, having one normal and one mutant allele, have serum α_1-antitrypsin activities midway between that of the homozygous deficient and normal individuals. The heterozygous state for any one of the mutant alleles that reduce activity exists in 3 to 5 percent of the population, while the homozygous state is quite rare.   The heterozygous state in combination with environmental factors can increase the risk of emphysema and predispose to the development of COPD. Alpha$_1$-antitrypsin deficiency can render that person more sensitive to cigarette smoke. It can be screened for at the DNA level. Thus, the gene is frequent enough to qualify for a screening program in the general population. To avoid damage to their lungs, such individuals should never smoke or be in polluted environments.   It would be difficult to justify workplace screening, as reducing the environmental causes is beneficial to all.   Air pollution is unhealthy for all workers.   Once the workplace has been cleaned up as far as is feasible, worker protective devices are also possible. In some workplaces after these steps are taken, screening could be considered, provided identified workers may be transferred to other employment without loss of pay or other detriment.

Antibiotic-Induced Deafness

The aminoglycosides are a class of antibiotics that include streptomycin, kanamycin, gentamicin, tobramicin, and neomycin and whose use can lead to hearing loss.   Some patients have developed aminoglycoside antibiotic induced deafness after treatment with conventional doses over a short period. This, along with the fact that family aggregation of this type of deafness has been reported, indicates that some subjects may have a genetically determined susceptibility to this class of antibiotics. An autosomal dominant inheritance may be involved (Hu et al. 1991).   The gene's low frequency and irregular expression make it an unsuitable candidate for screening even in the unlikely event that it will be mapped.

Creutzfeldt-Jakob Disease

Creutzfeldt-Jakob disease is a rare degenerative brain disease caused by a slow viral infection. A progressive dementia occurs, accompanied by a loss of control of the subject's involuntary and automatic movements. The disease is most common in adults in their fifties, and death usually occurs within two years after the diagnosis has been made. No means of treatment is known. It has been postulated that the development of this disease in some people is due to a sequence variation in one of their protein genes that had rendered them more susceptible to infection (Collinge et al. 1991). The putative gene would be unlikely to ever become a candidate for a screening program in the general population due to the very low frequency of this disease.

Discussion

Many of the common diseases in our society, such as cancers, psychiatric disorders, and heart disease, are multifactorial and caused by the interaction of genetic factors with each other and with environmental factors. With new methods being developed to identify genes and analyze DNA, researchers are beginning to identify some of the genetic factors involved in these diseases. However, these genes only confer susceptibility to the disease; they are insufficient to cause disease without the interaction of environmental factors. This interaction is not well understood and, although some environmental factors such as cigarette smoke and fatty diet have been identified for particular diseases, for most diseases they are not known.

The recognition of the genetic factors involved in multifactorial diseases presents the possibility of identifying susceptibility, with the aim of prevention or earlier treatment of the disease in question. These possible benefits come with the risk of possible harms. Unless the genetic information were protected, there could be discrimination against carriers of susceptibility genes by insurance companies, employers, or peers. Being identified as genetically susceptible could also have an adverse impact on the self-concept and sense of wellness of the identified individual, with a harmful focus on the risk of becoming ill. This paper studies the potential of screening programs for these susceptibility genes. It outlines what criteria characterize a susceptibility gene as suitable for mass screening, what susceptibility genes have been, or are likely to be, identified in the foreseeable future, and which, if any, of these genes might be suitable for population-wide screening.

To be a suitable candidate for population-wide screening, a gene that increases susceptibility to a disease should have the following characteristics:

(a)   Some form of intervention must be available that would prevent or reduce the severity of the disease. For example, screening for genes that increase susceptibility to IDDM would not be justified, since, at this time, almost nothing can be done to avert onset of the disease.

(b)   The gene to be screened for would have to increase susceptibility significantly — for example, it is not justified to screen for a gene that increases the probability of the disease occurring in a carrier only by 1 to 5 percent. Screening for a gene that is not certain to result in a disease in those carrying it, but only predicts a probability of getting the disorder, raises many serious concerns, and benefits should be estimated to outweigh the harms from careful pilot studies before population-wide screening is justified. These concerns are even more important if it is suggested in future that prenatal screening for susceptibility be done. At this time, there are no such disorders in which this is even suggested.

(c) Any susceptibility gene screened for should be frequent enough in the population to make the screening program worthwhile. It would not be justified to expend the resources required to detect 1 in 10 000 susceptible individuals, for example. A rate of 5 percent identified individuals has been suggested, but the optimal figure would depend on many other factors.

(d) The disorder would have to be severe enough to justify screening. Increased susceptibility to mild/trivial disorders would not be suitable, whereas increased susceptibility to severe, life-threatening disorders such as early coronary heart disease might be.

(e) The predictive value of the susceptibility gene should strike an optimal balance between allowing too many false positives, requiring additional testing and unnecessary anxiety for individuals, and too many false negatives, resulting in missed cases. Genetic heterogeneity, which is characteristic of multifactorial disorders, complicates the picture.

(f) The susceptibility gene must be identified by an alteration within the gene that can be detected by the appropriate probe. Genetic heterogeneity may require the use of several probes (as in cystic fibrosis), which increases cost. Genes that are detected by linkage or association with outside markers (such as polycystic kidneys) are not suitable for mass screening, because they require analysis of families rather than individuals.

(g) There must be clear benefits, and the cost of the program must be low enough to justify spending the funds on it, rather than some other program. The test must be simple, inexpensive, and reliable. The estimation of cost must include: the expense of the test, the cost of the necessary public education, the provision of counselling services, and the costs of the recommended preventive strategies. In addition, the anxiety caused by the testing, ensuring informed consent, and the protection of privacy must be taken into account. It is essential that other ramifications, including procedures to protect against discrimination against carriers of susceptibility genes by employers, insurers, government agencies, or peers, also be dealt with.

Review of the susceptibility genes so far identified has shown that none fulfils all of the criteria for a successful population-wide screening program, although some may be useful for testing family members related to affected individuals with a mutation.

Susceptibility genes are difficult to identify; the search requires the study of many large families, usually on a "needle-in-a-field-of-haystacks" basis (i.e., with few clues as to where to look among thousands of possible places). A few people have a change within the responsible gene itself that can be detected by DNA analysis. Susceptibility genes do not identify those who will get the disease, only those with increased susceptibility to it. By definition, they do not have high predictive value; they simply change the probability of becoming affected with a particular disorder. Thus, it is not surprising that no mass screening programs have been established for susceptibility genes. It is important to note that the increased knowledge that will come from the Human Genome Project is also very unlikely to identify any genes that are more eligible than those already known. However, widespread screening has the potential for commercial profit. There is much research occurring in the United States in this area, by pharmaceutical companies, to identify genes relevant to common diseases with the stated intention of finding therapeutic agents by a better understanding of the disease process. Many feel that there will be pressures for population-wide screening as a result. It is therefore important that guidelines be put in place and criteria be met before implementation is specified (Holtzman 1989).

It is also very unlikely that genes will be mapped that enhance "desirable "qualities such as longevity, intelligence, or kindness. Whatever genetic basis there may be for such traits must involve large numbers of genes, each of small effect, which are not likely to be amenable to mapping.

There are very serious issues, applying not only to susceptibility genes but to some single genes with regular expression, some of which are suitable for mass screening. These include possible discrimination against carriers of susceptibility genes by employers, insurers, government agencies, or peers. The subject needs serious discussion and recommendations about what social measures can and should be taken to protect from discrimination the carriers of genes causing disorders. This, however, falls beyond the scope of the current project. The objective of the current project was to describe what currently can be done and what is on the horizon with regard to screening for susceptibility genes.

Prenatal diagnosis is an area in which screening for susceptibility genes might become technically possible, which is relevant to reproductive technologies and so comes within the mandate of the Royal Commission. So far, prenatal diagnosis is done only in cases where the fetus is diagnosed as having a high probability of a serious disorder. Most of these disorders are present at birth, or appear in early childhood. Recently, predictive testing by DNA analysis has made it possible to identify individuals who carry a gene that will result in disease later in life, Huntington disease being the classical example. Prenatal diagnosis is therefore possible for such conditions. There is considerable concern, among geneticists and others, about the morality and legality of doing prenatal diagnosis for a gene that will result in a disease that will appear only in later life (Cooke 1993). Because of this concern, guidelines are being developed (Harper et al. 1990). It has not been seriously proposed to test prenatally for a gene that does not predict a disease of late onset with a high degree (e.g., 95 percent) of confidence, but only indicates a somewhat increased probability of its occurrence. There are serious misgivings about this possibility, and some geneticists feel strongly that it is inappropriate (Harper and Clarke 1990). Nevertheless, the possibility exists, and the number of potentially eligible diseases where susceptibility genes can be detected will increase.

The idea of doing prenatal diagnosis for the gene for a disorder that, if found, may result in abortion of a fetus that, if it survived, may never become affected by that disorder seems unjustified. Geneticists and others debate the question of how serious a disorder should be to justify prenatal testing for it. At this time there appears to be a consensus among many of those working in this area that undertaking prenatal testing for genes that simply increase susceptibility to a disease is not justified, and should not be done. There is a need for greater public awareness and debate on many of the issues raised.

Summary

An increasing number of genes are being identified by DNA analysis that increase susceptibility to a given disorder; that is, the gene carrier has an increased probability of developing the disorder. Concerns are being expressed that population-wide screening programs could be introduced to identify such individuals with the aim of making preventive measures available to them, but also with the possible undesirable risk of making them susceptible to discrimination by employers, insurers, government agencies, or peers.

When measured against the criteria for a successful population-wide screening program, none of the susceptibility genes identified so far would qualify, largely because of low predictive value, small effect, and genetic heterogeneity. It is unlikely, therefore, that population-based screening programs will be developed for genes that simply increase susceptibility to disease.

On the other hand, some susceptibility genes are suitable for testing families of affected individuals with the mutation, and a few are being used in this targeted way. Without appropriate protection of genetic information, this could lead to discrimination against carriers of such genes, just as they may for single-gene disorders with high penetrance, such as Huntington disease. Insurance companies already use the family history to adjust premiums of those at increased risk because of affected relatives, even without genetic screening. Ways to reconcile the rights and responsibilities of the various parties concerned will have to be developed.

The question has been raised whether society would approve of doing prenatal diagnosis to detect genes that have only an increased probability, not a certainty, of causing a serious disorder. Most geneticists would not approve, and existing guidelines suggest that it is not ethical. It might be concluded that prenatal testing for susceptibility genes is one possible use of prenatal diagnosis that has so many pitfalls and so few benefits that it should not be permitted.

Bibliography

Arnett, F.C. 1986. "HLA Genes and Predisposition to Rheumatic Diseases." *Hospital Practice* (Office Edition) 21 (15 December): 89-100.

Atkin, N.B., and M.F. Fox. 1990. "5q Deletion: The Sole Chromosome Change in a Carcinoma of the Bladder." *Cancer Genetics and Cytogenetics* 46: 129-31.

Ayesh, R., et al. 1984. "Metabolic Oxidation Phenotypes as Markers for Susceptibility to Lung Cancer." *Nature* 312: 169-70.

Babu, V.R., et al. 1989. "Chromosome 21q22 Deletion: A Specific Chromosome Change in a New Bladder Cancer Subgroup." *Cancer Genetics and Cytogenetics* 38: 127-30.

Baisch, J.M., et al. 1990. "Analysis of HLA-DQ Genotypes and Susceptibility in Insulin-Dependent Diabetes Mellitus." *New England Journal of Medicine* 322: 1836-41.

Baker, S.J., et al. 1989. "Chromosome 17 Deletions and p53 Gene Mutations in Colorectal Carcinomas." *Science* 244: 217-21.

Baron, M., et al. 1987. "Genetic Linkage Between X-Chromosome Markers and Bipolar Affective Illness." *Nature* 326: 289-92.

Berger, C.S., et al. 1986. "Chromosomes in Kidney, Ureter and Bladder Cancer." *Cancer Genetics and Cytogenetics* 23: 1-24.

Blum, K., et al. 1990. "Allelic Association of Human Dopamine D2 Receptor Gene in Alcoholism." *JAMA* 263: 2055-60.

Bodmer, W.F., et al. 1987. "Localization of the Gene for Familial Adenomatous Polyposis on Chromosome 5." *Nature* 328: 614-16.

Bos, J.L., et al. 1987. "Prevalence of Ras Gene Mutations in Human Colorectal Cancers." *Nature* 327: 293-97.

Breckenridge, W.C. 1990. "Lipoprotein (a): Genetic Marker for Atherosclerosis?" *Canadian Medical Association Journal* 143: 115.

Cloninger, C.R. 1987. "Neurogenetic Adaptive Mechanisms in Alcoholism." *Science* 236: 410-16.

Cohen, A.J., et al. 1979. "Hereditary Renal-Cell Carcinoma Associated with a Chromosomal Translocation." *New England Journal of Medicine* 301: 592-95.

Collinge, J., M.S. Palmer, and A.J. Dryden. 1991. "Genetic Predisposition to Iatrogenic Creutzfeldt-Jakob Disease." *Lancet* (15 June): 1441-42.

Cooke, M. 1993. "Ethical Issues of Prenatal Diagnosis for Predictive Testing for Genetic Disorders of Late Onset." In *Technologies of Sex Selection and Prenatal Diagnosis*, vol. 14 of the research studies of the Royal Commission on New Reproductive Technologies. Ottawa: Minister of Supply and Services Canada.

Detera-Wadleigh, S.D., et al. 1989. "Exclusion of Linkage to 5q11-13 in Families with Schizophrenia and Other Psychiatric Disorders." *Nature* 340: 391-93.

Egeland, J.A., et al. 1987. "Bipolar Affective Disorders Linked to DNA Markers on Chromosome 11." *Nature* 325: 783-87.

Fearon, E.R., et al. 1990. "Identification of a Chromosome 18q Gene that Is Altered in Colorectal Cancers." *Science* 247: 49-56.

Forrester, K., et al. 1987. "Detection of High Incidence of K-ras Oncogenes During Human Colon Tumorigenesis." *Nature* 327: 298-303.

Gavish, D., E.A. Brinton, and J.L. Breslow. 1989. "Heritable Allele-Specific Differences in Amounts of apoB and Low-Density Lipoproteins in Plasma." *Science* 244: 72-76.

Harper, P.S., and A. Clarke. 1990. "Should We Test Children for 'Adult' Genetic Diseases?" *Lancet* (19 May): 1205-1206.

Harper, P.S., M.J. Morris, and A. Tyler. 1990. "Genetic Testing for Huntington's Disease: Internationally Agreed Guidelines Are Being Followed." *British Medical Journal* 300: 1089-90.

Hegele, R.A., et al. 1986. "Apolipoprotein B-gene DNA Polymorphisms Associated with Myocardial Infarction." *New England Journal of Medicine* 315: 1509-15.

Holtzman, N.A. 1989. *Proceed with Caution*. Baltimore: Johns Hopkins University Press.

Hu, D.N., et al. 1991. "Genetic Aspects of Antibiotic Induced Deafness: Mitochondrial Inheritance." *Journal of Medical Genetics* 28: 79-83.

Kelsoe, J.R., et al. 1989. "Re-evaluation of the Linkage Relationship Between Chromosome 11p Loci and the Gene for Bipolar Affective Disorder in the Old Order Amish." *Nature* 342: 238-43.

Kennedy, J.L., et al. 1988. "Evidence Against Linkage of Schizophrenia to Markers on Chromosome 5 in a Northern Swedish Pedigree." *Nature* 336: 167-70.

Knudson, A.G., Jr. 1979. "Persons at High Risk of Cancer." *New England Journal of Medicine* 301: 606-607.

Kok, K., et al. 1987. "Deletion of a DNA Sequence at the Chromosomal Region 3p21 in All Major Types of Lung Cancer." *Nature* 330: 578-81.

Langlois, S., J.J. Kastelein, and M.R. Hayden. 1988. "Characterization of Six Partial Deletions in the Low-Density-Lipoprotein (LDL) Receptor Gene Causing Familial Hypercholesterolemia (FH)." *American Journal of Human Genetics* 43: 60-68.

Leppert, M., et al. 1986. "A DNA Probe for the LDL Receptor Gene Is Tightly Linked to Hypercholesterolemia in a Pedigree with Early Coronary Disease." *American Journal of Human Genetics* 39: 300-306.

—. 1987. "The Gene for Familial Polyposis Coli Maps to the Long Arm of Chromosome 5." *Science* 238: 1411-13.

Marx, J.L. 1985. "The Cytochrome P450's and Their Genes." *Science* 228: 975-76.

—. 1991. "Gene Identified for Inherited Cancer Susceptibility." *Science* 253: 616.

Mendlewicz, J., et al. 1987. "Polymorphic DNA Marker on X Chromosome and Manic Depression." *Lancet* (30 May): 1230-32.

Mowat, M., et al. 1985. "Rearrangements of the Cellular p53 Gene in Erythroleukaemic Cells Transformed by Friend Virus." *Nature* 314: 633-36.

Murray, R.F., Jr. 1986. "Tests of So-Called Genetic Susceptibility." *Journal of Occupational Medicine* 28: 1103-1107.

Omenn, G.S. 1982. "Predictive Identification of Hypersusceptible Individuals." *Journal of Occupational Medicine* 24: 369-74.

Ordovas, J.M., et al. 1986. "Apolipoprotein A-1 Gene Polymorphism Associated with Premature Coronary Artery Disease and Familial Hypoalphalipoproteinemia." *New England Journal of Medicine* 314: 671-77.

Pathobiological Determinants of Atherosclerosis in Youth (PDAY) Research Group. 1990. "Relationships of Atherosclerosis in Young Men to Serum Lipoprotein Cholesterol Concentrations and Smoking: A Preliminary Report." *JAMA* 264: 3060-61.

Prochazka, M., et al. 1987. "Three Recessive Loci Required for Insulin-Dependent Diabetes in Nonobese Diabetic Mice." *Science* 237: 286-89.

Robbins, S.L., R.S. Cotran, and V. Kumar. 1984. *Pathologic Basis of Disease.* 3d ed. Philadelphia: W.B. Saunders.

Robertson, M. 1989. "False Start on Manic Depression." *Nature* 342: 222.

Rotter, J.I., and E.M. Landaw. 1984. "Measuring the Genetic Contribution of a Single Locus to a Multilocus Disease." *Clinical Genetics* 26: 529-42.

Sherrington, R., et al. 1988. "Localization of a Susceptibility Locus for Schizophrenia on Chromosome 5." *Nature* 336: 164-67.

Silverberg, E., and J. Lubera. 1987. "Cancer Statistics, 1987." *CA: A Cancer Journal for Clinicians* 37: 2-19.

Steiner, D.F., et al. 1990. "Lessons Learned from Molecular Biology of Insulin-Gene Mutations." *Diabetes Care* 13: 600-609.

Takahashi, T., et al. 1989. "p53: A Frequent Target for Genetic Abnormalities in Lung Cancer." *Science* 246: 491-94.

Taylor, S.I., et al. 1990. "Mutations in Insulin-Receptor Gene in Insulin-Resistant Patients." *Diabetes Care* 13: 257-79.

Todd, J.A. 1990. "Genetic Control of Autoimmunity in Type 1 Diabetes." *Immunology Today* 11: 122-29.

Tsai, Y.C., et al. 1990. "Allelic Losses of Chromosomes 9, 11, and 17 in Human Bladder Cancer." *Cancer Research* 50: 44-47.

Utermann, G. 1990. "Coronary Heart Disease." In *Principles and Practice of Medical Genetics.* 2d ed., ed. A.E.H. Emery and D.L. Rimoin. Edinburgh: Churchill Livingstone.

Vadheim, C.M., D.L. Rimoin, and J.I. Rotter. 1990. "Diabetes Mellitus." In *Principles and Practice of Medical Genetics*. 2d ed., ed. A.E.H. Emery and D.L. Rimoin. Edinburgh: Churchill Livingstone.

Vogel, F., and A.G. Motulsky. 1986. *Human Genetics: Problems and Approaches*. 2d ed. Berlin: Springer-Verlag.

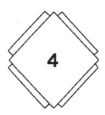

4

Preference for the Sex of One's Children and the Prospective Use of Sex Selection

Martin Thomas

Executive Summary

This report describes the results of empirical research into the potential use of sex selection methods by Canadians.

A predictive model incorporates data on the following variables: preferences for the sex of one's children, public awareness of sex preselection and fetal sexing methods, willingness to use preselection or abortion for sex selection, the reliability of the methods, et cetera.

Method reliability was determined by reviewing the relevant professional literature. The evidence appears to indicate that most preselection methods are probably ineffectual.

Data on attitudes were obtained from a national survey conducted for this purpose. They reveal no aggregate sex preference among women and a very slight pro-son bias among men. They indicate conclusively that the desire to have at least one child of each sex is by far the most pervasive and deeply held value with regard to children's sex. With few exceptions, it is the only motive for which preselection would be attempted. Roughly one-quarter of all respondents can imagine doing so.

Almost no respondents would use abortion for sex selection, notwithstanding the almost perfect reliability of fetal sexing methods.

This paper was completed for the Royal Commission on New Reproductive Technologies in May 1992.

The predictive model illustrates the redundancy of factors that virtually preclude maldistribution resulting from sex selection. These factors include a negligible aggregate sex bias and the ineffectiveness of preselection methods that people are willing to use.

Introduction

Purpose

This report describes the results of research into the implications of the possible use of various sex selection methods by Canadian residents. The report describes empirical evidence pertaining to the relevant variables and provides predictions based on extrapolations from the data. Of necessity, these inferences about future events and outcomes will be guided not only by the applicable data presented here, but also by assumptions about the relevance of other variables, for example, those concerning either human behaviour or possible changes in technology. These assumptions will be considered explicitly.

Sex maldistribution resulting from opportunities for the selection of the sex of one's children has extremely adverse potential implications for the most fundamental aspects of our society. Consequently, there is deep concern on the part of scholars, social policy planners, and lay people about these potential effects if people are free to use sex selection as they wish, when improved techniques are developed and become widely available. However, there is also a legitimate and abiding concern about the prospect of attempted government regulation of this practice or any other aspect of reproductive behaviour.

The ongoing debate about the use of sex selection has been based not only on differences in ethical positions concerning the social consequences of sex maldistribution, but also on differences in assumptions about factual issues, such as the nature and extent of maldistribution likely to result from the use of sex selection. It is important that the empirical questions be rigorously and systematically examined so that the ethical arguments will be informed and more easily resolved.

The causal link between maldistribution and social consequences is only one of many that are relevant to the issue of sex selection. There is a series of causal relationships, beginning with preference for the sex of one's children, knowledge of available sex selection methods, and access to those methods, through willingness to use sex selection and the reliability of methods used, to possible sex maldistribution and the social consequences of that maldistribution.

Much of the published writing on these issues, especially the work that is primarily theoretical, has focussed only on the last of these links, seemingly on the premise that opportunities to select the sex of one's children would inevitably result in a disproportionate number of males being born. That assumption has been made almost routinely and often uncritically. But virtually no evidence pertinent specifically to the Canadian population has been provided to justify such an assumption, or any assumption, about the direction and extent of sex maldistribution likely to result from the availability of sex selection methods.

Drawing inferences about the connection between preference for the sex of one's children and social consequences, after studying only the link between maldistribution and social consequences, is less than optimal. At best it is potentially inefficient, in that the research enterprise is wholly dependent on a premise that may prove to be false. At worst it is potentially harmful, in that it may foster a view of either societal risk, or the absence of risk, that is false. Sex maldistribution may occur, but neither its magnitude nor its direction — much less its potential consequences — should be taken for granted if empirical evidence can be obtained.

The study of individuals' preferences for the sex of their children, their awareness of opportunities for sex selection, and their willingness to attempt it should precede any assumptions about future frequency or methods of use. Furthermore, information on the probable frequency of use and the reliability of methods most likely to be used should precede consideration of the severity and direction of maldistribution. Finally, evidence concerning the nature of that maldistribution, if any, ought to precede any analysis of its social consequences.

This is not to say that no scientific research should proceed unless the antecedent causal link has been verified. Rather, it is to say that if assumptions are questionable and empirically verifiable, the argument in favour of attempting verification becomes all the more compelling. The logically prior questions in this instance, which deal with preference, knowledge, willingness, reliability, et cetera, are clearly empirically verifiable.

Scope

Methods of Sex Selection

Five approaches to affecting the likelihood of having a child of one sex or the other are available. The first two, because they involve actions taken prior to conception, are often referred to as "preselection" methods. They are

1. sex preselection in which fertilization of the ovum occurs *in vivo*, and there is an attempt to influence the type of sperm cell involved in fertilization;

2. sex preselection in which fertilization of the ovum occurs *in vitro*, and an embryo of the desired sex is implanted in the mother;

3. sex selection by abortion after identification of the fetus' sex;

4. selective adoption, based on the sex of the baby; and

5. giving up one's biological child for adoption, based on its sex.

Not all of these methods are considered in detail in this report. Preselection *in vivo* is explicitly considered, since it is directly relevant to advances in reproductive technologies that have made it, if not a highly reliable option at present, then one that at least holds promise. This portends a higher incidence of preselection attempts in the coming years, as the reliability and availability of preselection methods improve and as public awareness and acceptance of them increase. The reliability of sex selection techniques is critical in attempting to predict maldistribution, and opinion concerning the reliability of the various preselection methods varies considerably.

This report also includes an evaluation of the reliability of the prominent, popular, or credible methods of sex preselection for inclusion in the predictive model. This is based on a review of the professional literature on sex preselection.

The second approach, *in vitro* fertilization (IVF), has been employed with limited success to achieve conception when that would otherwise have been problematic, but rarely, if ever, has it been used primarily for the purpose of sex selection. If natural conception were not a problem, this method could be used as a method of preselection, but it would not be very useful. Sex could be determined with perfect reliability, but achieving a viable pregnancy *in vitro* would still be difficult. This method is extremely unlikely to be preferred by prospective parents, not only because of its ineffectiveness, but also because of its intrusiveness, inconvenience, and expense. Consequently, public attitudes concerning IVF for the sake of sex selection will not be a focus of this research.

The third approach, abortion, is also relevant to reproductive technology and is explicitly considered in this report. Future technical advances may mean that fetal sexing will be done with greater rapidity, ease, economy, and comfort to the mother, and/or earlier in the pregnancy, probably leading to its increased use. This may result in the more frequent use of abortion as a method of sex selection. Because of the fairly broad consensus on the reliability of various methods of fetal sexing, a critical review of this literature was not undertaken.

Adoption is not directly related to advances in reproductive technologies, has no effect on sex maldistribution, and is not a primary focus of this research. However, some attitudinal data concerning willingness to adopt under various circumstances have been collected to improve the interpretability of the corresponding data on willingness to use either preselection or fetal sexing and subsequent abortion.

The final category is not relevant to the question at hand. Furthermore, the frequency with which people in this country are willing to give their children up for adoption based on their sex preferences is assumed to be so small that any societal effect would be trivial.

Attitudinal Data

This report relies heavily on data from original survey research on Canadians' attitudes concerning preferences for the sex of their children. The correlates of different sex preference patterns are identified, and the preferences of Canadians are compared to those in other societies. The data on sex preferences are not method-specific but are critical to understanding and estimating potential use of both preselection methods and methods of fetal sexing and selective abortion.

The survey also examines attitudes with regard to the use of sex selection and awareness of available methods. With specific regard to preselection methods and their future use in Canada, this research describes Canadians' awareness of the most prominent preselection techniques and the circumstances under which they would be used, relating the demographic characteristics of diverse groups to their awareness of and willingness to use preselection methods. The survey also provides some evidence, for various methods, of the frequency and the success rates of previous attempts at preselection by Canadians. It was recognized at the outset, however, that the sample probably would not identify more than a handful of Canadians who had previously attempted either preselection or selection by abortion.

With respect to sex selection by abortion, the report provides an estimate of Canadians' awareness of fetal sexing methods and their willingness to submit (or to have their female partners submit) to various fetal sex determination techniques for the purpose of sex selection by abortion.

The attitudinal and method reliability data for both kinds of sex selection are incorporated in the predictive model to estimate their possible impact on the magnitude and direction of sex maldistribution.

A Predictive Model: The Consequences of Opportunities for Sex Selection

A predictive model, incorporating variables relevant to the use of sex selection and permitting an estimate of its consequences, was developed. Although it is presented initially in a rudimentary form, it is adaptable according to the characteristics of the data available.

A prediction of the direction and magnitude of sex imbalance resulting from the availability of sex selection techniques requires the following kinds of data:

1. the proportion of pregnancies that are planned;

2. the birth sex ratio in the absence of sex selection attempts;

3. the proportion of the population that intends to have a child or children, is able to do so, is aware of the availability of sex

selection techniques, has sex preferences (such that if they were acted on, the birth ratio would be different from what it is currently), and is willing to use specific sex preselection techniques to achieve the sex mix preferred;

4. the reliability of each of the techniques that might be used in attempts to create females; and

5. the reliability of each of the techniques that might be used in attempts to create males.

One recently published paper dealing with sex selection has predicted the extent of future sex imbalance by integrating these disparate variables, but it described data gleaned from a variety of previously published papers, obtaining preference data from one sample, willingness data from another, et cetera.[1] The accuracy of such an approach is certain only to the extent that the interrelatedness of the variables is known. Since little information is available on the interrelatedness of all of those variables — for example, between preference and willingness — a predictive model would be more effective if it incorporated data for all of those variables for a single population. This is all the more important since there are few data on any of these variables for Canadians, much less, data on all of them derived from a single sample. Data for these variables were obtained through the use of population surveys, and are incorporated in the predictive model.

The logic of the predictive model is not complicated; it is simply that the proportion of newborns of one sex can be estimated by adding the proportions of newborns of that sex from categories that are mutually exclusive and that together comprise all births. The four categories are (a) births from unplanned pregnancies, (b) births from planned pregnancies not involving sex selection, (c) successful attempts to select that sex, and (d) failed attempts to select the other sex. These categories simply reflect the axioms that pregnancies are either intended or not, that those not intended do not involve attempts at preselection, that those intended may or may not involve attempts at preselection, that attempts at sex selection are directed either toward having a son or toward having a daughter, and that sex selection attempts are either successful or unsuccessful.

To simplify the description of the model and to clarify the mathematical relationships among variables, the categories are also described symbolically. (The formula can be used to calculate the proportion of either males or females; it is set up to calculate the proportion of births that are females.) The following symbols are used:

F	=	the proportion of newborns who are female
I	=	the proportion of all births resulting from pregnancies that are intended
$(1 - I)$	=	the proportion of all births resulting from pregnancies that are not intended

S	=	the proportion of planned pregnancies that involve sex selection
(1 – S)	=	the proportion of planned pregnancies that do not involve sex selection
FN	=	the proportion of newborns who are females, when sex selection is not attempted
SF	=	the proportion of sex selection attempts that are intended to produce females
(1 – SF)	=	the proportion of sex selection attempts that are intended to produce males
RF	=	the proportion of attempts to select females that are successful
RM	=	the proportion of attempts to select males that are successful
(1 – RM)	=	the proportion of attempts to select males that are unsuccessful, i.e., result in the birth of a female

Therefore, the proportions of females born in each of the four categories can be expressed symbolically as follows:

(1 – I)(FN)	=	the proportion of females born as a result of unplanned pregnancies
(I)(1 – S)(FN)	=	the proportion of females born as a result of planned pregnancies without sex selection
(I)(S)(SF)(RF)	=	the proportion of females born as a result of successful attempts to select girls
(I)(S)(1 – SF)(1 – RM)	=	the proportion of females born as a result of unsuccessful attempts to select boys

The predictive equation, which sums these expressions, can be represented as follows:

$$F = (1 - I)(FN) + (I)(1 - S)(FN) + (I)(S)(SF)(RF) + (I)(S)(1 - SF)(1 - RM)$$

This is the most elementary representation of the model. But even in this form, it can be used to illustrate the limited impact of each of the separate variables, such as sex preference, on the predicted sex maldistribution.

There are possible circumstances, any of which would, axiomatically, effectively preclude a maldistributive effect. One of these circumstances is independent of sex selection method; no maldistributive impact is likely if the overall preference ratio is neutral, regardless of the characteristics of the methods available. The other circumstances are method-specific. For example, if an available method is ineffective in attempts to select both females and males, no maldistributive effect could occur as a result of its use, regardless of the values of the other relevant variables. Also, a lack of awareness of, or willingness to use, a specific method would preclude any change in the sex ratio at birth as a result of its availability. The essence of these points is that the model reflects a reality in which many of the relationships among relevant variables are multiplicative, and therefore that maldistribution is unlikely to occur unless all of the relevant variables have values that support it.

Some possible refinements to the model are discussed in a subsequent section, where the model is applied to the data.

The Effectiveness of Sex Preselection Methods

Relevance

Models designed to accurately predict sex maldistribution must incorporate data on the reliability of the methods by which sex selection is attempted. The importance of the reliability of the various methods of sex selection, whether involving preselection or sex determination during pregnancy, followed by abortion, is self-evident. However, most of the writing on sex maldistribution has paid little attention to the literature on technique reliability. As noted earlier, inferential leaps frequently have been made from research findings on preference patterns directly to projections of sex maldistribution. The intent of this section of the report is to obtain estimates of the reliability of various methods of preselecting the sex of one's children. These estimates are derived from a critical review of the relevant scholarly literature.

The focus is on contemporary methods described in the professional literature rather than on traditional or folk methods. This is not a review of all of the published research into all aspects of each of the various methods of preselection; the purpose is limited to ascertaining the best evidence on reliability rates for those methods most likely to be used. (For recent comprehensive reviews that are comparable or broader in scope, see Levin[2] or Zarutskie et al.[3])

In some ways, the data on method reliability are even more important than the preference data. For example, if all preselection methods were completely unreliable, sex preference patterns would become moot. On the other hand, even if aggregate preference patterns were sex-neutral, the fact that individuals have significant differences in preferences and might be willing to act on them means that the *differential* reliability in attempts to create females and males might be extremely important.

With respect to the reliability of methods of fetal sex identification during pregnancy, the literature is fairly clear and consistent, although there is some uncertainty with regard to specific techniques. There is virtual unanimity on the reliability of amniocentesis, and there is consensus that the reliability of chorionic villus sampling (CVS) is close to 100 percent. Less agreement exists on the reliability of ultrasound imagery at various stages of fetal development, especially prior to the second trimester. One technique under development that permits a determination of fetal sex identifies fetal cells in a sample of maternal blood. This promises facile, safe, inexpensive, and highly reliable fetal sex determination.

With respect to reliability estimates for sex preselection methods, somewhat less consensus has been achieved among scientists. This section of the report will review and summarize the available evidence concerning these estimates.

Preselection Method Classification

A variety of sex preselection methods, with notable similarities among some of them, have been studied. For the purpose of this paper, distinctions will be made among methods according to whether they rely on the following:

1. the external separation of sperm cells (into groups that carry X or Y chromosomes respectively) prior to insemination;

2. variations, either naturally occurring or induced, in the chemical or biological characteristics of the prospective mother; or

3. the control of other variables related to the different characteristics of X- and Y-bearing sperm cells.

To a considerable degree, similarities in the approaches used to evaluate the reliability of the preselection methods, and in the methodological problems encountered in trying to do so, parallel this classification system.

Methodological Problems in Assessing Effectiveness

For each method, or group of methods, there are problems encountered in drawing accurate inferences about their reliability. These difficulties refer both to methodological shortcomings in published studies of reliability and to differences among these studies that militate against effective comparison. With regard to the weaknesses in individual research projects, some of the methodological problems include the following:

1. the failure to effectively control the effects of extraneous and possibly intervening variables;

2. the use of small samples;

3. the absence of a coherent theoretical explanation for the findings, increasing the likelihood that findings may be spurious; and

4.   a higher rate of publication of positive findings, thereby spuriously increasing the stated effectiveness of the method.

Factors that limit comparisons among papers describing preselection methods include the following:

1.   the use of different methods to measure the characteristics and behaviour of sperm cells;

2.   the use of different methods to measure the occurrence of ovulation;

3.   the failure to describe methods in enough detail to allow replication, or even to permit useful comparisons with other research efforts; and

4.   the differences among research projects with regard to the control of possibly intervening variables.

Methods That Rely on Sperm Separation

Since the characteristics of the sperm cell determine the sex of the fetus, separating sperm cells into fractions richer in one type or the other, and using artificial insemination with the fraction corresponding to the preferred sex, seem likely to result in an increased rate of offspring of that sex. A number of different methods have been attempted (both for human and animal sperm cells), with wide variation in effectiveness. Generally, these sperm separation techniques depend on (alleged) differences between X- and Y-bearing spermatozoa with respect to size, mass, density, motility, longevity, or electrical charge.

Sperm Identification Methods

Theoretically, there are two methods by which the effectiveness of separation techniques can be evaluated. One is to use selected samples in attempts to cause pregnancies, and to measure the extent to which the results deviate from chance. The second approach is to identify specific sperm cells in separated samples in a laboratory as being either X- or Y-bearing, and thereby estimate the proportion of cells of each type in each sample. Although the former approach must be used ultimately if the technique is to be considered effective, as a practical matter the second approach is used initially to identify promising techniques. As a result, considerable effort has been devoted to cell identification, and a number of different methods have been developed.

The different methods used to identify X and Y spermatozoa may not be equally reliable, and not all research projects to determine whether sperm separation techniques are effective use the same sex identification method(s) to check results. That is, different reliability rates reported for different preselection methods may actually reflect variation in the accuracy with which the sperm cells are identified. Because of the importance of this issue, a brief review of the measurement methods is in order to facilitate subsequent discussion.

Staining (F-Body Test)

Treating sperm with quinacrine dihydrochloride, which stains the distal end of the long arm of the Y chromosome, is the most common method of identifying Y-bearing sperm. Under fluorescent microscopy, spermatozoa with a Y chromosome show a bright fluorescent dot (F-body), while X-bearing spermatozoa do not. This technique is used frequently to identify Y-bearing spermatozoa, though its accuracy is an issue of some debate among researchers. Barlow and Vosa[4] suggested that the F-body test tends to underestimate the number of Y sperm, while Gledhill[5] noted that the method indicates that approximately 5 percent of spermatozoa have two Y chromosomes, a considerably greater number than is indicated by the more reliable cytogenetic evidence. Another researcher commented on reliability problems having to do not with the accuracy of the staining method but with the limitations of the technician doing the counting.[6] Thomsen and Niebuhr[7] reported errors in both directions, as did Beatty,[8] who contended that some F-bodies do not represent Y chromosomes, and some Y chromosomes do not show up as F-bodies.

Gledhill, who is sceptical about the validity of the F-body test, argues strongly for the use of other confirmatory methods in conjunction with that test in evaluating sperm separation or enrichment methods.[9] But most studies of the effectiveness of external separation methods have used only the F-body test, perhaps because it is relatively easy, fast, and inexpensive.

Fertilization of Non-Human Eggs

An alternative method of sperm identification is the sperm penetration assay. Human sperm are joined with zona-free hamster eggs (see, for example, Chaudhuri and Schill[10]). The eggs are then karyotyped to identify the sex of the sperm. Some debate has occurred about the accuracy of this method, although it is usually regarded as reliable. However, the method is expensive and labour-intensive, and can provide assessment of only small numbers of sperm.

DNA Probes

The hybridization of Y-chromosome-specific deoxyribonucleic acid (DNA) probes is another method of sperm identification that may prove to be accurate (see, for example, Deininger et al.[11] and Sarkar[12]). West et al., using the DNA probe on unseparated sperm, reported that 46.7 percent of spermatozoa were labelled, a result close to the proportion of spermatozoa carrying Y chromosomes.[13] Although this technique involves much smaller sample sizes than the hundreds of sperm common in the F-body test, it is regarded as being highly reliable.

Microscopy

Shettles claimed to be able to distinguish between the two types of sperm cells using phase contrast microscopy.[14] This finding was not in agreement with the work of other researchers at the time,[15] and also was unsupported by the subsequent use of electron microscopy.[16] Microscopy is not considered to be a valid method of identifying the sex of individual cells. This is noteworthy, in part, because one prominent preselection method is based on Shettles' published findings.

Miscellany

A few studies have compared methods. Ueda and Yanagimachi obtained similar results by F-body scoring and by chromosome analysis after fertilization.[17] In contrast, Beckett et al. studied three of the techniques of Y sperm identification discussed above.[18] They viewed the F-body test as less reliable than either DNA probes or fertilization of hamster eggs.

Other methods have been developed that are not relevant here since they have not been used in attempts to evaluate the reliability of sperm separation methods.

Albumin Density Gradient Separation

The premise on which the albumin density gradient separation technique is based is that Y-bearing sperm have superior motility. Since the Y chromosome contains less genetic material than the X chromosome, there is a slight difference in mass between the two types of sperm cells. Roberts suggested that this mass differential allows Y-bearing spermatozoa to swim more quickly than X-bearing spermatozoa.[19] Ericsson et al. carried out experiments in which sperm were layered over media consisting of various concentrations of liquid bovine serum albumin (BSA) and allowed to swim through.[20] The initial objective of the separation was to select for spermatozoa with high motility. Ericsson's vague claim was that the concentration of Y sperm was increased from 48 percent to *as much as* 85 percent in some experiments. He reported recovery of 44 percent of live sperm from the final fraction, but this was variable. Although Ericsson's early work was pioneering, a number of shortcomings of the research, including the unreliable method of identifying spermatozoa with X and Y chromosomes, severely limit its value today. Attempts by other researchers to replicate Ericsson's studies have provided mixed results.

This technique has been used in various clinical settings. Beernink and Ericsson reported 66 males born from 84 conceptions (79 percent) in attempts to preselect males in one multicentre study,[21] and Corson et al. reported 28 successful efforts to preselect boys from 35 conceptions.[22] As a result of Y enrichment of sperm followed by artificial insemination, Dmowski et al. found that 6 of 8 fetuses produced were male.[23]

However, another clinical study reported no higher rate of males born as a result of the use of Ericsson's technique. Jaffe and colleagues used the albumin gradient filtration separation for patients who wanted a male child.[24] The success rate was 56.5 percent in the experimental group subjected to the separation procedure (13 males out of 23 pregnancies), and 60 percent in the control group (14 males out of 23 pregnancies), a difference contrary to the direction hypothesized.

If the clinical results were truly a result of the Ericsson technique, one would expect that laboratory evidence would indicate consistent separation of X and Y spermatozoa. If, on the other hand, there is no consistent proof of the effectiveness of the separation technique, one would be forced to conclude that separate confounding factors (such as timing of insemination or drugs given to the parents), and not the separation technique, were causing the varied sex ratio.

Quinlivan et al. reported an increase in Y-bearing spermatozoa from 52 percent to 74 percent following separation using BSA, with a reported recovery rate of approximately 35 percent of the original number of spermatozoa.[25] Using a variation on Ericsson's technique, with BSA replaced by human serum albumin (HSA), Dmowski et al. carried out Y enrichment of sperm prior to insemination.[26] They showed an average increase in the percentage of Y-bearing sperm from 46 percent to 71 percent in (male partners from) 20 couples with normal fertility, and from 45 percent to 65 percent in (males from) subfertile couples (n = 17). For these findings, there was no control group of untreated sperm.

In contrast, a number of other studies have not supported the findings of Ericsson's group. Studies by Evans et al. showed no separation of the two kinds of sperm cells using Ericsson's method.[27] Ross et al. demonstrated an increased percentage of motile sperm after using the technique, but no increase in the percentage of F-body spermatozoa.[28] Similarly, Ueda and Yanagimachi reported a non-significant increase in the percentage of F-body-positive sperm.[29] After using Ericsson's technique, Brandriff et al. reported a *reduction* in the percentage of Y-bearing sperm, opposite to the direction hypothesized.[30] Importantly, however, when a DNA probe was used as a marker, it showed no separation of X- and Y-bearing sperm that had been treated by the albumin density gradient technique.[31]

In conclusion, the evidence is mixed, but it appears improbable that methods like the one described by Ericsson can be used at present to preselect male children. Of some concern is Ericsson's failure to conduct true controlled studies of his method, although he would argue that those who do not attempt preselection constitute a control group. Some commentators have noted that Ericsson apparently has a significant financial interest in defending his patented and franchised method from criticism.

It is important to note that since abnormal sperm are likely to move more slowly than healthy sperm, use of the albumin density gradient separation method will leave abnormal Y-bearing sperm in the sample of primarily X-bearing sperm. Consequently, the fraction containing a larger proportion of sperm having X chromosomes should not be used for insemination, to avoid increasing the probability of fertilization by abnormal sperm. Thus, this method is not recommended for the preselection of daughters.

Sephadex Gel Filtration Technique

This technique to produce fractions rich in X-bearing spermatozoa, which could be used for daughter preselection, was also developed accidentally. Steeno et al. were developing a method to improve overall motility.[32] They suspended sperm in a solution and filtered it (using a Sephadex G-50 column). They discovered that in the fractions of the filtrate, only about 5 percent carried a fluorescent Y-body, and they reported an enhancement of X-bearing sperm to 74 percent of sperm in the final fraction.

Only one study has reported no X-bearing sperm enrichment following Sephadex separation. Beckett et al. analyzed sperm samples before and after the Sephadex treatment using three of the methods discussed earlier: the F-body test, chromosomal analysis after sperm fusion with hamster oocytes, and DNA probes for Y chromosomes.[33] They reported no consistent enrichment in X-bearing sperm as a result of the use of the Sephadex technique.

In contrast, four studies, including the one by Steeno et al., provided evidence of the effectiveness of this technique in both laboratory assessment and clinical use. Quinlivan et al. reported an increase in the percent of spermatozoa without Y-bodies from 60 percent before separation to 74 percent afterwards.[34] They also noted a wide variation in the degree of separation achieved depending on which sample was being used. Specifically, the decrease in Y-bearing sperm ranged from 6 percent to 22 percent. Corson et al. subsequently confirmed the findings of Steeno's team, reporting 8 females out of 11 offspring (a 73 percent success rate) when the Sephadex technique was used with artificial insemination.[35]

Geier et al. also reported on the clinical use of the Sephadex G-50 technique with artificial insemination, using Clomid® to induce ovulation.[36] Of the 21 viable infants born, 17 were female (81 percent), and among the miscarriages where sex determination was possible, 3 out of 4 were female. This was an overall rate of 80 percent. The authors cautioned that it was not possible to determine the extent to which the successes were due to the use of the Sephadex method, to the use of Clomid®, or to an interaction effect.

In summary, using the Sephadex technique in conjunction with Clomid® in attempts to preselect a daughter appears to provide the desired result approximately 70 to 80 percent of the time.

Electrophoresis

Daniell et al. based their research on the idea that X- and Y-bearing sperm respond differently to electrical fields.[37] They ran an electric current through a sperm sample and found that the cathode fraction contained 76 percent X-bearing sperm, while the anode fraction contained 77 percent Y-bearing sperm. To my knowledge, this study has not yet been replicated, and the technique has not been clinically tested.

This "convection counter streaming galvanization technique" allows accumulation of both X- and Y-bearing spermatozoa simultaneously. That factor may be of value in fertility clinics where one technique could be used to select for children of either sex, potentially reducing equipment expense, staff training, and space requirements.

Shishito et al. subjected semen from 11 individuals to electrophoresis. They reported that Y-bearing spermatozoa (F-body stained) were primarily attracted to the anode (61 percent were Y), while 89 percent of the spermatozoa at the cathode were X-bearing spermatozoa.[38] Engelmann et al. based a different technique — free-flow electrophoresis — on the same theory of separation based on different electrophoretic mobility.[39] They continuously injected a fine stream of pretreated sperm into a separation chamber while applying an electrical field to the system. They reported that the sperm near the anode end consisted of approximately 62 percent Y-positive sperm, while sperm nearer the cathode end contained a mean of about 15 percent Y-positive sperm. This was in contrast to a mean percentage of 44.4 percent in untreated sperm. These results are very close to those reported by Daniell et al.

The present utility of this method appears to be somewhat limited by its adverse effect on the viability of sperm cells.

Swim-Up

Check et al. used a relatively new technique to select for male children.[40] This technique involves centrifugation of sperm cells, after which they are allowed to swim up through a medium. This is followed by sample collection and further purification. They reported 81 percent male offspring (17 out of 21) resulting from insemination with this method. In an unfortunate oversight, the authors neglected to report the ratio of X- to Y-bearing spermatozoa (prior to insemination), which would have been easy to obtain, and which would have provided strong confirmatory or disconfirmatory evidence. One potentially confounding variable was the fact that all women inseminated were being treated with either clomiphene citrate or human gonadotropin, drugs associated with a higher rate of *female* offspring. Furthermore, there was no control of the effect of timing of insemination: all subjects were inseminated twice, at precisely the same time intervals, and at the same times with respect to ovulation.

As noted above, Chaudhuri and Yanagimachi reported that chromosomal analysis following a two-step "swim-up" technique produced a spermatozoa sex ratio of 1.34.[41] This is in contrast to the general sex ratio of human spermatozoa determined by chromosomal analysis, reported to be 0.74,[42] 0.89,[43] and 0.93[44] (the widely recognized human *birth* sex ratio in recent decades is approximately 1.06 in Europe and North America, indicating that 106 males are born for every 100 females). Therefore, this study suggests that using the swim-up technique to select spermatozoa for high motility results in the enrichment of Y-bearing spermatozoa.

Engelmann et al. carried out a study of four different sperm separation methods.[45] Following application of a swim-up separation technique, they reported a statistically significant but minor increase in the percentage of F-body spermatozoa from 44.7 percent to 49.5 percent ($p < 0.0025$).

Centrifugation methods, whether used in conjunction with filtration methods or not, are based on the assumption of a difference in mass or density between X- and Y-bearing spermatozoa. (The researchers generally refer to differences in mass, but centrifugation would not be effective unless there were a difference in density.) Such a difference does exist, but it is so slight that the likelihood of its being effectively exploited by centrifugation is extremely small. As is the case with some of the other methods described, centrifugation takes a heavy toll on healthy spermatozoa of both types.

Other Sperm Separation Techniques

The study by Engelmann et al., alluded to earlier, examined the effectiveness of three sperm separation methods in addition to the swim-up technique: Percoll gradient centrifugation, Sperm Select, and the Migration-Sedimentation technique.[46] They reported that these techniques also significantly increased the percentage of Y-bearing spermatozoa. The results showed increases from 44.8 percent to 50.2 percent, 45.5 percent to 49.8 percent, and 45.5 percent to 48.0 percent (all $p < 0.0005$) for the three techniques respectively. The slight and virtually identical changes reported by Englemann et al. for these three methods, as well as for the swim-up method, are so unlikely as to suggest that some general aspect of the handling of the sperm during the experiment may have affected X- and Y-bearing spermatozoa differentially. Differential filtration[47] and laminar flow column separation[48] have also been hypothesized, but no further studies have been reported since the publications first describing them.

Methods That Rely on Differential Hospitality to X- and Y-Bearing Spermatozoa

A number of techniques are based on the differential hospitality of the mother's body to the two kinds of sperm cells. These differences may be either naturally occurring or artificially induced.

Ovulation-Inducing Agents

A number of studies suggest that the use of clomiphene citrate (or Clomid®), which was developed as an ovulation-inducing drug, may increase the probability of having a female child. Sampson et al. reported that for artificial insemination with donor semen, 53.9 percent of 89 clomiphene-induced pregnancies resulted in daughters, compared to 39.4 percent of 162 pregnancies that were not clomiphene-induced.[49]

The female-promoting effect seems to have occurred even in conjunction with the albumin density gradient method, which, as discussed earlier, reportedly improves the chance of having a male child. Beernink and Ericsson used the albumin density gradient technique prior to insemination of women who were also given either clomiphene citrate or human (menopausal) gonadotropin.[50] They reported that five out of six babies were female.

Jaffe et al. employed albumin density gradient separation with artificial insemination.[51] Patients desiring a male child had no additional treatment, while patients preferring a female child were treated with clomiphene citrate and human (chorionic) gonadotropin at specific points in the cycle. Once again, male preselection was not successful, but for those desiring a female, the success rate was 78.6 percent (11 out of 14) for the treatment group and 35.3 percent (6 out of 17) for the control group.

James meticulously considered all the research available at the time on the sex of offspring following ovulation induction by either clomiphene citrate or chorionic gonadotropin, or the two in combination.[52] He reported 1 401 females and 1 207 males produced through natural insemination. This represents a birth sex ratio of 0.85, compared with the normal birth sex ratio of 1.06, a highly significant difference. James concluded that the sex of offspring may be partially controlled by the mother's gonadotropin levels at the time of conception.

Other research fails to confirm that clomiphene citrate improves the chance of conceiving a female. The largest body of data was described by Corson et al.[53] More than 2 000 Clomid®-induced pregnancies occurred under a variety of conditions (e.g., coitus, artificial insemination) with no deviation from the expected sex ratio except in the case of multiple births, which show an increased number of males. The authors argued that clomiphene citrate had no effect on the sex ratio and that results suggesting otherwise were aberrations, possibly due to small sample size.

That argument may be correct, but it should be noted that the data used by Corson's research team came from the investigational files of a pharmaceutical firm whose economic interests seemingly coincided with the findings reported. Corson et al. also studied the effect of clomiphene citrate administered in conjunction with (menopausal) gonadotropin and again found no significant effect.

In summary, both clomiphene citrate and human gonadotropin appear to be related to the conception of females. The evidence suggests that the effect of each is similar, and that it shifts the birth ratio from 106:100 to approximately 85:100.

Diet

Alterations in the sex ratio of both animal and human populations have been associated with changes in mineral intake in various circumstances. Stolkowski and Lorrain describe the manipulation of maternal diet prior to conception to affect the sex of offspring.[54] They extend the argument of Lyster and Bishop, who believed that the main factor in determining the sex of children is the ratio of potassium to calcium and magnesium in the diet.[55] Stolkowski and Lorrain, and

Stolkowski and Choukroun,[56] added sodium to the equation and expressed the ratio in the following manner:

$$R = [(Na^+) + (K^+)] / [(Ca^{++}) + (Mg^{++})]$$

They allude to work by Duc alleging that values of R greater than 4.0 indicate an improved chance of having a male, R values less than 2.8 favour females, and values between 2.8 and 4.0 are likely to result in the birth of approximately equal numbers of males and females.[57] Of the 36 couples studied by Stolkowski, who used this technique, 31 (86 percent) conceived a fetus of the desired sex. Similarly, of the 224 couples studied by Lorrain, 181 (81 percent) conceived a fetus of the desired sex. Astonishingly, the paper did not divulge the absolute numbers of males and females intended or conceived; as a result, it was not possible to determine the effectiveness of this technique in attempts to preselect children of each sex.

Stolkowski and Choukroun carried out a trial in which the mineral intake of women's diets was regulated for one and a half menstrual cycles prior to conception, in accordance with the theory described above.[58] Drug supplements were given to maintain the specific mineral levels. Out of 46 live births (excluding one set of male/female twins), 39 (83 percent) were of the sex desired and 7 were not. In that paper, the number of subjects desiring sons or daughters was reported, and the success rates in attempts to select children of each sex were similar.

These two studies suggested that dietary mineral composition might influence the sex of offspring in humans. However, in addition to the shortcomings noted previously, there was no reported follow-up to verify that patients were following the prescribed diet, or measurement of serum ionic concentrations to ensure that the mineral concentrations intended had been attained. Further, there was no control group, nor any controls for confounding variables such as timing or frequency of intercourse. Finally, there have not been many other attempts to study this method empirically.

The technique has enjoyed wide popular acceptance in France and increasing acceptance in English-speaking countries since the publication of a book in English describing this method.[59] If diet did work as a method of sex preselection, it would be a convenient and inexpensive method that could be implemented with little or no physician intervention. It is, in other words, the kind of method that large numbers of people would be willing to use. However, there is still considerable uncertainty concerning whether diet really does affect the probability of conceiving either a male or a female, nor is there anything close to unanimity on the specific ways in which diet might have such an effect, if it does.

pH

Shettles stated that Y-bearing spermatozoa are less tolerant of low pH (acidic) environments, and X-bearing sperm intolerant of a high pH.[60] As a result, one element of Shettles' method of sex preselection requires the female to douche just prior to intercourse with an alkaline solution if a son is desired, or with an acidic solution for a daughter. Shettles' view was probably based on research done decades earlier; it has never been confirmed.

Diasio and Glass carried out a thorough and convincing study of the effect of pH on X and Y spermatozoa.[61] They filled capillary tubes with solutions of pH 7.3, 7.9, and 8.4, corresponding to the pH levels of the cervical mucus throughout the reproductive cycle, and another at pH 6.5. They placed the capillary tubes into semen samples. They found no differences in the percentage of spermatozoa positive for the F-body among these four samples, nor did the samples differ from a fresh sample. The authors conclude that X- and Y-bearing spermatozoa are not differentially affected by pH, at least not within this range of pH values.

Similarly, Downing et al.[62] found that X- and Y-bearing spermatozoa did not differ in their reactions to environments of pH 5.2 and 8. (For more information on this issue see Broer et al.[63]) In summary, there is no reason to believe that acidity of the vaginal environment will have a significant differential effect on X- and Y-bearing spermatozoa.

Antigen-Antibody Reaction

Immunology may provide another method of sex selection. The prospective mother would be "vaccinated" with an antigen located on the Y chromosome, after which she would manufacture antibodies. The antibodies would be activated by the presence of Y chromosomes at any time in the future. In theory, all of the Y-bearing spermatozoa would be destroyed before having an opportunity to fertilize the egg.

The technique, which could be used only to select for females, is still considered experimental, with no publications describing human studies to date. Studies with mice have shown a modest alteration from 53 percent males in the control group to 45 percent males in the "vaccinated" group.[64] One issue of importance is the reversibility of such a technique. In the absence of a method to reverse the effects, the use of this technique would be appropriate only if the mother were certain that she would not want to have a male child in the future.

Methods That Rely on Timing of Insemination Relative to Ovulation

It has been theorized that insemination on specific days relative to the day of ovulation may influence the probability of fertilization by X-bearing or Y-bearing sperm. Unfortunately, almost all of the studies are retrospective, and therefore the reliability of the data is suspect. Most importantly, determination of the time of ovulation is difficult and not consistent for all research into the effect of timing on sex selection.

Clearly, in attempts to determine the importance (for sex selection) of the timing of insemination relative to ovulation, the sensitivity and validity of measurement of the time of ovulation are critical. It is important to keep in mind the purposes for which the determination of ovulation time is needed. The kinds of methods that could be used in a laboratory environment differ greatly from those that would be appropriate for prospective parents attempting preselection without the assistance of a health professional. A variety of methods have been used to determine the point of ovulation in clinical research, and they differ with respect to validity, reliability, and sensitivity. Three methods are used most frequently in research:

1. The most complex method, which requires laboratory tests, measures the level of luteinizing hormone (LH) in the blood or urine. Researchers have found that a sudden surge in LH level is followed about 32 hours later by ovulation.[65]

2. Another method involves observing daily change in the cervical mucus through the cycle. The fertile period is considered to commence with a change from low to increased mucus production. The day on which increased amounts of mucus are highest has been shown to be a fairly reliable indicator of ovulation.[66] Hilgers and Bailey estimated that in 95.4 percent of cycles, ovulation occurred within –2 to +2 days of the peak mucus symptom.[67]

3. The third method is measurement of the female's basal body temperature (BBT). Daily measurement shows some random fluctuation in BBT, but no sustained change. Near ovulation, the BBT will have a sustained rise of approximately 0.5 to 1 degree. Hilgers and Bailey reported that ovulation occurred an average of 1.5 days prior to the BBT rise.[68]

Measuring the LH level is the most sensitive of these methods of determining time of ovulation — measuring to within hours — and if that degree of sensitivity is needed, it is probably the most valid and reliable of them. The LH method also has the significant advantage of signalling the occurrence of ovulation well in advance of the event. This issue is of some importance since at least one of the timing theories requires insemination prior to ovulation in attempts to obtain females. On the other hand, the BBT and cervical mucus methods have the advantage of being employable without the assistance of a physician, and with minimal training of the potential parents. Since the research indicates much greater public acceptance of preselection methods that can be used without medical assistance, having an effective non-medical indicator of time of ovulation is extremely important.

Timing: The Shettles Method

Kleegman was one of the first to suggest that timing intercourse relative to ovulation could possibly be used for sex selection.[69] In studying 130 births, she explained that of couples who had intercourse 2 to 24 hours before ovulation, 77.6 percent had sons, and of those having intercourse 36 or more hours before ovulation, 73 percent had daughters. The small sample of those having intercourse from 2 to 8 hours after ovulation all had girls. In summary, more males resulted from intercourse near ovulation, while more females resulted from intercourse temporally distant from ovulation.

Shettles used this information in developing multiple factor recommendations on choosing the sex of one's children.[70] Shettles stated that since the Y-bearing sperm were smaller, they would be able to swim faster; thus, if intercourse took place near to ovulation, those sperm would more likely be the ones to reach the egg first. However, if intercourse occurred long before ovulation, the Y-bearing sperm would swim faster but then die before ovulation, leaving the slower-moving but hardier X-bearing sperm waiting around until ovulation occurred. Shettles reported that, using the method as directed, of 22 attempts to create males 19 were successful, and of 19 attempts to create females 16 were successful. Other elements were added to the theory, including acidity of the vagina, the position during coitus (deep penetration to improve odds of having a son), and whether the woman experienced orgasm(s) (orgasm associated with improved odds of having a son).

Since then, however, there has been widespread controversy regarding Shettles' method and findings. More recent research reveals flaws in the premises on which the method is based. First, Diasio and Glass found that there was no difference in the ratio of X- to Y-bearing sperm migrating through solutions of various pHs.[71] Second, research using scanning electron microscopes does not show a bimodal distribution of sperm size.[72] Most important, with minor exceptions, researchers have not been able to replicate Shettles' findings. For example, Simcock studied 73 women using a modification of Shettles' methodology.[73] This included timing of intercourse and acidic or alkaline douche, but excluded coital position and orgasm in the woman as variables. The results, contrary to the direction hypothesized, did not differ significantly from those expected by chance.

In North America, the Shettles method has almost certainly enjoyed greater publicity and use than any other preselection method. It was first described in popular magazines more than 20 years ago and in a number of successful books intended for the mass market. However, numerous empirical studies have produced findings that either failed to support, or contradicted, Shettles' theory. That is not to say, however, that timing is irrelevant in sex preselection.

Timing: The Guerrero Method

Guerrero developed a theory of timing for sex selection that has been supported in recent research.[74] He analyzed records of BBT, intercourse, and outcome of pregnancies for 875 births. BBT was used as an indication of ovulation, with the day before the temperature rise indicating day 0 (the day of ovulation).

Guerrero described a dramatic trend in which the percentage of male births was higher the further from ovulation (in either direction) that insemination had occurred. Specifically, from eight days prior to ovulation until the day of ovulation, the percentage of resulting male births declined. Beginning one day after ovulation, the trend shifted, and for the next two days, the percentage of males born increased for fertilizations on days +1 to +3. (The data suggest that fertilization never occurred more than three days after ovulation.) Plotting "percentage of births that are male" against "days relative to ovulation" provides what has been called Guerrero's "U-shaped curve."

Ostensibly because of small sample sizes, Guerrero combined the data for days +2 and +3. This decision obscured the fact that the raw data for day +2 differ slightly from the described trend. Considering that this group consisted of only 23 males out of 39 births, compared to the total sample size of 875 subjects, the lack of consistency may well be the result of random error, and Guerrero's decision to group the data is not entirely unreasonable. Nevertheless, this "blip" in the data is worth noting, because there is no generally accepted theory of why timing is a relevant variable. In the absence of such a theory, it is especially important that the data not be presented in a way that hides inconsistencies. In the as-yet-undiscovered causal mix of factors that determine the sex of a fetus, the "blip" may prove to be the impact of a relevant variable.

The use of Guerrero's prescription for sex selection appears to have an inherent sex bias. Using the ovulation prediction methods most likely to be used in attempts at preselection, it is relatively easy to identify ovulation once it has occurred or even the day before, through a change in the LH level, temperature (BBT), and cervical mucus methods, as described above. Thus, it is relatively simple to identify the optimal time for the conception of a female child. However, there are no such easily used markers for the days most effective for the conception of a male child, and specifically no indication of which days are too near to those that are equally likely to produce a daughter or a son. For a male child, a couple must depend on patterns identified in previous menstrual cycles to determine the best days for insemination.

Harlap studied the sex of 3 658 children born to Jewish women who claimed to have observed the ritual avoidance of sexual contact for seven days after menstruation.[75] She reported that a higher proportion of female children was conceived as a result of the resumption of intercourse on or near the day of ovulation, and that the proportion of males born was higher when intercourse was resumed either one or two days before ovulation, or two days after ovulation. This research tends to support Guerrero's "U-shaped curve" of high male to female ratio before and after ovulation, and low male to female ratio near ovulation. As was the case with Guerrero, a very small percentage of the total number of births (102 out of 2 766) were the result of intercourse two or more days after ovulation; thus, the increase in the proportion of males may be due to errors in counting days or determining the dates of ovulation. However, it is certainly possible that there are factors as yet unknown causing this pattern.

The Guerrero hypothesis is further supported by evidence from Perez et al.[76] Reporting research on 52 pregnancies resulting from failures of natural family planning, they found that intercourse on the day of the mucus peak (day 0) and on the previous day resulted in female babies 63 percent of the time. They described these two days as being the "most fertile days." Of pregnancies resulting from intercourse on the days before (days −6 to −2) or after (+1 to +3) this time (termed the "less fertile days"), 76 percent were male.

Timing: Summary

France et al. have recently published a paper that brings together much of the research on timing for sex selection.[77] In a meticulous study, they used all three of the methods described above (LH levels in the urine, BBT, and cervical mucus) to determine the point of ovulation in a prospective study of 33 pregnancies. (Note that most of the other research has been retrospective.) Considering the methods individually, there were strong indications that male births resulted from insemination one to five days before ovulation, with a peak about three days before ovulation; female births resulted from insemination from three days before ovulation to one day after ovulation, with a peak at the day of ovulation. This trend is similar but not identical to that reported by Guerrero.

France et al. followed guidelines set out by Shettles (intercourse far from ovulation for females, near ovulation for males), resulting in only 39 percent of the couples having a baby of the desired sex. Although there is no effectiveness rate reported by France et al. for a study of intercourse far from ovulation to create a male child and intercourse near ovulation to create a female child, one plausible inference based on their findings is a 61 percent success rate of achieving the desired sex.

Based on these findings, it would appear that one way to improve the effectiveness of sex selection may be to avoid insemination on days −2 and −1, since on these days similar proportions of both sexes are conceived. The percentage of males conceived as a result of intercourse up to day −3, and of females conceived through intercourse on day 0 and after, is much larger than it is on the two intermediate days. Of course, following that course of action may also lessen the likelihood of conception occurring.

A research paper by Vear was originally viewed as providing support for Shettles' theory.[78] However, I believe that it actually supports the contrary view of Guerrero, France et al., and Harlap. Vear explained that female offspring (eight in total) were the result of intercourse up to one day before ovulation, as indicated by an increase of 0.5 to 1.0 degrees Centigrade in BBT. In addition, males were the result of intercourse one day after the rise in BBT. France explained that ovulation occurred the day before the BBT rise, not the day of the rise as stated by Vear. Thus, when the studies are compared using the day of the rise in BBT rather than the expected date of ovulation as the point of comparison, the results are consistent.

The research described here represents an extremely small part of the body of work on timing of insemination relative to ovulation. It suggests some statistical relationship between timing and the sex of the fetus, but the causal link is undefined. Obviously, timing is not a direct causal agent, but is likely related to changes in women's bodies that render them more or less hospitable to the different kinds of sperm cells. Some have argued that different secretions at different points in the cycle give a temporary and brief physical advantage to the more motile sperm cells. Others argue that changing chemical characteristics of the environment (gonadotropin, pH, potassium, calcium, etc.) differentially affect either motility or viability.

The empirical evidence strongly suggests the existence of a more complex causal model than has been tested previously. It is likely that there are multiple factors at work, and since not all of them have been controlled in empirical studies, the effects of each have been masked.

Whether there is one important causal variable or more, it is likely that there are intervening variables that have not yet been identified, which also mask the effect of the most important determinants of fetal sex. It appears that much work has to be done before a comprehensive theory describing the determinants of fetal sex is formulated. The development of a reliable method of sex preselection based on that theory is, of course, even more remote.

Conclusion

Of the possible methods of sex preselection that have been described, perhaps three or four have been used with any frequency. Of these, only the least commonly used, sperm separation techniques, probably have an impact. In other words, it is likely that the overwhelming proportion of people who have some preference for the sex of their children have not acted on those preferences, and of the few that have acted on their preferences, almost all used methods that do not work. The set of individuals created by the intersection of groups of those who have preferences, and those who are willing to use the specific techniques that happen to be effective, is almost empty.

There is an indeterminate but significant number of Canadians who have tried to preselect the sex of their children using "home" methods. These include some of the methods described above, such as timing, douching, and diet, as well as more exotic folk recipes having to do with phases of the moon, direction of the wind or of the bed, et cetera. We have no way of knowing what proportion of these would-be parents would have opted for the more effective (albeit more invasive) techniques if they had realized that what they were attempting was ineffectual. Of course, approximately half of those people are certain that the techniques they tried were absolutely reliable (and they are much more likely to inform their friends of their experiences than are parents who were less fortunate in their preselection attempts).

It is clear from this review that the unreliability of the methods likely to be favoured by potential users greatly reduces the likelihood, in the short term, of any sex maldistribution resulting from sex preference. It may be that in the future, reliable, safe, and easily used methods of sex preselection will become available. What the likely sex distribution effects would be if such methods were available to Canadians can be determined only through surveys of Canadians' sex preference patterns and willingness to use preselection, issues that are addressed in subsequent sections of this report.

Previous Research on Attitudes Concerning Sex Preselection

Preferences for the Sex of One's Children

Prior to the 1970s, when medical knowledge about sex preselection began to advance rapidly, most of the social scientific research on sex preference focussed on fertility, rather than on preselection. Preference patterns were considered pertinent only to predicting number of children, since it was known that dissatisfaction with the current sex mix of one's children would tend to result in additional conception attempts.

Beginning more than 50 years ago, research efforts on sex preference used "parity progression ratios," relating the sexes of existing children to decisions to have additional children. (At that time, avoiding pregnancy after having a child of the desired sex was the only "selection" method generally available.) These behavioural studies, many with very large samples, documented a male-female ratio for the last child that was higher than for previous children, and by inference, a preference for male children.[79]

That body of research, although interesting, is flawed, in that the decision to have additional children is constrained by many factors unrelated to sex preference. Because these extraneous factors have random effects on the sex of children, the data on last-child sex ratio almost certainly have underestimated preference for males at the time that research was conducted. That is, if the sex ratio is partly a consequence of parental preference and partly the result of random factors that favour neither sex, then the ratio will inevitably underestimate the extent of parental sex bias.

More recently, research has tended to focus directly on stated preferences for the sex of one's children. Although this approach provides more accurate information about parents' intentions and motives than the study of parity progression ratios did, some questions remain about threats to the validity of these data. For example, the ability of attitude surveys to provide accurate predictions of behaviour diminishes as the time frame expands. Bennett has argued that the accuracy diminishes further if the respondent is required to indicate preferences in scenarios that are not only temporally distant, but also hypothetical.[80] On the other hand, some empirical research, designed specifically to measure the relationship between attitudinal measures (of sex preference) and behaviour (concerning the first-born child), reveals the two to be very closely related.[81] In any case, the body of recent survey research on this topic is rich in scope and detail, and the fact that the findings are consistent within societies enhances its credibility.

In developed Western societies, including Canada, there is evidence of a fairly consistent pattern of preference for more male than female children, but the difference is not very great.[82]

Williamson's thorough review of more than 50 studies of sex preference revealed that the respondents' preference ratios for all future children ranged from 51.5:48.5 to 54:46.[83] (Preference patterns are often described in terms of the percentages of each sex that are preferred, or similarly, in a ratio that sums to 100, as in this case. The figure representing the percentage of males is listed first. Another commonly used form is to express a ratio with the second term, representing the relative number of females, equal to 1. Thus, the equivalent of 54:46 is 1.17:1.) The dominant characteristic of surveys of sex preference is that most respondents want a balance of sons and daughters. Demographers have often noted that what most people claim they want is a three-child family with an equal number of boys and girls![84]

Even women have exhibited a mild pro-son bias. A typical finding, for example, is that although almost 70 percent of women consider it important to have at least one son, 60 percent consider it important to have one or more daughters. Men and women differ in the degree to which they prefer male children, with men generally having much stronger pro-son preferences.[85] One study of childless couples found that the women had an overall preference ratio of approximately 52:48. The comparable figure for men was 54:46. Fidell et al. authored one of the few research projects that found little or no difference between the preference patterns of male and female respondents (710 university students).[86]

Recent evidence strongly suggests that the preference for sons, on the part of both men and women, may have diminished in recent years.[87] In replicating Dinitz's work[88] done 20 years earlier, Peterson and Peterson found that there had been a significant decline in pro-male preferences for an only child.[89]

Interestingly, the available evidence indicates that children's aggregate preferences for future children are not skewed, although their individual preferences are. Almost half of the children surveyed did indicate a preference — for a child of their own sex.[90]

For both men and women, the son preference is markedly stronger for the first-born than it is for subsequent children.[91] Among childless women, the mean preference ratio for their expected first-born child is 65:35, and potential fathers' preferences are even more extreme. Even among those groups or individuals who express no overall sex preference, there is often a clear preference with regard to first-born children.[92] And even more extreme attitudes exist with regard to the preferred sex of an only child.[93]

It is common knowledge that nationality and culture are strongly related to sex preference.[94] The overwhelming preference for male children in some societies is well documented, with female infanticide and a host of other, only slightly less horrific, practices having been poignantly described, especially with reference to some Asian societies.

Even among the countries of northern Europe, and within English-speaking North America, there are significant differences.[95] Social class is very weakly related to sex preference, with the middle class showing the least pro-male bias, and those with low socioeconomic status manifesting the most. The correlation between parents' education level and male preference is generally negative.[96] A relationship appears to exist between religion and stated sex preference, with Catholics more interested than Protestants in having boys. The data on Jews, derived from relatively small samples, suggest a strong preference for male children. Those with no religious affiliation are the least likely to indicate any sex preference for their children.[97] Since social class, education, religion, and ethnicity variables are inter-related, the relationship of each with children's sex preference is confounded.

These findings of a pro-son preference refer only to families that expect to have their own biological children. With respect to adoptions, the preference is for females, even within groups who tend to have a strong pro-male preference. The research indicates that of the prospective adoptive parents who express a preference for the sex of their children, 70 percent or more would prefer daughters.[98] But even among adoptive parents, there is a preference for sons if they expect to have only one child.[99]

A tendency exists to express satisfaction with gender(s) previously obtained, although that preference does not necessarily extend to future children. Women are more likely than men to display this response pattern, perhaps reflecting the fact that women are less strongly committed to one sex than the other, or perhaps that mothers develop closer bonds with their young children than fathers do.

To summarize these findings, recent survey research conducted in the United States and Western Europe over the past few decades is fairly consistent in its findings: there is a slight but pervasive preference for male children. Preferences concerning first-born children are more strikingly pro-male, and the preferred sex of an only child is even more skewed. The desire for at least one male is more common than the corresponding preference for a female. For all of these preference patterns, men tend to show more pro-male bias than women do, but the research indicates that women also have some pro-male bias. There is some evidence that pro-male bias is slowly diminishing among both men and women. Social class is weakly related to sex preference, religion and national origin more strongly so.[100]

To my knowledge, there is no published evidence of sex preference for the entire Canadian population, but some work done in smaller geographical areas has been published in professional journals.

Public Awareness of Preselection Methods

There have been very few attempts to measure public awareness of preselection methods, and the validity of the findings is questionable, since it appears that respondents may claim considerably more knowledge of preselection than is warranted. For example, Markle and Nam found that 76 percent of the subjects in their student sample claimed to have heard of sex preselection methods.[101] When the students were asked about the source of their information, 60 percent identified the mass media, 26 percent referred to school, and the rest mentioned personal sources. However, when asked to be more specific about sources, many were so vague in their responses that the researchers concluded they were not being truthful.

More recently, Ullman and Fidell reported relatively detailed information about subjects' (self-proclaimed) knowledge of specific sex selection techniques.[102] Approximately two-thirds of their subjects were aware of sperm separation methods; half had heard about timing of intercourse relative to ovulation; approximately half were informed about the possibility of abortion for sex selection; and about one-quarter claimed they had heard about hormonal or chemical interventions. On the basis of Markle and Nam's findings, it seems likely that these numbers are gross exaggerations of the level of public information; one wonders whether a random sample of physicians would be as well informed as these subjects claimed to be.

Even if there were valid data on public knowledge, their utility in predicting possible use of preselection would be somewhat limited, since knowledge levels may change rapidly over time depending on the kind of attention given to the subject by the mass media.

There is very little evidence with respect to Canadians' knowledge of sex selection methods. Farr cites a national survey conducted in 1990 in which Canadians were asked whether they were "aware of anything that can be done to human sperm in a lab to improve the chances of having a boy or a girl."[103] Seventy-two percent answered that they were not.

Willingness to Use Sex Preselection

This issue has not been researched as extensively or as successfully as preferences for the sex of one's children, but a substantial body of research exists, most of it conducted in the United States. In much of this research, the samples have consisted exclusively of university students, especially those at large public universities. As a result, the samples have tended to consist disproportionately of those who are middle-class and unmarried. Since the research indicates that these groups are relatively unlikely to be interested in preselection, much of this research may have slightly underestimated public willingness to use preselection.

Adelman and Rosenzweig found that the majority of (white, married) respondents approved of sex selection for others, with non-intrusive forms of preselection (such as timing of intercourse) considered acceptable, and more intrusive forms, such as artificial insemination and abortion, regarded almost unanimously as unacceptable.[104] Matteson and Terranova also found a widely held belief that preselection methods should be available to everyone,[105] and Hartley described an approval rate of 66 percent among California university students.[106] But other researchers have reported great variation in public approval of the use of sex selection. Pebley and Westoff, who wrote specifically about instability in this value, stated that 37 percent of their respondents expressed approval and 59 percent, disapproval.[107]

Although the proportion of those "approving" of sex selection for others is of some importance and interest, it is less relevant to the question of maldistribution than the proportion of people who are willing to use specific sex selection methods themselves.

Two-thirds of Hartley and Pietraczyk's sample of California students generally supported the position that sex selection technology be made available to all parents who wanted to use it, and 45 percent said they might use it themselves.[108] No other researchers have reported this high a level of willingness to use sex selection, although some other findings were similar. Fidell et al. found that approximately 40 percent of their sample of university students would use sex selection methods,[109] and Ullman and Fidell report that 37 percent of respondents claim they would use sex selection methods, but only 10 percent would use chemical or hormonal interventions, and fewer than 1 percent would use abortion.

The students in Markle and Nam's sample were less enthusiastic about the use of sex selection: 41 percent gave general approval to its use, and 24 percent said they would use it themselves (although the latter figure declined markedly when even moderately intrusive methods were described).[110] Similarly, 24 percent of both male and female students who participated in Gilroy and Steinbacher's research indicated a willingness to use sex selection.[111] Steinbacher and Gilroy interviewed women experiencing their first pregnancy and found that willingness to use preselection is higher among older respondents, blacks, and non-Catholics.[112] They also found that of those who were willing to use preselection, equal numbers preferred daughters and sons. When the students in Markle and Nam's sample were asked whether they would be willing to use sex selection if their previous children were all of one sex, their receptivity increased dramatically to 62 percent.[113]

A study conducted for the U.S. government described a hypothetical situation in which a safe sex selection product had been developed.[114] Only 19 percent of the respondents said they would use the technique if it became available. Interestingly, 38 percent of the subjects thought the product should be banned by the government, a reflection of the fact that only 12 percent thought it would have a beneficial effect on society, while 52 percent expected its effect to be detrimental.

Studies that asked couples, rather than individuals, about their willingness to use preselection reached slightly different conclusions. One study with a relatively middle-class, well-educated sample revealed that 60 percent were willing to use preselection for their second child if the first was not the preferred sex.[115] (Subjects were not asked about subsequent children.) In another study, with a slightly more representative sample, almost two-thirds of the 127 couples expressed willingness to use preselection.[116]

Previous research provides clear evidence that generalized questions about willingness to use sex selection techniques are much more likely to elicit positive responses than are questions describing specific techniques, even when the techniques described are fairly innocuous. Approval in principle, especially among university students, remains high and may be increasing, and while there is no increase in individuals' willingness to use preselection methods themselves, there is a decline in the pro-son bias of those who would do so.

Summary

Preferences for the sex of one's children have been widely studied, especially in the past two decades, but little information is available on the attitudes of Canadians. Although research methods have differed, the data for specific societies at similar times have been similar, heightening the credibility of the findings. There are clear differences among societies, even among those that are culturally or religiously similar, and generalizing to a society like Canada's from the findings of research conducted elsewhere is risky.

There appears to be a trend in the United States and some European countries of declining sex bias on the part of future parents.

Occasional misinterpretation of the empirical findings, especially by those not doing research in the field, has probably perpetuated misconceptions about preferences for the sex of children, willingness to use sex selection methods, and resulting attempts at sex selection. These kinds of errors, among others, have been made:

- It has often been assumed that the set of responses to the question "which sex would you prefer your next child to be?" can be used to deduce what the overall preference pattern is. It cannot, especially if some or all of the respondents have not yet had their first child.

- It is inappropriate to infer that those who have preferences are aware of the possibilities of sex selection; or that those who are aware of it, and approve of it in principle, are willing to use it themselves; or that expressions of personal willingness to use sex selection will translate into attempts.

- Frequently, findings from a non-representative sample, such as a university student sample and/or a geographically limited one, have been generalized to the general population. Students are certainly not representative of the general population with regard to sex preferences and willingness to use sex selection; they are probably not representative either with respect to knowledge of sex selection methods. Few of the previous research efforts have used randomly selected national samples — most of the national data have come from regular omnibus surveys that are limited in what they can tell us about people's sex preferences or willingness to use sex selection.

- Many have assumed, implicitly, that single people's sex preferences and willingness to use sex selection will remain unchanged after marriage, unmoderated by the views of their marriage partners. However, for all preferences expressed prior to marriage to be translated into attempts at preselection during marriage, everyone who had a preference prior to marriage would have to find a partner with identical values concerning the sex of children and the use of preselection methods, or one who was completely passive about both issues.

- The values of those who are childless concerning sex preference and willingness to use sex selection will probably be affected by the children they ultimately have.

In conclusion, based on the results of population surveys, a mild pro-son bias exists in most Western societies. However, there is a logical and empirical chasm between individual expressions of preference for the sex of one's children and subsequent attempts to select their sex. The causal bridge consists of a number of links, some thought to be weak, and others of unknown strength. As described earlier, a single-sample survey of public knowledge and attitudes concerning the relevant variables is the optimal way of determining the individual and collective strengths of these links. The following two sections of this monograph describe the characteristics and results of such a survey.

Survey Method

Sampling

Most of the data used in the following analysis were obtained through mailed questionnaires. Two separate samples were created.

Sample #1

For the primary sample, the target population was the set of all Canadians who intend to have one or more children in the future, whether or not they have any currently. The sample was generated through preliminary screening surveys using random selection methods. Specifically, separate screening surveys were conducted at approximately the same time in late 1991 and early 1992 by four professional polling organizations. Two of the surveys were telephone surveys, with the phone numbers generated by random digit dialling. The others were door-to-door surveys using conventional polling methods for the random selection of residences.

One of the objectives of using both door-to-door and telephone surveys was the minimization of the effects of slight sampling biases inherent in each approach. The purpose of using more than one polling organization for both telephone and door-to-door screening was partly to minimize potential "house" effects (although I had no prior knowledge of such effects for the four organizations), and partly because no single "omnibus" survey would provide enough cases. Omnibus surveys generally reach between 1 000 and 1 500 households, only a small proportion of which would have respondents who plan to have children and are willing to fill out a written questionnaire.

Primarily because of cost considerations, the screening questions were appended to existing national omnibus surveys rather than being stand-alone surveys. Although some control was lost, the effect of the variability in sampling procedures is as likely to have been positive as negative, as suggested above. Furthermore, because the information collected by the screening surveys was very limited and elementary, any inconsistencies in interviewing styles were unlikely to have had any adverse effects.

In all of the screening surveys, subjects were asked whether they intended to have children in the future, and, if they answered affirmatively, whether they would be willing to receive a written questionnaire dealing with issues such as parents' preferences for the number and sex of their children. Only those who responded affirmatively to both questions were sent written questionnaires.

These respondents did not explicitly commit to answering the written questionnaire, but only to receiving one. The use of this kind of non-committal language in the screening survey probably meant slightly higher costs and an increase in sample size by getting marginally interested people to consider the questionnaire. It would result in a lower return rate if return rate were defined as the number of returned questionnaires as a percentage of those sent. On the other hand, it probably would have a very slight positive effect, if response rate were defined as the number of questionnaires returned as a percentage of the number of subjects sampled (by the screening surveys).

One thousand one hundred and twenty-four questionnaires were mailed. Five hundred and two completed questionnaires were returned.

Unfortunately, the screening surveys did not provide the language preferences of the respondents. The procedure followed in mailing the written questionnaires was to send English-language questionnaires to all subjects outside Quebec and a second one in French if the surname suggested that the subject might be a francophone. Similarly, all those with Quebec addresses received a French-language copy; Quebec residents whose surname suggested non-francophones also received an English-language version.

All of the subjects were asked (in the written questionnaires) whether their spouses or partners, if any, would also be willing to complete one. This was intended primarily to allow attitudinal comparisons between partners, but it provided some additional potential benefits: it increased the total number of respondents, tended to equalize the number of males and females who responded, and tended to ameliorate one of the biases of both random digit dialling and door-to-door surveys — specifically, the slight over-representation of those living alone rather than in family units or other groups.

It is not possible to determine precisely whether the sample is representative of the population, because the target population is all Canadians who intend to have children at some time in the future, and there are no data available on the demographic characteristics of such a population. It is possible to identify the population parameters for a particular age group — for example, all those between the ages of 18 and 40 — but that proves to be not very useful, since age subgroups differ greatly with respect to their intention to have children.

Nevertheless, it is feasible to evaluate sample representativeness. With respect to some variables, such as sex or language, the distribution for the target population should not differ greatly from the entire Canadian population. In the case of other variables, such as education and marital status, the direction of the differences between the target population and the general population is clear, and its magnitude may also be roughly estimated. This approach will alert us to serious deviations from representativeness.

Given the current research topic, the most important variable to consider in evaluating representativeness is the sex of the respondents. The sex ratio for the general population is approximately 49:51, with females being more numerous, and in all probability the distribution for those of childbearing age is very similar. (The population under age 18 has a slightly higher proportion of males, and the population of those past their childbearing years has a much higher proportion of females.) Since females respond to surveys at a significantly higher rate than males (often at a 60:40 ratio), there was concern about even more extreme unrepresentativeness on a survey dealing with reproductive issues. Fortunately, the sample consisted of 45 percent males, a slight and manageable deviation from probable proportions in the target population.

With respect to the two dominant language groups, the sample was fairly representative, with 76 percent of the respondents being anglophone and 24 percent francophone.

Previous methodological research has indicated that foreign-born subjects are much less likely to respond to surveys. This was a serious concern at the outset, especially given the use of only two languages in the survey and the fact that some of the issues addressed were "culturally sensitive." The problem proved to be much less serious than had been anticipated. Nine percent of the respondents were foreign-born, as were approximately 29 percent of their mothers and 28 percent of their fathers. Nine percent is certainly smaller than the true proportion of the entire Canadian population that is foreign-born, but probably close to the proportion of the foreign-born population that is of childbearing age.

Approximately 59 percent of the respondents claimed to be married or living with someone in an intimate relationship, which is slightly lower than for the entire adult population (65 percent) but more closely representative of the target population, which has a relatively large proportion of people in their twenties.

In addition to being asked their own sex, the subjects were also asked to indicate the sex of their partners, a question that was answered by virtually all respondents. Fewer than two percent of responses indicated a homosexual relationship. In part, this reflects the fact that a smaller proportion of homosexuals than heterosexuals intend to have children, and that given the nature of the screening questions, people who did not intend to have children were unlikely to have received a questionnaire.

Sample #2

The second sample consisted of university students, who were targeted for a number of reasons. A large proportion of them intend to have children at some point in the future; in most cases, they have not yet begun child-rearing and their preference patterns are not coloured by children already born; they generally respond at a relatively high rate to attitude surveys; and, most importantly, students and others in their age cohort tend to be under-represented in random samples of the general population, because they often live either in family units or in shared accommodations with other students. Sample #1 is much more important to the analysis, both because of its representativeness and because of its size. The student sample was used primarily to identify gross differences between the student population and the general population.

The sampling method for the student sample was two-stage cluster sampling. Eight Canadian universities were selected, such that they were diverse and roughly representative of all Canadian universities with respect to size and location. One hundred students were randomly selected from each of these universities. The written questionnaire used in the student survey differed very slightly from the one used for sample #1, with most of the differences pertaining to vocation and education.

The following description and analysis refer to data from the general population sample unless otherwise indicated.

Response Rate

Because the time available was severely limited, only one mailed reminder was sent to all subjects, approximately one week after the questionnaire had been sent. This had implications for total sample size and response rate. The final sample size was not adversely affected, since the probable reduction in the number of responses was offset by a larger initial mailing (made possible by the savings resulting from limiting the number of reminders and the larger-than-expected sample generated by the screening surveys).

The effect of using a single reminder notice probably was significant for response rate but is unlikely to have significantly affected sample representativeness. The use of multiple reminders does increase total response rate. However, at issue here is not the difference in numbers between those who are willing to answer questionnaires and those who refuse to do so; rather, it is whether the small number of subjects who would have responded *only* after repeated prompting differ significantly in their sex preferences and attitudes toward sex selection from those who responded without receiving multiple reminders. Although there is no way of knowing with certainty, it is assumed that the threat this posed to sample representativeness was extremely slight.

Measuring Knowledge of Preselection Methods

If one wants to predict the consequences of access to sex preselection methods, it is important that both knowledge of available sex selection methods and willingness to use them be measured accurately. Unfortunately, a methodological problem arises from attempts to measure both of these elements in the same questionnaire. The provision of accurate descriptions of the various methods of preselection is necessary to measure willingness in a meaningful way; it is not useful to ask subjects about their willingness to use a technique if they have no information about it. Unfortunately, if descriptions of techniques were provided, they would almost certainly compromise the data on prior knowledge of those methods. The following approaches to solving the problem were employed.

A subsample (of approximately 15 percent) of subjects was surveyed in two phases, the first phase asking about knowledge of available techniques, and the second inquiring about willingness to use specific techniques. This subsample provided a validity check on the knowledge level as measured for one-phase subjects. This approach probably resulted in additional expense, a slightly smaller number of respondents (because some subjects who responded to the first questionnaire may not have answered the second), and invalidity (because some respondents to the second mailed survey may not have been the same persons as those who responded to the first).

For the remaining 85 percent of those sampled, two steps were taken to try to minimize the potential invalidity of the "knowledge of sex selection methods." First of all, the descriptions of the various preselection and fetal sexing methods were not made evident at the outset but were contained in closed envelopes (identified only by a number), which subjects were asked not to open until they reached the point in the questionnaire that specifically asked them to do so.

Second, after questions were asked about knowledge of techniques, hypothetical and existing techniques were described, and respondents were emphatically told to regard the techniques as possibly fictitious. Willingness to use preselection was then measured with respect to all of the methods described. This approach not only avoided compromising the "knowledge" data, but also facilitated the measurement of public willingness to use techniques that hold some promise of becoming available in the future. There was potential invalidity in that some respondents might have assumed that the "possibly hypothetical" techniques do exist, and then "cheated" on the questions about their knowledge of preselection.

A personal interview or telephone survey that would have allowed sequential questioning, first on knowledge and then on willingness, could have been used to solve the problem. However, because of the cost, and because written questions are often more effective when complicated information has to be provided to the respondent prior to questions being answered, this was not an optimal solution.

It was decided that awareness of sex selection methods could not be measured with a high degree of validity using short answers. All of the coding of these written answers was effected by a single coder, working closely with the primary investigator.

In the two-phase subsample, the first phase included requests for demographic information, questions about sex preference, and questions concerned with knowledge or opinions about preselection and fetal sex determination methods. The second phase provided respondents with easily understood factual information about these issues and asked which methods of sex selection or preselection would be acceptable to them under specific circumstances.

The one-phase survey included all of the questions that were in the two-phase survey and no others.

Reporting Statistical Results

This research is primarily exploratory and descriptive and does not employ formal tests of hypotheses. Nevertheless, measures of the probability that the findings occurred by chance may be useful to the reader and are provided when deemed appropriate. The specific probabilities, rather than the achievement of thresholds, will be reported, except that computed values less than 0.001 will not be reported precisely, but simply as $p < 0.001$.

Survey Results

The survey was designed primarily to produce data about three variables critical to predicting maldistribution resulting from the availability of sex selection methods: preference for the sex of one's children, awareness of the sex selection methods available, and willingness to use any of those methods in specific situations. The survey findings will be discussed for each of those issues in turn.

For the sake of clarity and brevity, the findings from the student survey will not be presented with the results from the primary survey but will be briefly described at the end of this section.

Preferences for the Sex of One's Children

Variables

Because preferences concerning the sex of one's children are multi-dimensional, data from a variety of variables are required to describe the full range and mix of preferences.

The written questionnaire asked respondents who intended to have children to describe their sex preferences, if any, for up to five future children, as well as the total number of daughters and the total number of sons they would consider ideal. The difference between the total number of daughters and the total number of sons they wanted to have was used as a measure of overall sex preference.

The questionnaire also posed a series of questions concerning importance to the respondents of different dimensions of sex preference:

- the importance of having at least one daughter,
- the importance of having at least one son,
- the importance of having at least one child of each sex,
- the importance of having an equal number of children of each sex,
- the importance of having a daughter first, and
- the importance of having a son first.

These scales produced interval data by using five-point numerical scales with verbal descriptions provided only for the extreme positions of "not important" and "very important." The purpose of this mix of questions was to determine not only the direction of different kinds of sex preferences, but also the intensity with which each of those views is held.

Respondents were also asked about their perceptions of their partners' preferences on each of these six issues, measured on similar scales.

Finally, the subjects were asked to describe, in an open-ended answer, any other aspect of their preferences for the sex of their children that they felt had not been covered adequately by the previous questions.

Sex Preference: Direction

One way of describing the extent of preference for daughters or sons is to examine the proportion of the population that would prefer to have an equal number of both sexes and the proportions that would like to have more children of one sex than of the other. These data were generated in two forms: first of all, for future children only, and secondly, for the total number of children intended, including those already born. As will be seen, differences in responses to these two questions are useful in interpreting preference patterns.

With respect only to children intended in the future, the data show clearly that the pervasive preference pattern is the desire for an equal number of daughters and sons, with approximately 71 percent of the respondents considering that as optimal. Even more important is the fact that the remaining respondents are virtually equally divided between preferences for a greater number of daughters and a greater number of sons. As indicated in Table 1, approximately 14 percent of the sample want more daughters than sons, and 15 percent prefer a greater number of sons. Those who want to have more boys than girls tend to be slightly more skewed, or extreme, in their aggregate preference distribution than those who prefer more girls. Once again, these data refer only to future children desired.

Table 1. Preference for the Sex of One's Children

Percentage who would prefer:	Future children only	Current and future children
More daughters	13.5	16.3
An equal number of each	71.2	64.6
More sons	15.3	19.2
Total	100.0	100.1

The comparable data for all children wanted, including those already born, provide similar results, but show a slightly stronger pro-son bias. Approximately 65 percent prefer an equal number of males and females, with almost 20 percent wanting more sons than daughters and roughly 16 percent wanting a greater number of daughters.

Two differences between the data for these two slightly different variables are important with respect to understanding the preference of the respondents, and are considered in some detail.   The first pertinent difference is the percentage wanting an equal number of children of each sex: 71.2 percent versus 64.6 percent (see Table 1). This difference is attributable largely to the inclusion in the former sample of those who do not intend to have any more children; if they are excluded, the percentage wanting an equal number of each sex drops from 71.2 percent to approximately 68 percent. The slight remaining difference is attributable to the fact that some respondents already have two or more children of the same sex, and are not willing to have four or more children for the sake of achieving balance.

The second difference, which is more subtle, is the difference in the apparent extent of pro-son bias. The data for the two variables differ slightly in comparing the number of respondents who want more daughters with the number who want more sons. With respect to future children only, the difference in percentage points is 1.8; concerning present and future children, the difference is 2.9. This apparent inconsistency may be partly an artifact of a slightly atypical characteristic of the sample. Specifically, although the sample appears representative with respect to the various demographic variables previously considered, it is not perfectly representative with respect to the sexes of the children the respondents already have. Of the set of respondents' first children, more than 52 percent were boys, and the same was true for the set of second children. In fact, 52.8 percent of all of the respondents' children were boys (n = 459). (Consideration is given later to whether this maldistribution could be partly the result of previous attempts at sex selection or preselection.)

It is worth noting, in this context, that the birth sex ratio in North America is not exactly 50:50, but approximately 51.5:48.5. (It is widely believed, as a result of the examination of spontaneous abortuses, that the conception ratio is even more skewed, but that disparity is reduced by a higher fetal mortality rate for males.) In any case, the disparity at birth is definitely reduced by higher male mortality rates in infancy, in early childhood, and for all age cohorts until and including old age. Although the 52.8:47.2 ratio for children reported in this sample is atypical, this deviation from the norm is slight — only about half as large as it initially appears to be.

At the moment, we are concerned with the significant deviation from 50:50, because previous research informs us that parents, and especially mothers, tend to express satisfaction with the sex(es) of whatever children they have. Regardless of preference patterns prior to the birth of their children, the parents' expressed preferences tend to change after their children are born to conform to the sex(es) of those children. Therefore, a sample like this one, with a disproportionate number of boys already born, may provide misleading information about overall sex preferences in the population if subjects are asked about the total number of daughters and sons they would like to have.

The preceding interpretations of the differences between the two related variables suggest that the data describing preferences for future children are likely to be a slightly better indicator of sex preferences than are the corresponding data on all children intended, including those already born.

However, there is another plausible interpretation of the data, which points in the opposite direction. Given that the majority of the respondents' existing children are males (as shown above), and given that a balance between the number of male and female children is a widespread value, one could reasonably conclude that the data on preferred sex(es) of future children, which seemingly indicate a sex-neutral position, are in fact masking a slight pro-son preference. That would happen if either some of those whose answers indicated a pro-daughter position were really opting for balance after having had sons, or some of those who really had a son preference expressed what appeared to be a neutral position for future children, because they already had more sons than daughters.

It is not possible to definitively separate these effects, all of which probably are operant to some degree. Fortunately, the conclusions point in opposite directions, minimizing the possible error. In addition, since the data sets are not too dissimilar, interpolation of the numbers is a reasonable, if imprecise, method of resolution.

One other piece of information should be considered in this regard: the overall sex preference pattern of those who have no children, a group that is not subject to the contradictory biases affecting those who are already parents. A remarkable 82 percent of this group would prefer to have an equal number of girls and boys. Approximately 8 percent would prefer to have more daughters, and the remaining 10 percent would prefer more sons. For this group, the overall preference ratio is approximately 51:49.

In spite of these minor difficulties in interpreting some of the data, they are, overall, consistent and conclusive. They indicate that the dominant preference value is the desire to have an equal number of children of each sex. Of the small number of respondents who prefer to have more of one sex than the other, there is a very slight preference for a larger number of males. These conclusions are similar to the findings of other research efforts in North America in recent years, although the current findings depict slightly less pro-son bias than most of the previous work did.

Intensity

Although these kinds of data on overall preference patterns are interesting, they are of limited utility because they fail to measure the intensity with which respondents' views are held, an issue that is critical in determining whether individuals would act on their preferences. Data have been collected which describe the importance that respondents attach to various sex preference principles. One of those principles is the desire to have an equal number of daughters and sons. Given the previous finding that a large majority of respondents would prefer to have an equal number of daughters and sons, it is surprising how unimportant they consider this issue to be. With the value "1" representing "not important" and "5" corresponding to "very important," the mean score for this variable was 1.6.

The data on the proportion wanting an equal number of sons and daughters, and the slight importance respondents attach to that principle, are not contradictory.   Examination of the data for a related principle, "having at least one child of each sex," clarifies the issue. The mean value for this variable is slightly over 3.0.   Apparently, a large majority of prospective parents would prefer to have exactly the same number of children of each sex, but few regard this as an important issue.   What almost all prospective Canadian parents want, and feel strongly about, is having at least one child of each sex.

Since the nature of a preference and the importance one attaches to it are obviously independent, perhaps other principles, a preference for sons, for example, might be regarded as very important by the respondents who want more sons than daughters. A less extreme principle than "having more sons than daughters," and one to which many more respondents are likely to subscribe, is "having at least one son." The mean values for this and its companion variable, "having at least one daughter," are both approximately 3.2.

The data for each of these two variables would be misleading if considered on their own, but their meaning is clear if they are viewed together and in conjunction with the corresponding statistic on "having at least one of each." It becomes evident that the high score for "at least one son" does not reflect a pro-son bias, any more than the virtually identical score for "at least one daughter" represents a pro-daughter orientation. Rather, they both reflect part of the intensely held value of having at least one child of each sex. The logic of these questions is such that whatever importance one attaches to having at least one child of each sex, one should attach at least as much importance to the two separate issues, "having at least one daughter" and "having at least one son." The data reveal that there is very little sentiment for "having at least one son" beyond the value placed on "having at least one of each," and the same is true of the desire to "have at least one daughter."

First-Born

Preference patterns for the sex of the first-born child are considered to be an important issue, in part because of the commonly held view that many intellectual and emotional advantages accrue to first-born children. (This hypothesis is not generally supported by recent research.)

The data considered here describe the preferred sex of the first child for those respondents who intend to have children but do not yet have any. A slight majority of these respondents have no preference with respect to the sex of first-born children, with the rest tilting in favour of sons over daughters, 26 percent to 21 percent respectively. Once again, this kind of preference data is most meaningful if the intensity with which the values are held is also considered. Interestingly, the companion variables, "having a son first" and "having a daughter first," obtained mean values of only 1.8 and 1.7 respectively on the five-point importance scales. Although the slight difference is also in a pro-son direction, compounding the bias reflected in the numbers of first-born sons and first-born daughters wanted, the extremely low scores suggest that sex selection of first children would not be very common unless an effective method were available that had no unattractive features (cost, intrusiveness, inconvenience, delay, etc.).

Determinants of Sex Preferences

Sex

It is a cliché that preference for male children is much stronger among prospective fathers than among mothers, but, as noted earlier, most of the previous research has indicated that women, married or unmarried, also tend to have pro-son preferences.

The women who participated in this research do *not* want to have more sons than daughters. Nor are they likely to consider having at least one son, or having a son as their first-born, to be more important than the corresponding values with regard to daughters. The attitudes of women respondents are, in the aggregate, almost perfectly sex-neutral, with just slightly more importance attached to having at least one daughter than to having one or more sons.

One interesting feature of these data is the very slight difference between women and men. Table 2 summarizes and compares the sex preference patterns of women and men. The relationship between sex of the respondent and the desire to have more children of one sex than the other, although evident, is extremely weak. Unlike women in the sample, men do indicate a slight pro-son bias. On average, they want more sons than daughters, they place more value on having at least one son than on having at least one daughter, and they are likely to consider it important to have a boy as their first child. But each of these biases is slight, and it is clear that for men, as for women, biases in favour of either sex are trivial compared to the value of having at least one child of each sex.

Table 2. Mean Sex Preference Values, by Sex and Marital Status

	Mean importance of having:					
Sex/marital status	At least one daughter	At least one son	At least one of each sex	An equal number of each	A daughter first	A son first
All females	3.24	3.11	2.94	1.43	1.72	1.78
All males	2.96	3.22	3.01	1.55	1.56	1.92
Married females	3.30	3.12	2.83	1.34	1.70	1.75
Unmarried females	3.18	3.11	3.05	1.52	1.73	1.80
Married males	2.84	3.12	2.89	1.48	1.49	1.89
Unmarried males	3.07	3.32	3.13	1.62	1.63	1.95

Although the groups of female and male respondents are characterized much more by attitudinal similarities than by differences, when the combined effect of sex of the respondent and other related variables is considered, some subtle statistical relationships can be identified.

Impact of Partner's Values

Regarding the effect of sex and marital status on sex preference, married women and men attached the same importance to having a son (3.1), while unmarried men saw this issue as being somewhat more important than unmarried women did (3.3 and 3.1 respectively). Although the difference is not very great, the finding is interesting because it suggests that the attitudes of people on issues like these may shift when they enter intimate relationships, with men especially moving in the direction of their partner's position. This is consistent with findings in the professional literature concerning attitudes in other substantive areas. It is interesting in the present context because it suggests that if some single heterosexual males, for example, hold relatively extreme views, those views are likely to be moderated by contact with their ultimate partners in child-planning and child-rearing.

Respondents were advised that they could answer the questionnaire on their own, or in conjunction with their partners, as they preferred. They were asked to indicate which alternative they had chosen; the importance of an accurate response here was emphasized. Interestingly, 91 percent of the respondents chose to answer on their own, rather than consulting with their spouse/partners. This issue is pertinent for some of the same reasons that marital status is. If there are differences between one's own views and the views of one's intimate partner, there is likely to be some narrowing of differences of opinion as the views of each party become known to the other.

The data indicate that the differences in expressed attitudes between those who answered on their own and those whose responses were a joint effort were narrow. Even when the groups were divided further according to sex, only a few noteworthy differences were apparent. With respect to the desire to have at least one son, for example, women expressing only their own views had a mean score of 3.1, in contrast to 3.3 for those who consulted their spouses. On this question, the differences between the two groups of men were negligible (both 3.1). On the question of the importance of having at least one daughter, there were no clear differences. That was also true for the issue of total number of children of each sex and for questions related to the sex of the first-born child.

Although the data on individual and joint responses have been provided, this does not constitute a rigorous test of the hypothesis that discussion among partners will moderate the relatively extreme views they might have had prior to consultation. The current findings are confounded by a number of variables, most notably the different personality characteristics of those who chose to consult with their partners and those who did not. Similarly, the fact that married and unmarried respondents have different preference patterns does not prove that marriage affects one's views, since they represent two separate samples.

There are additional data indicating the extent to which respondents' attitudes are linked to their partners' perceived values. It was noted earlier that the mean number of sons that males want is just slightly greater than the number of daughters they want. However, men who believe that their partners consider it very important to have at least *one* daughter indicate they would prefer to have more daughters than sons. There is a significant difference (of 0.5) in numbers of daughters wanted by men who think their partners see this issue as very important and those who believe that their partners consider it unimportant. There is a similar pattern among women with respect to the number of sons they want and their perceptions of their partner's concern with having even one son.

The correlation is even stronger between pairs of like variables, such as the importance respondents attach to having at least one daughter and their perceptions of their partner's values on the same issue ($r = 0.53$, $p \leq 0.001$). The link between desire to have a son and the perception of one's partner's position on that issue is similar ($r = 0.65$, $p \leq 0.001$). The correlation between the variables concerning having at least one child of each sex is comparable, as are the bivariate relationships for the pairs of variables concerning the sex of the first-born.

Although this is strong evidence of a "partner effect," it is not entirely conclusive. The statistical relationships may reflect nothing more than people's decisions to marry those who have similar values concerning the sex of their children.

However, the fact that three different kinds of comparisons all point to the existence of a partner effect, and that it is consistent with empirical and theoretical work in closely related areas, is compelling evidence of such an effect.

Age

Age and sex do not have any significant interaction effects, although age seemingly has an independent effect on the importance one attaches to certain preference values. For every "importance" variable considered, those who are older take more moderate positions. This trend is slightly more pronounced for males than for females. It is worth noting that, among women, the importance of having a son drops from 3.3 for those aged 25 and under, to 2.9 for those over 30. For men, the corresponding means are 3.5 and 2.9 respectively. Concerning having at least one daughter, older women see this as marginally less important than younger women do, while men differ more markedly according to their age (3.2 and 2.7).

Once again, the appropriate interpretation of the data is not entirely clear. Attitudinal differences at one point in time between two samples, which seemingly differ only with respect to the age of the subjects, may be attributed either to attitudinal changes that take place as people age, or to attitudinal differences between the two groups because they were socialized at different points in time. Repeated measurement at different points in time is the surest way of separating these effects.

Nevertheless, these findings concerning the effects of marriage and age are useful in attempts to interpret preference data for student populations, on whom much of the previous research on sex preference has been conducted.

Other Demographic Characteristics

There are a few other variables that appear to have some impact on preferences for the sex of one's children.

Anglophone and francophone respondents are quite similar in their response patterns, although the latter place somewhat more value on having at least one child of each sex ($p \leq 0.01$).

The respondent's level of education is rather strongly correlated with the perceived ideal mix of daughters and sons ($r = 0.33$; $p \leq 0.06$), with more highly educated respondents opting for a relatively equal distribution of sons and daughters.

The occupational status of the respondents is also related to their preferences. Higher-status respondents generally have more moderate attitudes, especially with regard to the issues of "having at least one son," and of having at least one child of each sex. There is a likelihood of interaction effects between occupational status and age, which appear to have similar effects on sex preferences. Occupational status is also correlated with level of education. This is not to argue that occupational status is spuriously related to preferences. Rather, it appears that social class, including both occupation and education dimensions, is related to attitudes concerning the sex of one's children. This is consistent with the results of previous research.

The single most surprising aspect of the data is that there is virtually no difference between the stated preference patterns of Canadian-born respondents and those of Canadian residents who were born in other countries. Admittedly, the foreign-born subsample is probably not perfectly representative of the population of foreign-born Canadians who intend to have children, since those who have integrated most completely into the society are more likely to have responded than are those who are still closely linked to other national or ethnic groups, and the latter are less likely to have relatively egalitarian attitudes with respect to the sex of their children. Nevertheless, the small differences between these two groups are interesting. Even for the "having a son first" variable, both groups have a mean score of 1.8.

With regard to the personal sexual orientation of the respondents, the small number of respondents who indicated they were homosexuals limits the kinds of inferences one could make confidently. Only about 1 percent of the respondents were male homosexuals, and even a smaller number were lesbians. With this caveat in mind, it can be noted that neither of these groups of respondents had response patterns that differed significantly from those of heterosexuals on any issue, including the desire to have children of one's own sex.

Sex of Children or Siblings

Previous research suggests that the expressed preferences of individuals who already have children tend to shift in the direction of the sexes of their existing children, and that this tendency is more pronounced for women. The current data are relevant to this hypothesis. They indicate clearly that of the subjects who already have at least one child, there is a tendency to place relatively high value on having a first child of the sex that was in fact obtained. For example, the importance of having a son first was rated 1.9 by those who did in fact have a son first, and 1.3 by those whose first child was a girl. The related question about a daughter first generated scores of 1.3 and 1.5 in the expected direction.

The second part of the hypothesis, that women are more likely than men to manifest this kind of behaviour, is not supported by the data. On the contrary, it is the men who appear to be more influenced by the sex of their first-born in describing how important it is to have a daughter or a son first.

The data collected are also pertinent to another hypothesis that some social scientists have advanced, that an individual's preferred mix of female and male children will tend to conform to the number of male and female siblings that person had while growing up. There is an extremely weak relationship between those two variables in the hypothesized direction. If the relative number of brothers and sisters one has is related to the stated importance of having at least one son, the relationship is a bit stronger ($p \leq 0.08$), but by no means conclusive.

Finally, there has been speculation, on theoretical grounds, that preference for the sex of one's first-born will tend to correspond to the sex of an individual's oldest sibling. The current data indicate that preference for a first-born son was unrelated to whether the respondent's oldest sibling was a brother or sister, or whether the respondent was the eldest. These variables were also unrelated to the importance attached to having a daughter first.

Summary

There is little doubt that the value held most strongly by the respondents was the desire to have children of both sexes. As noted earlier, responses to this question should be interpreted with reference to two others: one asking about the desire to have at least one son, and the other on the importance of having at least one daughter. Ratings on the two questions dealing with a single sex were in no instance significantly greater than the score on the question asking about having a child of each sex. This indicates clearly that people's expressed desire to have a child of a particular sex is almost invariably a reflection of the desire to achieve balance, to have children of both sexes. This is in accord with the customary findings of previous research.

In spite of a strong desire to have children of both sexes, respondents of various types simply do not consider it very important to have an equal number of children of each sex. The findings of this survey do differ slightly from the conclusions often drawn by other researchers. The current research reveals a very slight pro-male bias which is weaker than has usually been reported, but certainly not unique in the literature. However, the correlates of pro-son bias evident in this research are fairly consistent with those identified in earlier work: men showed slightly more bias than women; the bias is more prevalent among unmarried than married men and more common among those who are young; it is most evident with respect to preferences for the sex of a first-born child; and it is more evident among those with relatively low social status.

One interesting set of findings has to do with the effect of one's partner's views on one's own. The separate bits of evidence were not conclusive but, taken together, they strongly suggest that such an effect occurs, and that it can be significant. This is of obvious practical importance both because the overwhelming majority of attempts at preselection will involve couples rather than individuals, and because methods of preselection are likely to require the compliance of both partners.

There are two plausible explanations for the apparent differences between the current findings and those described in other published papers.

First of all, no national survey of Canadians' attitudes on sex preference had previously been conducted; any apparent inconsistencies are not between works that seek to generalize to a single population, but between works that refer to distinct populations possessed of manifest cultural differences. It is entirely possible that the attitudes of Canadians on questions of preference for the sex of their children are slightly more egalitarian than those of people in some other countries, including the United States, where much of the comparable work had been done. But even with that comparison, the difference is not extreme, or fundamental. It is one of degree, and the degree is slight. Furthermore, some comparable sex preference research done in other countries, notably Sweden, has provided evidence of little or no pro-son bias.

Another explanation of apparent differences between the current and previous findings is that the attitudes of North Americans are changing, with pro-son bias becoming less common and/or less extreme. Evidence of such a shift was cited earlier. The findings presented here may simply be the most recent to document such a trend.

Third, it is likely that most previous surveys used samples that were less representative than the national sample used in this research. Many of the earlier projects relied on samples that were either geographically limited, or homogeneous with regard to marital status, age, education, or social class.

These explanations are not incompatible, and it is likely that each has some merit. As additional attitudinal research on sex preference is done on the Canadian population and residents of other countries, the validity of each explanation will be clearer.

Knowledge of Sex Preselection Methods

Some of the problems involved in obtaining valid measurement of knowledge of preselection methods, especially in conjunction with attempts to measure willingness to use them, were described earlier. There is also a more fundamental problem of deciding exactly what to measure and how to interpret it. Is knowledge of preselection to be seen as accurate or correct information about the effectiveness of various preselection methods, or should it be defined as accurate information about the alleged effectiveness of specific methods as described by their proponents?

One's first reaction may be to select the definition that refers to the amount of accurate information that the respondent has. The alternative, defining knowledge as possessing a body of probably inaccurate information, may seem pointless, but the issue is not so clear-cut.

If there is little agreement among clinicians and researchers concerning the effectiveness of the various methods, how is one to measure the level of public knowledge about their effectiveness? Opinions about what does or does not work are likely to be characterized as accurate or inaccurate according to whether they conform with those held by oneself, especially given the lack of consensus among professionals. If the accuracy criterion were used, all respondents who admitted to being uninformed about preselection, and who didn't believe there was any reliable method available, would be labelled "knowledgeable," while those who were very well informed about Shettles' approach, and considered it effective, would be labelled "not knowledgeable." Of course, it would be unreasonable to expect many lay persons to be aware of the complicated claims and counterclaims that have appeared in the professional literature.

Respondents were asked to write descriptions of specific methods they considered effective. The responses were evaluated according to whether they accurately outlined specific methods of sex selection, as might have been described by the proponents of those methods. Respondents were not assigned a single score on level of information about preselection generally; rather, they were given one score for each of three basic approaches to preselection: timing, sperm separation, and body chemistry. The ordinal values assigned were "incorrect information," "minimal to moderate information" (which included anything from just the name of the method to some understanding of its application or logic), and "extensive information."

In addition to this open-ended question, subjects were also asked if they believed that sex preselection is possible, if they had heard of others using preselection, and if they themselves had previously attempted preselection.

Twenty-four percent of the respondents believed that sex preselection is possible, and 60 percent of these claimed they had heard about someone else trying preselection. It is difficult to compare these findings to previously published survey data on knowledge of preselection methods because so little work has been done, and the findings have not been consistent.

Fewer than one-third of those who thought that preselection is possible had even a rudimentary idea of how it might work. Of these, most had heard about timing methods, a smaller number knew about sperm separation, and one respondent thought that diet could determine fetal sex. Virtually all of these "informed" respondents had only minimal or moderate knowledge; only a handful were well informed about any method.

From a methodological point of view, it is extremely interesting and important that none of the respondents described a method similar to the methods presented to them as part of the attempt to measure their willingness to use preselection. These method descriptions were contained in sealed envelopes, which the respondents were asked not to open until directed to do so at a specific point in the questionnaire. The fact that not a single respondent described the fictitious method, and that very few respondents wrote answers that reflected extensive knowledge of the other method, suggests that very little cheating, if any, occurred, and that the potential threat to the validity of the "knowledge" data was minimized.

Willingness to Use Sex Preselection Methods

Prevalence
Descriptions of two preselection methods were provided with the written questionnaire. One was a sperm separation method (labelled Method E) having some similarities to the Sephadex and Ericsson methods discussed earlier, and the other was a fictitious method (Method F) based both on timing and the taking of pills during the month preceding the attempt at conception (see Appendix 1). (Method E is probably more similar to effective methods that might be developed in the foreseeable future than Method F.)

After the subjects had read the researcher-provided descriptions of possible preselection methods, they were asked if they could "imagine any situation" in which they might be willing to use a sex preselection method. Twenty-one percent answered that they could. Given the innocuousness of one of the described methods — the fictitious one — it is noteworthy that barely one out of five respondents thought they might use preselection under any circumstances. That provides a different perspective on the importance, or lack of importance, that individuals attach to sex selection, and it highlights the necessity of studying individuals' willingness to use specific preselection methods in specific circumstances, and not simply their preferences for the sex of their children.

But even that 21 percent figure may be a slight exaggeration. It appears that many of the respondents who stated that they would be willing to attempt preselection under some circumstances would not do so under ordinary circumstances. In response to the description of a variety of specific scenarios (i.e., combinations of existing daughters and sons), the percentage of respondents who said they would attempt preselection did not exceed 11 percent for any single scenario. And the percentage of future parents who thought they might use preselection in any of those scenarios, using either method, to select either sex, was only about 19 percent.

The slight discrepancy between the 21 percent and 19 percent figures is probably attributable to the fact that a limited number of scenarios were described. It is likely that some respondents would not use preselection for any of those scenarios, but might do so in other circumstances — for example, to avoid passing on a sex-linked genetic disease, or after having had four children of the same sex.

Table 3 describes the different scenarios and the percentages of respondents who would be willing to use either preselection method if no other were available. First of all, the data are informative with respect to the total number of respondents willing to use preselection. Thirteen percent of those who said they intended to have children would try to preselect a daughter using Method E, if no other method were available, in at least one of the scenarios described. Approximately 14 percent would be willing to use that method in an attempt to preselect a son. Seventeen percent would use Method F to preselect a daughter, and a similar number would use that method to preselect a son.

It is noteworthy that there is so great a difference between the percentage of respondents who would use preselection in any single scenario to select a specific sex, and the percentage of those who would use that method to select that sex in any of the scenarios. That means there is only a moderate amount of overlap among the groups of respondents who would try to preselect a son as their first, second, third, or fourth child. The same can be said of those who would attempt to preselect daughters.

For example, a slight majority of those who would preselect the sex of a child after having one child of the opposite sex would also preselect after having two of that sex. (The pattern exists regardless of the sex of existing children.) And almost half of those who would preselect after two same-sex children would also be willing to do so after three of the same sex. But there is not a great deal of overlap between those who would attempt preselection after their first child and those who would preselect after three same-sex children. All of this suggests that those who might use preselection would do so as part of reasoned family planning, taking into consideration the number and sex of existing children, rather than using the technique repeatedly simply to preselect a child of a particular sex.

Additional information with respect to motives for the use of preselection is provided below.

Table 3. Willingness to Use Preselection Methods E and F in Specific Scenarios

Currently have:	Would use method E to preselect (%)		Would use method F to preselect (%)	
	A daughter	A son	A daughter	A son
No children	1.0	1.7	1.8	3.1
One daughter	0.6	6.9	0.7	9.7
One son	6.1	0.6	8.9	1.0
Two daughters	0.0	8.7	0.4	10.5
Two sons	8.0	0.3	9.7	0.3
One daughter, one son	0.3	0.7	0.4	0.9
Three daughters	0.2	6.1	0.3	7.2
Three sons	5.6	0.3	7.1	0.3
Two daughters, one son	0.0	1.3	0.3	1.9
Two sons, one daughter	0.7	0.2	1.5	0.2
Total: any scenario	13.0	13.9	16.8	17.0
Total: % who would use each method in any scenario	15.2		18.1	
Total: % who would use either method in any scenario		18.6		

Sex Bias

The percentages of respondents who would use preselection in attempts to obtain daughters (any scenario), and those who would attempt to obtain sons, are very close to the percentage who would attempt either. That indicates, importantly, that the people who are willing to use preselection in attempts to select sons are, to a great extent, the same ones who would try to preselect daughters. This is especially interesting in view of the fact that, among those who would preselect a particular sex, there is relatively less overlap for different scenarios. It appears that a very large proportion of those who would attempt preselection in these scenarios is not motivated by a strong pro-daughter or pro-son bias, but is pursuing the objective of having *both* sons and daughters. The same pattern exists with regard to the use of Method F.

The data for individual scenarios reinforce that impression. The greatest incidence of willingness to attempt preselection occurs when the respondents already have one or more children of one sex and none of the other. For example, in the three scenarios (using Method E) that describe a family that already has two children, the number of respondents who would attempt preselection if they already had two children of the same sex (and were attempting to have one of the other) is roughly 10 times the number who would use preselection if they had only one child of each sex.

For all the Method E scenarios presented, respondents expressed willingness to use preselection in instances in which their existing children were all of one sex approximately 14 times as often as in instances in which they already had children of different sexes. If, for the sake of this comparison, one-child families are excluded (because they could not possibly have children of both sexes), the ratio would still be greater than 13:1. The data on the use of Method F are similar, with ratios of 10:1 and 9:1 respectively.

Even more important than the frequency of preselection under different circumstances is the nature of the selection attempts that would be made (i.e., male or female) if the existing children were of one sex. In virtually all such cases, and regardless of the sex of the existing children, the attempt would be to have a child of the opposite sex. The consistency of this pattern is remarkable; out of all instances of willingness to use Method E when existing children are of one sex, more than 98 percent would preselect a child of the other sex (p < 0.001).

It is also useful to consider the frequency of attempts to have daughters and attempts to have sons in comparable scenarios. For example, the intended sex of preselection attempts using either method if the parents already have one daughter can be compared to the intended sex of such attempts if they have a son. In this case, and for every pair of similar scenarios, where the sexes of existing children are the only difference, the sets of frequencies of prospective attempts to preselect each sex mirror each other almost perfectly.

The number of respondents who would want to use sex preselection for their first-born child appears to be quite low, considering that preferences for the sex of one's first-born child have been viewed as among the most strongly held of preference values. The number of attempts that would be made to select the sex of a first child does not come close to the number of attempts that would be made if the parents already have one or more children of only one sex. These data are unambiguous: having children of both sexes is much more highly valued than having children of one particular sex, and even more highly valued than being able to choose the sex of one's first child.

However, it is also important to know whether some respondents who are willing to use preselection are motivated by a preference for one specific sex, and, if so, whether those preferences cancel each other for the entire sample, or result in an aggregate preference for one sex or the other.

First, let us consider differences in the percentages of respondents favouring each sex in the corresponding pairs of scenarios described above. It was noted above that they mirror each other, but even slight differences can indicate a preference for one sex or the other. There is an extremely weak but fairly consistent pattern of preference for sons in these data. For each pair of scenarios, there are a few more respondents who would use preselection to select sons than those who would select daughters. The numbers are too small to be conclusive, but the consistent pattern among pairs of scenarios suggests that the apparent preference for sons is not random error. It appears that willingness to use preselection Method E in attempts to have sons is marginally more common than a corresponding willingness to preselect daughters, with the difference generally representing less than 1 percent of respondents.

With regard to the critical "no children" scenario, the differences are extremely small when Method E is the only one available, but more substantial when the less intrusive Method F can be used. There appears to be more demand elasticity for this scenario than for any other, where elasticity refers not only to cost, but to the entire set of issues on which Methods E and F differ. This provides further support for the view that most of those who do have a sex preference do not feel very strongly about it. Expressed as percentages, the difference between the number who would select daughters and those who would select sons is proportionately large, but so few of the respondents would even consider using preselection in this circumstance that the difference is inconsequential.

The trends described above with respect to Method E are also evident in the data for Method F. The one important difference, as expected, is that people are more willing to attempt preselection using Method F. Roughly 30 percent to 50 percent more people are willing to use Method F than Method E in any specific scenario.

Extraordinary Circumstances

Respondents were also asked whether they would use either of the preselection methods if they learned that the sex ratio for recent births was skewed (ostensibly as the result of others using some kind of sex selection method). The question is intriguing because it is directly relevant to the issue of the social consequences of a maldistribution based on sex. Would opportunities for sex preselection create a homeostatic system, in which every sex maldistribution was soon corrected by the deliberate reproductive behaviour of adults? Some biologists have argued that any perceived maldistribution of this type would trigger an impulse in many people to have children of whichever sex was less common.[117] Westoff and Rindfuss also argue that "a surplus of male births ... would be followed by a wave of female births to achieve balance, and the oscillations would eventually damp out."[118]

One theoretical explanation is that there is a primal need to try to perpetuate the species, and that this need would be served by having children in the minority group. It may be likely that people would behave in that manner, but not necessarily because of the kind of biological determinism that Dawkins has described.[119] When faced with a future population consisting disproportionately of one sex or the other, prospective parents who are even mildly homophobic can be expected to prefer to have children of the minority sex, so that their children will have more "opportunities."[120]

The data, which reflect respondents' views of their probable behaviour if they were to become aware of maldistribution while planning their next child, are summarized in Table 4. First of all, concerning frequency of use of preselection when more children of one sex than the other are born, it is evident that willingness to use preselection increases as the maldistribution does. The number of respondents who would use preselection in a 70/30 distribution is approximately double the number who would do so if the distribution were not skewed.

Even more important than the frequency of use of preselection in these extreme situations is the nature of the preselection decisions made. These data also reveal a surprising level of responsiveness to the hypothetical maldistribution in births. Through the range of five different hypothetical distributions of female and male births, with an increasing proportion of male births there is a consistent increase in the proportion of prospective parents who would preselect daughters ($p < 0.001$).

Table 4. Responsiveness to Perceived Skewed Birth Ratio by Those Willing to Use Sex Preselection

Perceived percentage of male newborns	30.0	40.0	50.0	60.0	70.0
Mean percentage of daughters planned	39.2 (n = 79)	45.3 (n = 53)	53.8 (n = 39)	58.0 (n = 50)	61.6 (n = 73)

These data are probably of limited relevance in Canada, where, even if there were reliable preselection methods available, the prospects of extreme maldistribution appear to be slim. But the implications of these data are interesting in their applicability to other societies. Since data of this type have not previously been collected, we have no way of knowing with certainty that the various incentives operant on this sample of subjects, whether biological determinism, homophobic opportunism, or otherwise, would also affect those whose cultures are more characterized by sex bias than Canada's is.

Values of Those Willing to Use Preselection

Those who claim they would be willing to use preselection, and those who say they would not, do not differ significantly with respect to the sex preferences they describe. For four of the six preference variables described earlier, as well as the relative number of daughters and sons wanted, the differences between them are non-existent or trivial. For the two preference variables that specifically refer to boys, the differences are greater, but slight.

There is another set of variables relevant to the issue of willingness to use preselection. The subjects who had indicated a willingness to use preselection were asked about the importance of various characteristics of preselection methods. The issues or characteristics described, and the importance that respondents attached to them, are described in Table 5.

Table 5. Issues Relevant to the Choice of a Sex Preselection Method

Issues	Issue importance* to respondents**	
	Female	Male
Risk of failure; having a baby of the "wrong" sex	2.14	2.35
Financial cost of the procedure	4.00	3.47
Feeling it might make the pregnancy less romantic	2.87	2.78
The lack of privacy if a doctor had to be involved	2.87	2.74
How much it would delay the pregnancy	2.61	2.18
How much it "interferes" with a natural process	3.27	3.21

* From five-point interval scale where 1 represents "not important" and 5 represents "very important."
** n = 176.

Interestingly, these prospective users of preselection methods were not especially concerned about method reliability, giving it a mean importance score of 2.2, the lowest score of any of the issues raised. This is consistent with the data, which revealed that even when preferences are held, respondents do not place a great deal of importance on having a child of the preferred sex. The most important issue rated, by far, was the cost of the procedure, with a mean score above 3.8. Both women and men were also worried about the extent to which preselection would interfere with a natural process. These findings are extremely important given the likelihood that the next effective preselection method will probably be a sperm separation method — flow cytometry — requiring both great expertise and the use of expensive equipment, and interfering significantly and conspicuously in the customary method of conception.

On the other hand, the data indicate that if an inexpensive method were developed that was also non-intrusive, it would probably be fairly widely used, even if it provided only a marginal improvement in the likelihood of obtaining children of the sex desired.

The differences between male and female respondents on the importance of these issues are interesting. Women are more concerned about all of the issues except one: "the chances of having a baby of the 'wrong' sex," about which men were much more concerned.

Previous Preselection Attempts

Three respondents claim that they had previously attempted preselection. Of these, only one achieved a pregnancy, allegedly a successful attempt to preselect a son. None of these respondents made a second attempt to preselect the sex of one of their children.

Knowledge of Fetal Sex Determination Methods

There is more respondent awareness of fetal sex determination than was the case for preselection methods, probably because the former methods are widely used for purposes other than sex selection. Approximately 63 percent of the respondents who intend to have children believe that "it is possible for a pregnant woman, either with or without the help of her doctor, to accurately predict the sex of her expected baby." But the majority of those who think it possible have no knowledge at all about how it is done. The knowledge that does exist is almost exclusively of two methods: amniocentesis and ultrasound imagery. However, a large majority of our respondents consider these methods, coupled with deliberate termination of the pregnancy, to be completely unacceptable as a sex selection method.

CVS is virtually unknown. It is reasonable to assume that as CVS and the test of maternal blood become more commonly used, public knowledge of them will increase. Although increased knowledge might lead to increased use, there is scarcely any doubt that the primary reason respondents are reluctant to use fetal sexing and abortion as a method of sex selection has little to do with their feelings about fetal sexing, but a great deal to do with their feelings about abortion for the purpose of sex selection.

Willingness to Use Abortion for Sex Selection

When asked whether they could imagine *any* circumstances, not necessarily for sex selection, in which they would be willing to have an abortion (or approve of their female partner having an abortion), 70 percent answered affirmatively. But when asked whether they could imagine any situation under which they would do so for the sake of sex selection, fewer than 4 percent said they could.

The few respondents who answered yes to the second question were asked to open the envelopes containing descriptions of fetal sexing methods. The techniques described for the respondents included amniocentesis (labelled Method A), a test under development that identifies fetal cells in a maternal blood sample (Method B), CVS (Method C), and ultrasound imaging (Method D). The various methods were labelled only as methods A, B, C, or D and not by the more descriptive "amniocentesis," etc.

The descriptions of fetal sexing methods provided to the subjects indicated that one important difference among the methods was whether findings would be available by the twelfth week, or early enough to permit an abortion to be done quickly and relatively easily without inducing labour. (See these descriptions in Appendix 1.)

None of the handful of respondents who were willing to abort a fetus based on its sex was willing to do so if it was to be his or her first child. In fact, the *only* situations in which respondents were willing to use abortion for the sake of sex selection were those in which there were one or more existing children all of the same sex, and the fetus was also of that sex.

A second important finding is that no respondent was willing to use either of the methods of sexing if they did not provide results by the twelfth week. That is, none was willing to use either amniocentesis or ultrasound for fetal sexing with the intention of aborting for sex selection after the twelfth week, regardless of the number or sex of existing children.

CVS was slightly more acceptable as a method of sexing. One respondent would abort a female fetus if he already had a daughter, and one with a son would prevent the birth of a second. Three or four respondents were willing to use CVS for sexing and would be prepared to abort if the fetus was the same sex as two existing children, but would not use it in any other circumstances.

Note that neither CVS nor amniocentesis is routinely available to pregnant women in Canada.

The blood test and subsequent abortion would have been used as a sex selection method by only one respondent in *any* situation in which the fetus was the same sex as existing children. The advent of this safe and reliable test providing early indications of fetal sex apparently would have negligible impact on people's willingness to use fetal sexing and abortion for the sake of sex selection.

The reliability of fetal sexing methods is sufficiently high that if there were public knowledge of them and willingness to use them, and payment for routine fetal sexing by provincial health programs, their impact would be significant. But the impact would be nothing more than many people attempting to have children of both sexes. Although fetal sexing techniques may improve, and knowledge of them may increase, there is no reason to anticipate a significant change in the current negligible willingness to use abortion for sex selection; in the absence of such a change, there will be no widespread use of abortion for that purpose.

Results of the Student Survey

Now that the relevant variables and issues have been defined, and the findings described for the primary sample, the findings for the student sample can be described briefly in a comparative manner. The results of the student survey provide additional support to the findings that have been presented. In spite of the differences in sample characteristics with respect to age, marital status, et cetera, the findings are similar.

The overall preference ratio for the student sample is 55:45. The importance that the students attach to specific issues is summarized in Table 6. Clearly, the student sample differs from the primary sample only slightly.

A significantly larger proportion of students (28 percent) could imagine themselves attempting preselection, and the scenarios in which they were willing to do so were familiar: they were motivated almost exclusively by the desire to have at least one child of each sex. Willingness to use either method to select either sex was approximately 3 percent higher than it was for the primary sample.

None of the female students was willing to use abortion for sex selection, and only one male student would agree to his partner having an abortion for that reason.

Table 6. Mean Sex Preference Values (Student Sample)

Importance of having:	Mean score
At least one daughter	2.9
At least one son	3.1
At least one of each sex	2.9
An equal number of each	1.5
A daughter first	1.5
A son first	1.8

In general, the student respondents were similar to those in the larger sample with respect to their knowledge and values. If compared to the subsample of unmarried respondents from the primary survey, the differences are negligible.

Application of the Model

The predictive model described earlier can be applied to the collected data, although the clarity and meaning of that information may appear to have rendered the model superfluous. The data have provided an unambiguous and detailed picture of the attitudes of Canadians on the related issues of preference for the sex of their children, awareness of both preconception and post-conception sex selection methods, and willingness to use those methods. The absence of significant aggregate sex bias, coupled with a limited awareness of effective sex selection methods and an almost unanimous unwillingness to use them, portend neither widespread use of sex selection nor significant maldistribution.

Although some of the implications of those data appear to be clear, the relationship between preference patterns and maldistribution may not be exactly as expected. Furthermore, not all of the data for the variables that comprise the model are conclusive, and some assumptions still have to be made. The formal model is used to clarify the combined effect of these variables, to provide slightly greater precision than might otherwise be achieved, and, most importantly, to test the implications of alternative assumptions.

Refinement of the Model

The model was presented earlier in its most elementary form. The model is flexible, and a number of refinements are possible. Although some terms appear in more than one of the four expressions, improvements in measuring the variables in one category can be incorporated without necessarily affecting either the other categories or the basic structure of the model.

For example, if different methods are expected to be used that do not have exactly the same degree of reliability, the equation can be refined by replacing each expression that includes a reliability term (RF or RM) with a set of separate expressions, each representing a single sex selection method, and each having a unique reliability term (RF_j or RM_j). If this is done, each of these new expressions must include a unique term (TF_j or TM_j) representing "the proportion of attempts to sex select females (males) that use that technique." That is, for each sex selection method used, the equation will include an expression that represents the relative frequency of its use, multiplied by the probability that its use would result in the birth of a child of the desired sex.

A similar breakdown of the method/reliability expression into multiple expressions would be appropriate if the reliability rates of specific methods differed for attempts to select males and females, or if not all methods were expected to be used in selecting both females and males, et cetera.

The sum of all TF (or TM) terms should equal 1.0, but values of the individual RF and RM terms are independent of each other.

Variables

To reiterate, the model requires the following kinds of data:

* the naturally occurring birth sex ratio in the absence of sex selection attempts;

* the proportion of pregnancies that are planned;

* the proportion of planned pregnancies that involve sex selection using each of the available methods of sex selection (this is derived from evidence of a combination of individuals' sex preference, awareness of the availability of sex selection techniques, and willingness to use specific sex preselection techniques to achieve the sex or sexes preferred);

* the reliability of each of those techniques in attempts to create females; and

* the reliability of each of those techniques in attempts to create males.

Predicted values for each of these variables are described below. Because of the importance of not underestimating maldistribution, assumptions deliberately err in the direction of inflating the predicted male/female birth ratio.

Naturally Occurring Sex Ratio

The proportion of newborns who were females, during the past few decades in North America and Europe, has consistently been between 0.48 and 0.49, indicating the ratio that exists when sex selection is not being used. The ratio at conception — or primary sex ratio — must be even more skewed, since fetal mortality is known to be significantly higher for males. There are a number of plausible explanations for the fact that the ratio is not 50:50. (See Zarutskie et al.[121] or Chahazarian[122] for a comprehensive review of possible determinants identified in previous research.) For the sake of the predictive model used here, the assumption is that 51.5:48.5 is a very close approximation of what the naturally occurring birth ratio in Canada would be in the absence of any attempt at sex selection.

Proportion of Births That Are Planned

There are no truly reliable data available on the proportion of births that are planned, largely because of the problem of respondent dishonesty. For the sake of the predictive model, it will be assumed that 80 percent of all pregnancies resulting in births are planned, although the actual figure is almost certainly considerably lower.

Sex Preselection Method Reliability

The reliability of preselection methods was addressed at some length earlier in this report. The reliability values used in the predictive model are based on the conclusions drawn in that section. There is no strong evidence that any of the methods of preselection currently available accomplishes much more than raising the hopes of those who use it. The most likely exception is the use of the Sephadex sperm separation method in conjunction with the administration of clomiphene citrate in attempts to preselect daughters. Although the available evidence is not conclusive about reliability, 0.7 appears to be a reasonable estimate.

It may be that timing intercourse relative to the estimated time of ovulation also has some impact on the primary sex ratio, but the reported results are so contradictory and uncertain that no conclusion concerning method effectiveness can be drawn with confidence. Ironically, if Guerrero's findings are valid, it may be that most of those who have attempted to use the Shettles method during the past 25 years to preselect a child of a particular sex are likely to have increased the probability of having a child of the opposite sex.

Given this assessment of the reliability of the various preselection methods, the predictive equation initially omits preselection methods other than Sephadex/clomiphene citrate (SC) in attempts to select females. It is not necessary to consider attempts to preselect males using SC because the method is not expected to be used for that purpose.

Fetal Sexing Method Reliability

The information on fetal sexing contained in the method descriptions accompanying the questionnaires is thought to be accurate, and is used in the predictive model (see Appendix 1).

Prevalence of Sex Selection

The proportion of pregnancies that represents sex selection attempts is derived from the data on respondent willingness to use those methods. Because the respondents' expressions of willingness to use specific methods followed their being informed about them in detail, the use of willingness data as an estimate of projected use implicitly assumes perfect information about methods on the part of potential users of sex selection. This admittedly unrealistic assumption is likely to result in an exaggeration of the possible maldistributive effect of any preference bias.

With respect to the expected use of SC, a number of respondents were willing to use a sperm separation method. The method described for the respondents was probably more attractive than the SC combination in that it simply involves sperm separation and not the ingestion of drugs, an important issue for many potential users of preselection. Notwithstanding the fact that the respondent data on willingness to use a sperm separation method probably slightly exaggerate willingness to use SC, they are used in the model as an estimate of willingness to undertake this kind of preselection. This might trivially inflate the predicted number of attempts to preselect daughters.

Willingness to use preselection was approximately 20 times as common as willingness to use abortion as a method of sex selection. Furthermore, none of the respondents considered abortion acceptable unless the fetal sexing method provided results within the first 12 weeks of the pregnancy. Neither amniocentesis nor ultrasound imaging (followed by induced labour and abortion) was considered acceptable in any of the scenarios presented to the respondents, even when depicted as "the only method available." Therefore, both of these methods are excluded from the predictive model. Although it is likely that a sample of many thousands would reveal some willingness to use abortion in this way, there is no justification for assuming such willingness if it was not evidenced by any in our samples of almost 700.

The blood test described for respondents is not yet clinically available, and thus is obviously unknown to potential users of fetal sexing for sex selection.

The equation does include an expression reflecting public willingness to use CVS and abortion in attempts to sex select both males and females.

For the initial application of the model, we shall assume, as loosely suggested by the data, that 95 percent of all attempts to select females will utilize preselection, and 5 percent will depend on abortion. We shall also assume, far beyond what the data convey, since no effective preselection method is available to select sons, that use of abortion to select males will be approximately twice as common as similar attempts to select girls.

First Set of Assumptions

To reiterate, the predictive equation can be represented as follows:

$$F = (1 - I)(FN) + (I)(1 - S)(FN) + (I)(S)(SF)(RF) + (I)(S)(1 - SF)(1 - RM)$$

The third and fourth expressions will be expanded to provide separate expressions for SC (preselection) and CVS (selection by fetal sexing and selective abortion). Each of the new expressions includes a term for the proportion of attempts involving the use of this particular technique of sex selection to select females (TF) or males (TM), and a term for the reliability of this technique in attempts to select a female (RF) or a male (RM). Each TF (or TM) term is multiplied by the corresponding RF (or RM) term. However, there may be terms for a particular technique used to select one sex without corresponding terms for attempts to select the other sex using that particular technique.

To avoid making the formula more complex than is necessary, it includes only methods with some degree of reliability (different from the naturally occurring birth ratio). Thus, SF is defined as the proportion of all such sex selection attempts intended to result in a girl being born, TF_j is the proportion of SF that involves the use of technique "j," and RF_j is the reliability of method j in attempts to select daughters.

Incorporating the specific sex selection techniques that respondents are willing to use and that have some measure of effectiveness, the third expression can be represented:

$$[(I)(S)(SF)][(TF_{sc})(RF_{sc}) + (TF_{cvs})(RF_{cvs})]$$

and the fourth becomes:

$$[(I)(S)(1 - SF)][(TM_{cvs})(1 - RM_{cvs})]$$

The values of relevant variables will be incorporated into the predictive equation. The assumptions and conclusions about those values, which were drawn previously, can be summarized as follows:

1. 0.80 of all pregnancies will be intended;

2. 0.485 of all births resulting from unintended pregnancies will be girls;

3. 0.10 of all intended pregnancies will involve sex selection;

4. 0.90 of all sex selection attempts *using methods which are reliable* will be attempts to select girls;

5. 0.95 of all attempts (using reliable methods) to select girls will involve the SC method;

6. 0.70 is the reliability of the SC method in attempts to select girls;

7. 0.05 of all attempts to select girls will involve the CVS method;

8. 0.99 is the reliability of the CVS method in attempts to select girls;

9. all attempts (using reliable methods) to select sons will involve the CVS method; and

10. 1.0 is the reliability of the CVS method in attempts to select boys.

Based on these values, the equation takes the form:

$$
\begin{aligned}
F &= [(1.0 - 0.8)(0.485)] + [(0.8)(1.0 - 0.1)(0.485)] + \\
&\quad [(0.8)(0.1)(0.9)][(0.95)(0.7) + (0.05)(0.99)] + \\
&\quad [(0.8)(0.1)(1.0 - 0.9)][(1.0)(1.0 - 0.99)] \\
&= [0.097] + [0.349] + [0.051] + [0.000] \\
&= 0.497
\end{aligned}
$$

That is, the data from a sample of Canadians who intend to have children suggest that if they were perfectly well informed about opportunities for sex selection, and ultimately used it as often as they claim they would, the sex ratio of all Canadian children would be, coincidentally, approximately 50:50.

Second Set of Assumptions

Although the first set of assumptions was intended to be accurate, they may have erred in one direction or the other. Also, changing circumstances may result in a different scenario than the one described. It is useful to speculate about expected maldistributive effects if alternative assumptions are made. Values reflecting alternative assumptions can be incorporated easily into the model. It becomes apparent in doing so that the conclusions that have been drawn are fairly robust.

For example, let us assume that a safe, non-intrusive, inexpensive, and reliable method of preselection (such as Method F) has been developed that is equally effective (0.7) in selecting daughters and sons. Note that such a method would be much more popular than the Ericsson or SC methods, and only slightly less popular than a simple timing method (e.g., Guerrero). Assume also that 80 percent of pregnancies resulting in births are planned.

The total number of preselection attempts that might be made for each sex is estimated in the following manner: willingness to use preselection in each of the scenarios for Method F is multiplied by the probability of individuals ever finding themselves in the respective scenarios (e.g., the probability of having two girls first is approximately 0.25), and by estimating the proportion of possible sex selection attempts that would be obviated by previous successful attempts. Preselection would be attempted in approximately 10 percent of all pregnancies, and the overall preference ratio would be 50.6:49.4. (This estimate ignores the moderating effects of age, marriage, etc.)

The simplified form of the predictive equation can be used, both because the reliability rate is the same in attempts to preselect males and females, and because other possible methods can be excluded from the formula since they would be much less attractive than the hypothetical one described. Therefore, the predictive equation might look like the following:

$$
\begin{aligned}
F &= [(1 - I)(FN)] + [(I)(1 - S)(FN)] + \\
&\quad [(I)(S)(SF)(RF)] + [(I)(S)(1 - SF)(1 - RM)] \\
&= [(1 - 0.8)(0.485)] + [(0.8)(1 - 0.1)(0.485)] + \\
&\quad [(0.8)(0.1)(0.494)(0.7)] + [(0.8)(0.1)(1 - 0.494)(1 - 0.7)] \\
&= [0.097] + [0.349] + [0.028] + [0.012] \\
&= 0.486
\end{aligned}
$$

That is, given the assumptions made, 48.6 percent of newborns would be females and 51.4 percent would be males. This prediction reveals an overall preference ratio that is slightly *less* extreme than the current birth ratio of 51.5:48.5. Given the preference ratio that respondents described, and their stated willingness to use preselection, it appears that *the more reliable and popular the preselection methods available, the less the maldistribution that would result from their use.*

The two estimates of maldistribution are based in part on assumptions that are not completely verifiable, or are known to be exaggerations, or are based on circumstances that can be expected to change. Furthermore, the predictions ignore some relevant variables.

These omitted variables could be incorporated into the predictive model, but not without cost. Their explicit consideration would entail making further assumptions, since the magnitude of their effects is uncertain. Furthermore, in making the model more complex, clarity and interpretability would be sacrificed for a measure of unneeded precision. Making the model more sophisticated by including other variables that had been omitted would tend to reduce the predicted maldistributive effects of sex bias. However, it is informative to consider the likely effects of some of these variables and alternative assumptions. They are considered in greater detail in the following section.

Conclusion

Review of Findings

This research strongly suggests that there is little chance of sex maldistribution in Canada resulting from the availability of sex selection methods. The confidence that can be placed in this conclusion is heightened by the redundancy of factors that effectively preclude maldistribution. First of all, the aggregate sex preference ratio is almost perfectly neutral and, most pertinently, is less extreme than the existing birth sex ratio. Available evidence indicates that pro-son bias is diminishing, especially with respect to sex selection, and there is no reason to expect a sudden reversal of this trend. Secondly, the kinds of sex selection methods that significant numbers of people would be willing to use are ineffective at present, while those that appear to be effective are unacceptable to all but a handful of people.

However, an aggregate preference pattern that is sex-neutral does not ensure an equal distribution of female and male births in the long term. For example, if a society had two gender groups in intense competition and tenuous balance, each with an ardent desire for children of only its sex, and with the desires of one group offsetting the goals of the other, there would be great risk because of the situation's inherent instability. But the data indicate that, in Canada, it is not only the aggregate sex preference that is neutral; the great majority of individual preference patterns are sex-neutral as well.

It is difficult to imagine a set of circumstances that would suddenly change the deeply held value of having children of both sexes. The preference for exactly an equal number of children of each sex, although widespread, is not held so strongly, and may change more easily.

The fundamental conclusion of this research is that the sex ratio of births that would result from people using sex selection is probably *less* extreme than the existing birth sex ratio, and that would continue to be true even if equally attractive and reliable methods to select males and females were available. This conclusion is likely to be received sceptically, but it does not differ significantly from the findings of a great number of other recent research efforts, which have consistently shown that the dominant sex choice value is having children of both sexes, and that although there is a pro-son preference, it is weak. They have also demonstrated that the general unwillingness to use sex selection renders pro-son preferences inconsequential, or nearly so.

Conventional wisdom has been incorrect for a number of reasons — primarily because it has overestimated sex bias by falsely assuming that a large proportion of those with sex bias would attempt sex selection (and that none of those without bias would), and incorrectly assuming that reliable and acceptable techniques were available to potential users.

Nevertheless, there are some ways in which maldistribution could occur as a result of sex selection, and they must be considered.

It was contended earlier that a sex-neutral preference pattern "effectively precludes" maldistribution. That statement may be misleading. The absence of any sex bias, even of individual bias, does not logically preclude maldistribution; it simply makes such an outcome unlikely. The reason that this is so becomes clearer when one considers that the desire to have an equal number of children of both sexes does not render an individual unwilling to attempt sex selection. On the contrary, most who are willing to use preselection would do so to have an equal number of daughters and sons. Such attempts at sex selection could result in a skewed birth ratio if the reliability of the sex selection methods used differed for attempts to select females and attempts to select males. The greater the disparity in reliability levels, the greater the possible maldistribution.

Interestingly, this scenario has some similarities to the present situation. It appears there is currently no effective means of preselecting males, but there probably is a method of preselecting females with a reliability rate of approximately 0.7. This method, which involves drug-taking by the would-be mother, physical sperm separation prior to artificial insemination, and significant expense, is not popular, and is unlikely to become so.

Obviously, a problem might arise if a technique were developed that was highly reliable in preselecting one sex, but not at all reliable in preselecting the other. If such a method were also inexpensive and widely available, there would exist the potential for significant maldistribution. Although this scenario is unlikely, it is probably the most serious threat to the sex distribution status quo in Canada.

Possible Errors in Prediction

Although the evidence appears conclusive, the possibility of errors remains. Four kinds of errors or shortcomings in the research are considered: unrepresentativeness of the sample, invalid measurement of the variables, omission of relevant variables from the predictive model, and changes in relevant variables.

Sample Representativeness

This issue already has been addressed at some length. In almost all respects, the sample appears to be highly representative. Fortunately, the possible biasing effects of the minor deviations from representativeness are not all in the same direction.

Previous methodological research has indicated that recent immigrants are less likely to respond to written questionnaires, even if language is not a problem. The fact that preference patterns are extremely skewed in some countries from which immigrants to Canada have come raises concern that the extent of son preference may have been underestimated in this survey. The data on the percentage of foreign-born in the sample allay this concern considerably, although the possibility of sample bias based on ethnicity remains.

The effect of the surplus of unmarried females in the sample probably was slight. These respondents tended to have less pro-son bias than male respondents, but more pro-son bias than married women. Any effect it had probably would have been to understate preferences for sons.

The high number of sons already born to the respondents may have inflated the apparent pro-son bias, but only to a trivial degree, if at all.

Invalid Measurement

Some of the problems of inferring behaviour from responses to questionnaires, especially in an area such as this one, were touched on earlier. The critical variables in this research are sex preference patterns, willingness to use sex selection, and, to a lesser degree, awareness of sex selection methods. Considerable effort was made in this research to validly measure respondents' values and knowledge in these areas, and the entire questionnaire was extensively pretested.

With respect to preference, a number of questions dealing with different dimensions of the concept were included. The questions measured not only different dimensions of preference, but also the importance that respondents attached to them.

Willingness to use sex selection was measured with reference to specific methods. The techniques were described in detail and for different specific scenarios, including the issues of risk, reliability, discomfort, cost, et cetera. Although this is no guarantee of valid measurement, it provides a more valid measure of willingness to use sex selection methods than research that asks about willingness only in general terms. Although the questions were complex because of their detail, response patterns indicate strongly that the respondents made reasoned answers. There were many logically related questions that were likely to have revealed any inconsistencies in responses, but these kinds of anomalies were not found.

The most significant threat to validity in this kind of research is probably respondent dishonesty. There is no way of knowing with certainty whether some respondents deliberately understated a strong preference for children of one sex or the other, or lied in other answers, but the consistency of their answers within individual questionnaires provides encouraging evidence of respondent honesty and seriousness in completing the questionnaires.

Omission of Relevant Variables

As noted earlier, some variables were deliberately excluded from the predictive model. This was done because their expected effect would be to minimize predicted maldistribution, and there was a reluctance to sacrifice clarity and interpretability for the sake of strengthening an already compelling argument.

The model did not take into consideration the following facts or premises, among others:

- People tend to become satisfied with the sexes of the children they have, and place less value on a specific mix of children, or sequence, after having had children who don't fit that pattern.

- People's views on sex preference tend to moderate with age, and preferences held now are likely to decline in importance as time passes.

- The views of people entering into an intimate relationship are unlikely to coincide exactly with those of their new partners, and are likely to moderate as they become aware of their partners' views.

- If people's sex preferences or views about the use of sex selection do not moderate after marriage, the likelihood of their using sex selection will be diminished by the incompatibility of views between partners.

- It is highly significant that there is public sensitivity to maldistribution and a willingness to use sex selection to have children of the less prevalent group. This response pattern, which had not previously been measured, would not completely counteract a maldistribution in either direction, but would lessen it significantly. Whether this motivation is a function of social consciousness or some other factor is uncertain, but it does exist.

Predicted Consequences of Maldistribution

Whatever prediction of maldistribution is made, extreme or otherwise, it is important that any attempt to assess its social consequences compare the estimated birth ratio not to 50:50, but to the normal birth ratio in the absence of sex selection, or approximately 51.5:48.5. That is not to say that a birth ratio of 51.5:48.5 is necessarily preferable to one of 50:50, but rather that it is easier to analyze social change with reference to the status quo than with reference to a demographic arrangement that does not exist in this society.

Notwithstanding the fact that male births have outnumbered female births consistently for many generations, the current adult female population is slightly larger than the adult male population. This can be attributed to higher male mortality rates, beginning in infancy (or, as noted earlier, at conception), and extending through childhood and into adult life. (Reviews of the determinants of this difference in death rates generally lead to the view that the rate will continue to be higher for males, but that the disparity will diminish, largely because of narrowing differences in cardiovascular and lung cancer deaths.)

One implication of the higher male mortality rate is that a decline in the proportion of male newborns would ameliorate the maldistribution among those under age 40, approximately, and exacerbate it among those who are older.[123]

As indicated earlier, two scenarios, both implausible, engender risk of maldistribution. In one, a significant change from the existing aggregate sex preference is coupled with the availability of a preselection method that is reliable, inexpensive, and otherwise attractive to potential users. In the second, a preselection method that is attractive to users becomes available, but has grossly different reliability rates in attempts to select the two sexes (or is reliable only for the selection of a single sex). Although the second scenario appears to be far more plausible, its maximum potential impact is smaller.

The risk to our society, although slight, should not be ignored. It would seem appropriate to monitor the types of sex preselection methods that become available, so that if a cheap, reliable method of choosing only children of one sex were developed, the appropriate policy response could be implemented quickly. A number of policy options suggest themselves, some of which would have a very rapid impact, whereas the change in birth ratio that would occur as the result of the availability of a new preselection method would be gradual because most of the relevant variables would tend to change incrementally, and not all at the same time.

The issue of the pace of change is an important one if consideration is being given to appropriate policy response. The extreme improbability of sudden maldistribution obviates the need for any government intervention apart from monitoring relevant conditions. There is no clear and present danger.

It also seems appropriate to monitor Canadians' values on issues pertaining to sex selection, but this hardly needs to be done more than once a decade. It is somewhat more important to measure awareness of, and willingness to use, new preselection methods when they become available, especially if there were the promise of an attractive technique that was significantly more reliable for the selection of one of the sexes than the other.

One implication of these findings is that research into preselection methods with similar reliability rates for attempts to select either sex is to be preferred over research intended to perfect methods allowing preselection of only one sex. It suggests also that the second priority should be to support research into methods to preselect females. This should be done not only because the majority of newborns are males, but also because of the grossly disproportionate degree to which males are afflicted with inherited diseases, and the consequent need for women and their partners to be able to preselect daughters if they so choose. Some inherited diseases affect only daughters, or are more likely to affect them. Consequently, social benefits would also be derived from selection methods which increased the probability of having a son. However, the number of such diseases is much smaller than ones which affect boys exclusively or disproportionately. The greater social need is for a method that would permit the preselection of daughters.

There exists a justifiable fear of the adverse social consequences of gross sex maldistribution, specifically with respect to an excess of males. However, common assumptions concerning the patterns of sex preference, willingness to use sex selection, and other factors that determine the level of maldistribution are patently false.

There is no extreme pro-son bias and no pro-daughter bias. There is no widespread knowledge of specific sex selection methods or, generally, of their feasibility. There is no great desire to use preselection methods (which are, in any case, generally ineffective) and almost complete unwillingness to sex select by abortion.

One can conclude only that there is no impending sex maldistribution in Canada resulting from the use of sex selection or preselection methods.

Appendix 1.
Survey on Sex Preference and Sex Selection*

---

*   Editor's note: The questionnaire is not presented in the same format as the original because of
formatting constraints.

Dear

A couple of months ago, when you completed a nationwide telephone survey, you kindly agreed to answer a written questionnaire on people's values concerning the ideal number of children, preferences for daughters or sons, and related issues.

The questionnaire is part of research being done for the Royal Commission on New Reproductive Technologies. We appreciate your agreeing to participate in it, since it's extremely important that we collect data from as representative a group as possible. We'd also be very grateful if you could respond quickly. That would save us the expense of sending you reminder notices, and so on.

There are a few things I'd like you to know about the questionnaire.

1. *Your identity will be kept completely confidential.* Neither your name nor your address will be included with the questionnaire.

2. The questionnaire won't take long to complete. As you'll see, most of the questions don't require written answers and can be answered by simply putting an "X" in the appropriate set of brackets [ ]. But feel free to add written comments if you feel that the short answer doesn't express your views accurately or completely. Also, there is space at the end of the questionnaire for any additional comments you want to make.

3. You won't have to answer all of the questions. Watch for directions that tell you which question to go to next.

4. There are information sheets in separate sealed envelopes. Please do *not* open them until the instructions in the questionnaire ask you to.

5. If you have questions about this questionnaire, or about the research generally, you can write to me at York University, or phone me at (416) 736-5128, ext. 77272.

All of us at the Royal Commission on New Reproductive Technologies and York University who are involved in this research are truly grateful for your help. Thank you.

A Survey of the Preferences of Canadians Concerning the Sex of their Children

Conducted by:
The Institute for Social Research, York University, Toronto
as part of research for:
The Royal Commission on New Reproductive Technologies

March 1992

INSTRUCTIONS: You'll find information or instructions in other double-outlined boxes like this one. Also, watch for instructions that follow some of the questions, telling you which one to go to next. If you need more space for a written answer, please use the section on the back page. When answers have sets of brackets "[ ]", put an "X" inside the brackets beside the single best answer.

BACKGROUND INFORMATION

1. What is your sex?
    [ ] female
    [ ] male

2. In what year were you born? 19____

3. In the spaces below, write "sister," "brother," or "me" in the order in which you and any brothers or sisters you had were born. (For example, if you had one older sister, and two younger brothers, you would write: Sister, Me, Brother, Brother). Include everyone who was raised as your brother or sister, even if they were not "blood" relatives.

    _____ _____ _____ _____ _____ _____

4. In which countries were you and your parents born? (This refers to the parents who raised you.)

    (a) your country of birth? _____

    (b) your mother's country of birth? _____

    (c) your father's country of birth? _____

5. Which cultural or ethnic group(s), if any, do you feel closest to? _____

6. How important is it to you to have regular contact with people who have the same cultural or ethnic background as you do? (Circle any number between "1" and "5," where "1" means "not important" and "5" means "very important.")

not important				very important
1	2	3	4	5

7. With which religion, if any, do you identify most closely? _____

8. How important a role does religion play in your life? (Circle any number between "1" and "5".)

not important				very important
1	2	3	4	5

9. Which of the following statements best describes your level of formal education?
    [ ]   never attended high school
    [ ]   attended or currently attending high school or vocational training school
    [ ]   attended or currently attending university, community college, or technical school
    [ ]   received a university degree (degree(s) received: _____)

10. Which of the following categories best describes your usual occupation?
    [ ]   Farming, fishing, forestry, mining
    [ ]   Homemaking
    [ ]   Managerial or administrative (Junior level)
    [ ]   Managerial or administrative (Senior level)
    [ ]   Professional
    [ ]   Sales, service, clerical
    [ ]   Semi-skilled labour
    [ ]   Skilled labour; trades
    [ ]   Other: _____

11. In 1991, what was your approximate total household income (from all sources) before taxes?
    [ ]   less than $20,000   [ ] $60,000 - $79,999
    [ ] $20,000 - $39,999   [ ] $80,000 - $99,999
    [ ] $40,000 - $59,999   [ ] $100,000 or more

12. How many people, including yourself, were in your household during the past year? _____

FAMILY STRUCTURE AND SEX PREFERENCE

13. Have you ever had, or do you now have, any children? (That is, have you raised children which you considered to be a part of your family?)
    [ ] yes (If "yes," go on to the next question.)
    [ ] no (If "no," go to question 15.)

14. Put an "X" in each appropriate box to indicate the sex of each of your children (for up to five). If you've had more than five, please also write the total number of each sex in the last column.

	1st child	2nd child	3rd child	4th child	5th child	Total
daughter						
son						

15. Are you presently married, or living with someone in an intimate relationship?
    [ ] yes (If "yes," go on to the next question.)
    [ ] no (If "no," go to question 20.)

16. What is your partner's sex?
    [ ] female
    [ ] male

17. Is your partner also willing to complete and return a separate copy of this questionnaire?
    [ ] no
    [ ] yes (If (s)he has already received one, put an "X" here [ ]; if not, write her/his name and mailing address below.)

    _____

    _____

    _____

18. It's important that we know whether your answers reflect only your own values, or joint decisions of your partner and yourself. Although we prefer that your answers are based only on your own values, that's not a critical issue. What's critical is that we know what your answers represent.
    [ ] my answers reflect only my own values   (Go to question 19.)
    [ ] my answers reflect both my partner's values
         and my own   (Go to question 20.)

19. How important do you believe each of the following issues are to your spouse or partner?

	not important			very important	
having at least one daughter	1	2	3	4	5
having at least one son	1	2	3	4	5
having at least one of each sex	1	2	3	4	5
having the same number of daughters and sons	1	2	3	4	5
having a daughter first	1	2	3	4	5
having a son first	1	2	3	4	5

20. Would you like to have (more) children at some time in the future?
    [ ] yes (If "yes," go on to the next question.)
    [ ] no (If "no," go to question 44.)

21. Put "X"s in the boxes below to indicate whether you'd like boys, girls, or have no preference for the sex of children you'd like to have *in the future* (whether or not you already have children). If you plan to have more than five children, please also write in the total number in the last column.

Preferences	Planned future children					
	Next child	2nd future child	3rd future child	4th future child	5th future child	Total
I'd prefer a girl						
I'd prefer a boy						
I'd have no preference						

22. How important are each of the following issues to you?

	not important			very important	
having at least one daughter	1	2	3	4	5
having at least one son	1	2	3	4	5
having at least one of each sex	1	2	3	4	5
having the same number of daughters and sons	1	2	3	4	5
having a daughter first	1	2	3	4	5
having a son first	1	2	3	4	5

23. Is there anything else you can tell us about your preferences for the sex of your children that isn't explained in your answers to the previous questions?

_____

_____

SEX SELECTION

Sex Preselection

24. Do you believe there is anything which can be done *before* a woman becomes pregnant to increase the chances of her having a child of the sex she prefers?
    [ ] yes (If "yes," go on to the next question.)
    [ ] no   (If "no," go to question 29.)

25. Describe this method including your opinion of its accuracy and availability. If you know of more than one method, describe each one. (Use the back of the questionnaire if you need more space.) If you don't have any information about a preselection method, just write "no information."

_____

_____

26. Have you ever attempted to preselect the sex of one of your children?
    [ ] yes (If "yes," go on to the next question.)
    [ ] r.   (If "no," go to question 29.)

27. For each preselection attempt, which of the methods described in question 25 did you use?
First attempt method: _____
Second attempt method: _____

28. For each preselection attempt, check the box which most closely describes what happened.

First preselection attempt	**Second preselection attempt**
[ ] No pregnancy occurred.	[ ] No pregnancy occurred.
[ ] The pregnancy was not completed.	[ ] The pregnancy was not completed.
[ ] I wanted a girl and had a girl.	[ ] I wanted a girl and had a girl.
[ ] I wanted a boy and had a boy.	[ ] I wanted a boy and had a boy.
[ ] I wanted a girl and had a boy.	[ ] I wanted a girl and had a boy.
[ ] I wanted a boy and had a girl.	[ ] I wanted a boy and had a girl.

29. Have you ever heard of anyone (else) attempting to preselect the sex of their baby?
[ ] yes
[ ] no

Read the descriptions of sex preselection methods in envelope #1. Do *not* assume that methods like these are available; they may or may not exist. The next few questions ask whether you might use them *if* they were available. (If you'd like information on which methods, if any, really work, put an "X" in the following box [ ] and enclose a stamped, self-addressed envelope when you return your questionnaire.)

---

30. Can you imagine any situation in which you, or you and your partner, might use any of these methods of sex preselection, *if* they were available, to try to choose your baby's sex?
[ ] yes (If "yes," go on to the next question.)
[ ] no (If "no," go to the section "Sex prediction during ..." after question 33.)

31. After the description of each situation below, put an "X" in one of the four boxes in that row, to indicate what you think you would *probably* do.

Situations	Choices			
If sex preselection method "E" were the only one available, what would you probably do if:	I wouldn't want to have a (another) child	I'd want to have a child, but would not try to preselect sex	I'd try to preselect a girl, using preselection method "E"	I'd try to preselect a boy, using preselection method "E"
you didn't yet have any children?				
you already had one girl?				
you already had one boy?				
you already had two girls?				
you already had two boys?				
you already had a girl and a boy?				
you already had three girls?				
you already had three boys?				
you already had two girls and a boy?				
you already had two boys and a girl?				

Situations	Choices			
If sex preselection method "F" were the only one available, what would you probably do if:	**I wouldn't want to have a (another) child**	**I'd want to have a child, but would not try to preselect sex**	**I'd try to preselect a girl, using preselection method "F"**	**I'd try to preselect a boy, using preselection method "F"**
you didn't yet have any children?				
you already had one girl?				
you already had one boy?				
you already had two girls?				
you already had two boys?				
you already had a girl and a boy?				
you already had three girls?				
you already had three boys?				
you already had two girls and a boy?				
you already had two boys and a girl?				

Situations	Choices			
Assume that sex preselection method "F" were available to you. What would you probably do if, in planning your next child, you learned that of all babies born in the past few years:	I wouldn't want to have a (another) child	I'd want to have a child, but would not try to preselect sex	I'd try to preselect a girl, using preselection method "F"	I'd try to preselect a boy, using preselection method "F"
30% were girls and 70% were boys?				
40% were girls and 60% were boys?				
50% were girls and 50% were boys?				
60% were girls and 40% were boys?				
70% were girls and 30% were boys?				

32. How important would each of the following issues be in your choice of a sex-preselection method?

	not important			very important	
The risk of failure, of having a "wrong sex" baby	1	2	3	4	5
The financial cost of the procedure	1	2	3	4	5
Feeling it would make the pregnancy less romantic	1	2	3	4	5
The lack of privacy if a doctor had to be involved	1	2	3	4	5
Any delay in beginning the pregnancy	1	2	3	4	5
Not wanting to interfere with a natural process	1	2	3	4	5
Other: _____	1	2	3	4	5

33. Which statement most accurately reflects your views concerning the proper role of government with regard to sex preselection?
    [ ] Sex preselection, even if done by individuals at home, should be against the law.
    [ ] Sex preselection should be against the law unless there is a valid medical reason (such as a sex-linked genetic disease) for doing it.
    [ ] Sex preselection should not be against the law, since it harms no-one. But governments should not pay for it unless there is a valid medical reason.
    [ ] Sex preselection should not be against the law. It harms no-one and is a way for people to plan their families. Costs should be paid by provincial health insurance.

Sex prediction during pregnancy

34. Do you believe it is possible for a pregnant woman, either with or without the help of her doctor, to accurately predict the sex of her expected baby?
    [ ] yes (If "yes," go on to the next question.)
    [ ] no (If "no," go to question 36.)

35. Describe this method of sex prediction, including your opinion of its accuracy and availability. If you think there is more than one method available, describe each one. (Use the back of the questionnaire if you need more space.) If you don't have any information about methods of sex determination during pregnancy, write "no information."

_____

_____

_____

36. Can you imagine any situation — not necessarily for the sake of sex selection — in which you would be willing to have an abortion (or agree with your female partner's decision to have an abortion)?
    [ ] yes (If "yes," go on to the next question.)
    [ ] no   (If "no," go to question 40.)

37. Can you imagine any situation in which you would be willing to have an abortion (or agree with your female partner's decision to have an abortion) for the purpose of sex selection?
    [ ] yes (If "yes," continue.)
    [ ] no   (If "no," go to question 40.)

Please read the information on "Predicting a baby's sex during pregnancy" in envelope #2. Do *not* draw conclusions about whether methods like these are available; they may or may not exist. (If you want to know whether effective methods of predicting a baby's sex during pregnancy really exist, put an "X" in this box [ ] and enclose a stamped, self-addressed envelope when you return the questionnaire.)

---

38. After the description of each situation below, put an "X" in one of the four boxes in that row, to indicate what you think you would *probably* do.

Situations	Choices			
Imagine that you are pregnant (or that your partner is) and that sex prediction method "A" is the only one available. What would you probably do if:	I would have the baby	I'd have an abortion, but not for sex selection	I'd predict its sex and have an abortion if it were a girl	I'd predict its sex and have an abortion if it were a boy
you didn't yet have any children?				
you already had one girl?				
you already had one boy?				
you already had two girls?				
you already had two boys?				
you already had a girl and a boy?				
you already had three girls?				
you already had three boys?				
you already had two girls and a boy?				
you already had two boys and a girl?				

Situations	Choices			
Imagine that you are pregnant (or that your partner is) and that sex prediction method "B" is the only one available. What would you probably do if:	I would have the baby	I'd have an abortion, but not for sex selection	I'd predict its sex and have an abortion if it were a girl	I'd predict its sex and have an abortion if it were a boy
you didn't yet have any children?				
you already had one girl?				
you already had one boy?				
you already had two girls?				
you already had two boys?				
you already had a girl and a boy?				
you already had three girls?				
you already had three boys?				
you already had two girls and a boy?				
you already had two boys and a girl?				

Situations	Choices			
Imagine that you are pregnant (or that your partner is) and that sex prediction method "C" is the only one available. What would you probably do if:	I would have the baby	I'd have an abortion, but not for sex selection	I'd predict its sex and have an abortion if it were a girl	I'd predict its sex and have an abortion if it were a boy
you didn't yet have any children?				
you already had one girl?				
you already had one boy?				
you already had two girls?				
you already had two boys?				
you already had a girl and a boy?				
you already had three girls?				
you already had three boys?				
you already had two girls and a boy?				
you already had two boys and a girl?				

Situations	Choices			
Imagine that you are pregnant (or that your partner is) and that sex prediction method "D" is the only one available. What would you probably do if:	I would have the baby	I'd have an abortion, but not for sex selection	I'd predict its sex and have an abortion if it were a girl	I'd predict its sex and have an abortion if it were a boy
you didn't yet have any children?				
you already had one girl?				
you already had one boy?				
you already had two girls?				
you already had two boys?				
you already had a girl and a boy?				
you already had three girls?				
you already had three boys?				
you already had two girls and a boy?				
you already had two boys and a girl?				

Situations	Choices			
Imagine that you are pregnant (or that your partner is) and that sex prediction method "A" is the only one available. What would you probably do if you found out that of babies born in recent years:	I would have the baby	I'd have an abortion, but not for sex selection	I'd predict its sex and have an abortion if it were a girl	I'd predict its sex and have an abortion if it were a boy
30% were girls and 70% were boys?				
40% were girls and 60% were boys?				
50% were girls and 50% were boys?				
60% were girls and 40% were boys?				
70% were girls and 30% were boys?				

39. Which statement most accurately reflects your views concerning the proper role of government with regard to sex prediction during pregnancy?

    [ ] Sex prediction during pregnancy should be against the law in all circumstances, including the possible occurrence of a sex-linked inherited disease.

    [ ] Sex prediction during pregnancy should be against the law unless there is a valid medical reason for doing it (such as a possible sex-linked genetic disease).

    [ ] Sex prediction should not be against the law, but governments should not pay health care workers to do it for patients unless there is a valid medical reason.

    [ ] Sex prediction should not be against the law. It is reasonable for people to want to predict the sex of their children, and costs should be covered by provincial health insurance plans.

40. Imagine that you (or your female partner) are (is) pregnant, and have absolutely no desire to end the pregnancy prematurely. If an easy, inexpensive, safe and reliable method of sex-prediction were available, do you think you would want it, simply so that you would know whether you were going to have a girl or a boy?

    [ ]   I definitely would not want to know the baby's sex.
    [ ]   I probably would not want to know the baby's sex.
    [ ]   I probably would want to know the baby's sex.
    [ ]   I definitely would want to know the baby's sex.
    [ ]   Not applicable.

Adoption

> Please read the information on "adoption methods" in envelope #3. Adoption procedures are not exactly the same in every province or town, and they may be quite different in your community.

41. Assuming that you and your partner are able to have your own (biological) children, can you imagine any situation in which you would be willing to adopt a child?

    [ ]   yes (If "yes," go on to the next question.)
    [ ]   no   (If "no," go to question 43.)

42. After the description of each situation, put an "X" in the box that best describes what you would probably decide to do. (Put one "X" in each row of five boxes.)

Situations	Choices				
If you and your partner were able to have children, and if both adoption methods were available to you, what would you do if you (already) had	I wouldn't want another child	I'd want a child, but would not adopt one	I'd adopt a baby of either sex	I'd adopt only if certain I'd get a girl	I'd adopt only if certain I'd get a boy
no children?	N/A				
one girl?					
one boy?					
two girls?					
two boys?					
a girl and a boy?					
three girls?					
three boys?					

CONCLUSION

43. If you think that you might use any of the methods of sex selection described in this questionnaire, tell us which specific method you are most likely to use, and why.

   _____

   _____

   _____

44. In your opinion, what percent of Canadians:
   would prefer to have more daughters than sons? _____ %
   would prefer to have more sons than daughters? _____ %
   would prefer to have the same number of each? _____ %
   have no preference concerning the number of each? _____ %

45. In your opinion, what percent of Canadians:
   would prefer to have a daughter as their first child? _____ %
   would prefer to have a son as their first child? _____ %
   have no preference concerning the sex of their first child? _____ %

This is the end of the questionnaire. If you have any additions to your answers, or other comments, please write them in the space below. Thanks again for helping us with this research project. We do appreciate it.

_____

_____

_____

_____

_____

_____

_____

_____

_____

_____

_____

_____

METHODS OF SEX PREDICTION DURING PREGNANCY

A number of issues affect people's willingness to try sex-prediction during pregnancy for the sake of sex selection, including the number and sex of children they already have and hope to have.

Obviously their feelings about abortion would be an important issue. And, if they are willing to have an abortion for sex selection, one related issue is whether it's possible to get results by the twelfth week of the pregnancy. This is important because if an abortion is done by approximately the twelfth week, it can be done in a couple of hours on an outpatient basis in either a hospital or a clinic. But, if it's done after the twelfth week, the procedure generally followed is that the pregnant woman is injected with a drug which causes labour to begin; she delivers the fetus in the hospital, and usually has to stay there for a few days.

Another issue is the prediction method. How accurate, risky, uncomfortable, or expensive is it?

Finally, one other issue that most people don't think about now, but might be important if many parents used sex selection is the percent of all newborn babies of each sex. For example, if 80% of all babies born recently were of one sex — whether girls or boys — that might affect some people's decisions concerning which sex they wanted their child to be.

The methods described below are not listed in any particular order. Once again, do *not* assume that methods like these really exist.

Method "A"

A physician inserts a needle through the mother's belly, into the uterus, and into the fluid-filled sac which contains the developing baby (fetus). A small amount of fluid is removed, and then analyzed in a laboratory. The baby is not touched by the needle, and isn't harmed by the removal of the fluid. This is done around the sixteenth week of the pregnancy; results are obtained a few weeks later.

Accuracy in identifying a fetus which is female:	Virtually 100%
Accuracy in identifying a fetus which is male:	Virtually 100%
Risk to the fetus:	Fewer than 1% of all tests cause a miscarriage
Risk to the mother:	Almost none
Pain or discomfort to the mother:	Almost none
Results obtained by the twelfth week:	No

Method "B"

Blood is taken from a vein in the arm of the pregnant woman, and analyzed in a laboratory. This can be done at about the tenth week of the pregnancy, and results are obtained within two weeks.

Accuracy in identifying a fetus which is female: Virtually 100%
Accuracy in identifying a fetus which is male: Virtually 100%
Risk to the fetus: None
Risk to the mother: None
Pain or discomfort to the mother: Almost none
Results obtained by the twelfth week: Yes

Method "C"

A physician inserts a very narrow plastic tube in the vagina of the pregnant woman, up to the uterus. Some cells are removed and analyzed. Results can be obtained at approximately the twelfth week of the pregnancy.

Accuracy in identifying a fetus which is female: Virtually 100%
Accuracy in identifying a fetus which is male: About 99%
Risk to the fetus: About 2% of all tests cause a miscarriage
Risk to the mother: Almost none
Pain or discomfort to the mother: Slight
Results obtained by the twelfth week: Yes

Method "D"

A physician holds a camera-like device against the belly of the pregnant woman to get a picture of the developing baby. It looks something like a very fuzzy TV picture. It usually is clear enough to show whether the baby has a penis.

Accuracy in identifying a fetus which is female: Virtually 100%
Accuracy in identifying a fetus which is male: Approximately 95%
Risk to the fetus: None
Risk to the mother: None
Pain or discomfort to the mother: None
Results obtained by the twelfth week: No

METHODS OF SEX PRESELECTION

The preselection methods described on this sheet are used prior to the start of a pregnancy to try to affect the odds of conceiving either a female or a male child. Once again, do *not* assume that techniques exactly like these really exist.

A number of issues might affect people's willingness to try sex-preselection.

One might be the sex of children they already have and hope to have. Another is the method itself. How reliable, risky, expensive or time-consuming is it?

One other issue that most people don't think about now, but might be important if many parents used sex selection is the percent of all newborn babies of each sex. For example, if 80% of all babies born recently were of one sex — whether girls or boys — that might affect some people's decisions concerning which sex they wanted their child to be.

Method "E"

This method requires the help of a physician, and can be done by only a very small number of obstetricians who have the necessary specialized equipment. It's very unlikely that your family physician or obstetrician would be able to apply this method.

For three months prior to the time that she wants to become pregnant, the woman takes her temperature every morning and records the information. This will help to determine exactly when she is ovulating and most likely to become pregnant. On the day suggested by the temperature chart, a sperm sample is collected at home from the prospective father and placed in a sterile glass jar. This sample is taken to the physician's office. After the sample is "filtered" by the physician's equipment, it is placed in a tiny cup and inserted in the woman's vagina.

Success rate in attempts to have females:	Approximately 70%
Success rate in attempts to have males:	Approximately 70%
Pain or discomfort to the mother:	Almost none
Cost (not covered by insurance):	Approximately $1000 to $1500

Method "F"

For three months prior to the time that she wants to become pregnant, the woman takes her temperature every morning and records the information. This will help to determine exactly when she is ovulating and most likely to become pregnant. For one month prior to the time she wants to get pregnant, she takes a pill every morning. The pills have no side-effects. On the day indicated by the temperature chart, she has sex with her partner, or is artificially inseminated.

Success rate in attempts to have females:	Approximately 70%
Success rate in attempts to have males:	Approximately 70%
Pain or discomfort to the mother:	None
Cost (not covered by insurance):	Approximately $50 for pills

ADOPTION METHODS

The following brief description of adoption methods is not intended to include all of the details of the typical adoption. Also, these details often differ a great deal from province to province, and perhaps even from community to community.

The descriptions refer to adoptions within this country, and do not describe the adoption of children from other countries.

Public Adoptions

Public adoptions are supervised either by specific government agencies, or by a Children's Aid Society. A "home study" is done to determine the suitability of the adopting parent(s). Their suitability might be based not only on their values and behavior, but possibly also on issues such as their age, whether they are married, etc. The emphasis here is usually on finding appropriate parents for a specific child.

The cost to the adoptive parents varies; usually there is no necessary cost, but often the adoptive parents will choose to have a lawyer involved, and that may cost a few hundred dollars.

This process often takes many years, but usually is shorter if adoptive parents are willing to take a child having characteristics that are not in great demand. This generally includes children who are older, who have some kind of physical or emotional problem, or who are mixed race, etc. Requesting a child of a specific sex may delay the process further.

Private Adoptions

Private adoptions are often initiated by a physician or lawyer who knows both a woman who intends to give a child up for adoption, and a person or couple who wants to adopt. The question of the parent's suitability to adopt is much less important in private adoptions than in public ones. The emphasis here is usually on finding an appropriate child for specific parents.

The cost is generally a few thousand dollars, but there is a great deal of variation in cost. The adoptive parent(s) are not allowed to pay the birth mother for the baby, but may pay her for any expenses she had in bearing and having the child.

Private adoptions often take less time than public adoptions, but that depends partly on how many specific characteristics, such as sex or age, the adoptive parents insist on.

Acknowledgments

My thanks go to a number of people, without whom this work could not have been completed.

Shira Thomas, a medical student at McMaster University, co-authored the section dealing with the reliability of preselection methods and made many other valuable contributions. Primary research assistant Natalie Wallach's skill and dedication contributed immensely. David Northrup and his colleagues at York University's Institute for Social Research provided excellent advice from the earliest stages of the project, and effective management of the written survey. Professor Paul Laurendeau of York University translated the questionnaires into French. Michal Bornstein-Thomas, genetic counsellor at The Toronto Hospital, prepared lucid descriptions of fetal sexing methods for use in the questionnaire, and served as a reproductive technology consultant over the course of the project. Melanie Joyner, a graduate student in political science at York University, completed computer runs for statistical analysis of the data. I appreciate the efforts of administrative staff at York University, especially Esther Stoch of Accounting Services, and Noli Swatman and Gisela Birmingham of York's Office of Research Administration.

A number of scholars of sex preselection methods shared their views with me, including Sandra Carson, Mark Geier, Barton Gledhill, Raphael Jewelewicz, Landrum Shettles, and Paul Zarutskie. In addition, a number of anonymous referees of a preliminary draft of this report made comments that were extremely helpful.

At the Royal Commission, Dolores Backman, Neil Tremblay, Clarke Fraser, and Anne Marie Smart were unfailingly supportive and fair-minded.

Finally, my thanks and compliments go to all respondents to either the survey or the pretest for their unselfish participation.

To all of you, for your patience, interest, and cooperation over a lengthy project, I am deeply grateful.

Notes

1. M. Thomas, "The Impact of Gender Preselection on Gender Maldistribution," in *Feminist Research: Prospect and Retrospect*, ed. P. Tancred-Sheriff (Montreal and Kingston: McGill-Queen's University Press, 1988).

2. R.J. Levin, "Human Sex Pre-Selection," in *Oxford Review of Reproductive Biology*, vol. 9, ed. J.R. Clarke (Oxford: Clarendon Press, 1987).

3. P.W. Zarutskie et al., "The Clinical Relevance of Sex Selection Techniques," *Fertility and Sterility* 52 (1989): 891-905.

4. P. Barlow and C.G. Vosa, "The Y Chromosome in Human Spermatozoa," *Nature* 226 (1970): 961-62.

5. B.L. Gledhill, "Control of Mammalian Sex Ratio by Sexing Sperm," *Fertility and Sterility* 40 (1983): 572-74.

6. A.M. Roberts and H. Goodall, "Y Chromosome Visibility in Quinacrine-Stained Human Spermatozoa," *Nature* 262 (1976): 493-94.

7. J.L. Thomsen and E. Niebuhr, "The Frequency of False-Positive and False-Negative Results in the Detection of Y-Chromosome in Interphase Nuclei," *Human Genetics* 73 (1986): 27-30.

8. R.A. Beatty, "F-Bodies as Y Chromosome Markers in Mature Human Sperm Heads: A Quantitative Approach," *Cytogenetics and Cell Genetics* 18 (1977): 33-49.

9. Gledhill, "Control of Mammalian Sex Ratio."

10. J.P. Chaudhuri and W.-B. Schill, "A Possibility of Unbiased Sex Preselection in Humans by Enrichment of X or Y Chromosome Bearing Spermatozoa," *Andrologia* 19 (1987): 157-60.

11. P.L. Deininger et al., "Base Sequence Studies of 300 Nucleotide Renatured Repeated Human DNA Clones," *Journal of Molecular Biology* 15 (1981): 17-33.

12. S. Sarkar, "Motility, Expression of Surface Antigen, and X and Y Human Sperm Separation in *In Vitro* Fertilization Medium," *Fertility and Sterility* 42 (1984): 899-905.

13. J.D. West, K.M. West, and R.J. Aitken, "Detection of Y-Bearing Spermatozoa by DNA-DNA In Situ Hybridisation," *Molecular Reproduction and Development* 1 (1989): 201-207.

14. L.B. Shettles, "Human Spermatozoan Types," *Gynaecologia* 152 (1961): 153-62.

15. D.W. Bishop, "Biology: X and Y Spermatozoa," *Nature* 187 (1960): 255-56; V. Rothschild, "Biology: X and Y Spermatozoa," *Nature* 187 (1960): 253-54; C. Van Duijn, "Nuclear Structure of Human Spermatozoa," *Nature* 188 (1960): 916-18.

16. L.J.D. Zaneveld et al., "Scanning Electron Microscopy of Mammalian Spermatozoa," *Journal of Reproductive Medicine* 6 (1971): 147-51.

17. K. Ueda and R. Yanagimachi, "Sperm Chromosome Analysis as a New System to Test Human X- and Y-Sperm Separation," *Gamete Research* 17 (1987): 221-28.

18. T.A. Beckett, R.H. Martin, and D.I. Hoar, "Assessment of the Sephadex Technique for Selection of X-Bearing Human Sperm by Analysis of Sperm Chromosomes, Deoxyribonucleic Acid and Y-Bodies," *Fertility and Sterility* 52 (1989): 829-35.

19. A.M. Roberts, "Gravitational Separation of X and Y Spermatozoa," *Nature* 238 (1972): 223-25.

20. R.J. Ericsson, C.N. Langevin, and M. Nishino, "Isolation of Fractions Rich in Human Y Sperm," *Nature* 246 (1973): 421-24.

21. F.J. Beernink and R.J. Ericsson, "Male Sex Preselection Through Sperm Isolation," *Fertility and Sterility* 38 (1982): 493-95.

22. S.L. Corson et al., "Sex Selection by Sperm Separation and Insemination," *Fertility and Sterility* 42 (1984): 756-60.

23. W.P. Dmowski et al., "Use of Albumin Gradients for X and Y Sperm Separation and Clinical Experience with Male Sex Preselection," *Fertility and Sterility* 31 (1979): 52-57.

24. S.B. Jaffe et al., "A Controlled Study for Gender Selection," *Fertility and Sterility* 56 (1991): 254-58.

25. W.L.G. Quinlivan et al., "Separation of Human X and Y Spermatozoa by Albumin Gradients and Sephadex Chromatography," *Fertility and Sterility* 37 (1982): 104-107.

26. Dmowski et al., "Use of Albumin Gradients."

27. J.M. Evans, T.A. Douglas, and J.P. Renton, "An Attempt to Separate Fractions Rich in Human Y Sperm," *Nature* 253 (1975): 352-54.

28. A. Ross, J.A. Robinson, and H.J. Evans, "Failure to Confirm Separation of X- and Y-Bearing Human Sperm Using BSA Gradients," *Nature* 253 (1975): 354-55.

29. Ueda and Yanagimachi, "Sperm Chromosome Analysis."

30. B.F. Brandriff et al., "Sex Chromosome Ratios Determined by Karyotypic Analysis in Albumin-Isolated Human Sperm," *Fertility and Sterility* 46 (1986): 678-85.

31. S.A. Carson, "Sex Selection: The Ultimate in Family Planning," *Fertility and Sterility* 50 (1988): 16-19.

32. O. Steeno, A. Adimoelja, and J. Steeno, "Separation of X- and Y-Bearing Human Spermatozoa with the Sephadex Gel-Filtration Method," *Andrologia* 7 (1975): 95-97.

33. Beckett et al., "Assessment of the Sephadex Technique."

34. Quinlivan et al., "Separation of Human X and Y Spermatozoa."

35. Corson et al., "Sex Selection by Sperm Separation."

36. M.R. Geier, J.L. Young, and D. Kessler, "Too Much or Too Little Science in Sex Selection Techniques?" *Fertility and Sterility* 53 (1990): 1111-14.

37. J.F. Daniell et al., "Initial Evaluation of a Convection Counter Streaming Galvanization Technique of Sex Separation of Human Spermatozoa," *Fertility and Sterility* 38 (1982): 233-37.

38. S. Shishito, M. Shirai, and K. Sasaki, "Galvanic Separation of X and Y Bearing Human Spermatozoa," *International Journal of Fertility* 20 (1975): 13-16.

39. U. Engelmann et al., "Separation of Human X and Y Spermatozoa by Free-Flow Electrophoresis," *Gamete Research* 19 (1988): 151-60.

40. J.H. Check et al., "Male Sex Preselection: Swim-Up Technique and Insemination of Women After Ovulation Induction," *Archives of Andrology* 23 (1989): 165-66.

41. J.P. Chaudhuri and R. Yanagimachi, "An Improved Method to Visualize Human Sperm Chromosomes Using Zona-Free Hamster Eggs," *Gamete Research* 10 (1984): 233-39.

42. E. Rudak, P.A. Jacobs, and R. Yanagimachi, "Direct Analysis of the Chromosome Constitution of Human Spermatozoa," *Nature* 274 (1978): 911-13.

43. R.H. Martin et al., "The Chromosome Constitution of 1,000 Human Spermatozoa," *Human Genetics* 63 (1983): 305-309.

44. B.F. Brandriff et al., "Chromosomal Abnormalities in Human Sperm: Comparisons Among Four Healthy Men," *Human Genetics* 66 (1984): 193-201.

45. U. Engelmann, E.-M. Parch, and W.-B. Schill, "Modern Techniques of Sperm Preparation — Do They Influence the Sex of Offspring?" *Andrologia* 21 (1989): 523-28.

46. Ibid.

47. L.B. Shettles, "Separation of X and Y Spermatozoa," *Journal of Urology* 116 (1976): 462-64.

48. S. Sarkar, "Human Sperm Swimming in Flow," *Differentiation* 27 (1984): 126-32.

49. J.H. Sampson et al., "Gender After Artificial Induction of Ovulation and Artificial Insemination," *Fertility and Sterility* 40 (1983): 481-84.

50. Beernink and Ericsson, "Male Sex Preselection."

51. Jaffe et al., "A Controlled Study."

52. W.H. James, "The Sex Ratio of Infants Born After Hormonal Induction of Ovulation," *British Journal of Obstetrics and Gynaecology* 92 (1985): 299-301.

53. Corson et al., "Sex Selection by Sperm Separation."

54. J. Stolkowski and J. Lorrain, "Preconceptional Selection of Fetal Sex," *International Journal of Gynecology and Obstetrics* 18 (1980): 440-43.

55. W.R. Lyster and M.W.H. Bishop, "An Association Between Rainfall and Sex in Man," *Journal of Reproduction and Fertility* 10 (1965): 35-47.

56. J. Stolkowski and J. Choukroun, "Preconception Selection of Sex in Man," *Israel Journal of Medical Sciences* 17 (1981): 1061-67.

57. M. Cabut, "De l'influence des apports nutritionnels en ions K⁺, Na⁺, Ca⁺⁺, Mg⁺⁺ sur la sex-ratio chez l'homme. Étude rétrospective chez 102 femmes n'ayant que des enfants du même sexe" (M.D. dissertation, Université de Paris, Val-de-Marne, 1977).

58. Stolkowski and Choukroun, "Preconception Selection."

59. F. Labro and F. Papa, *Boy or Girl? Choosing Your Child Through Diet* (London: Souvenir Press, 1984).

60. L.B. Shettles, "Factors Influencing Sex Ratios," *International Journal of Gynecology and Obstetrics* 8 (1970): 643-47.

61. R.B. Diasio and R.H. Glass, "Effects of pH on the Migration of X and Y Sperm," *Fertility and Sterility* 22 (1971): 303-305.

62. D.C. Downing et al., "The Effect of Ion-Exchange Column Chromatography on Separation of X and Y Chromosome-Bearing Human Spermatozoa," *Fertility and Sterility* 27 (1976): 1187-90.

63. K.H. Broer, U. Dauber, and R. Kaiser, "Enrichment of X-Spermatozoa and *In Vitro* Penetration Through Cervical Mucus," *Andrologia* 9 (1977): 74-78.

64. D. Bennett and E.A. Boyse, "Sex Ratio in Progeny of Mice Inseminated with Sperm Treated with H-Y Antiserum," *Nature* 246 (1973): 308-309.

65. J.T. France et al., "A Prospective Study of the Preselection of the Sex of Offspring by Timing Intercourse Relative to Ovulation," *Fertility and Sterility* 41 (1984): 894-900.

66. E.L. Billings et al., "Symptoms and Hormonal Changes Accompanying Ovulation," *Lancet* (5 February 1972): 282-84.

67. T.W. Hilgers and A.J. Bailey, "Natural Family Planning. II. Basal Body Temperature and Estimated Time of Ovulation," *Obstetrics and Gynecology* 55 (1980): 333-39.

68. Ibid.

69. S. Kleegman, "Can Sex Be Predetermined by the Physician?" in *Proceedings of the Fifth World Congress on Fertility and Sterility: 16-22 June 1966, Stockholm*, ed. B. Westin et al. (Amsterdam: Excerpta Medica Foundation, 1967).

70. D.M. Rorvik and L.B. Shettles, *Your Baby's Sex: Now You Can Choose* (New York: Bantam Books, 1971).

71. Diasio and Glass, "Effects of pH."

72. Carson, "Sex Selection."

73. B.W. Simcock, "Sons and Daughters — A Sex Preselection Study," *Medical Journal of Australia* (13 May 1985): 541-42.

74. R. Guerrero, "Association of the Type and Time of Insemination Within the Menstrual Cycle with the Human Sex Ratio at Birth," *New England Journal of Medicine* 291 (1974): 1056-59.

75. S. Harlap, "Gender of Infants Conceived on Different Days of the Menstrual Cycle," *New England Journal of Medicine* 300 (1979): 1445-48.

76. A. Perez et al., "Sex Ratio Associated with Natural Family Planning," *Fertility and Sterility* 43 (1985): 152-53.

77. France et al., "A Prospective Study of the Preselection."

78. C.S. Vear, "Preselective Sex Determination," *Medical Journal of Australia* (19 November 1977): 700-702.

79. See, for example, H.L. Fancher, "The Relationship Between Occupational Status of Individuals and the Sex Ratio of Their Offspring," *Human Biology* 28 (1956): 316-22; D.S. Freedman, R. Freedman, and P.K. Whelpton, "Size of Family and Preference for Children of Each Sex," *American Journal of Sociology* 66 (1960): 141-46; L. Bumpass and C. Westoff, *The Later Years of Childbearing* (Princeton: Princeton University Press, 1970). For similar recent data on Canadians, see J. Chen and T.R. Balakrishnan, *Do Gender Preferences Affect Fertility and Family Dissolution in Canada?* Discussion Paper 90-7 (London: University of Western Ontario, Population Studies Centre, 1990).

80. N.G. Bennett, "Sex Selection of Children: An Overview," in *Sex Selection of Children*, ed. N.G. Bennett (New York: Academic Press, 1983).

81. N. Calway-Fagen, B.S. Wallston, and H. Gabel, "The Relationship Between Attitudinal and Behavioral Measures of Sex Preference," *Psychology of Women Quarterly* 4 (1979): 274-80.

82. This discussion will not focus on the large amount of research that has been done in Asian and other countries that are culturally dissimilar to Canada.

83. N.E. Williamson, *Sons or Daughters: A Cross-Cultural Survey of Parental Preferences* (Beverly Hills: Sage Publications, 1976).

84. G.S. Rotter and N.G. Rotter, "Preferred Family Constellations: A Pilot Study," *Social Biology* 19 (1972): 401-404; also see C.H. Coombs, L.C. Coombs, and G.H. McClelland, "Preference Scales for Number and Sex of Children," *Population Studies* 29 (1975): 273-98; S. Adelman and S. Rosenzweig, "Parental Predetermination of the Sex of Offspring. II. The Attitudes of Young Married Couples with High School and with College Education," *Journal of Biosocial Science* 10 (1978): 235-47.

85. See N.E. Williamson, "Sex Preferences, Sex Control, and the Status of Women," *Signs: Journal of Women in Culture and Society* 1 (1976): 847-62; A.R. Pebley and C.F. Westoff, "Women's Sex Preferences in the United States: 1970 to 1975," *Demography* 19 (1982): 177-89; E. Stark, "The Sexes: Boys 1, Girls 1," *Psychology Today* 19 (August 1985): 18.

86. L.S. Fidell, D. Hoffman, and P. Keith-Spiegel, "Some Social Implications of Sex-Choice Technology," *Psychology of Women Quarterly* 4 (1979): 32-42.

87. Consider the research findings of: F. Gilroy and R. Steinbacher, "Preselection of Child's Sex: Technological Utilization and Feminism," *Psychological Reports* 53 (1983): 671-76; R. Norman, "Sex Differences in Preferences for Sex of Children: A Replication After 20 Years," *Journal of Psychology* 88 (1974): 229-39; M. Hammer and J. McFerran, "Preference for Sex of Child: A Research Update," *Individual Psychology: Journal of Adlerian Theory, Research and Practice* 44 (1988): 481-91.

88. S. Dinitz, R.R. Dynes, and A.C. Clarke, "Preferences for Male or Female Children: Traditional or Affectional?" *Marriage and Family Living* 16 (May 1964): 128-30.

89. C.C. Peterson and J.L. Peterson, "Preference for Sex of Offspring as a Measure of Change in Sex Attitudes," *Psychology* 10 (2)(1973): 3-5.

90. R.E. Hartley, F.P. Hardesty, and D.S. Gorfein, "Children's Perceptions and Expressions of Sex Preference," *Child Development* 33 (1962): 221-27.

91. See R. Steinbacher and F.D. Gilroy, "Preference for Sex of Child Among Primiparous Women," *Journal of Psychology* 119 (1985): 541-47; M.E. Pharis and M. Manosevitz, "Sexual Stereotyping of Infants: Implications for Social Work Practice," *Social Work Research and Abstracts* 20 (1)(1984): 7-12; C.S. Rent and G.S. Rent, "More on Offspring-Sex Preference: A Comment on Nancy E. Williamson's 'Sex Preference, Sex Control, and the Status of Women,' " *Signs: Journal of Women in Culture and Society* 3 (1977): 505-15; A. Oakley, "What Makes Girls Differ from Boys?" *New Society* 46 (21-28 December 1978): xii-xiv; G.E. Markle, "Sex Ratio at Birth: Values, Variance, and Some Determinants," *Demography* 11 (1974): 131-42.

92. N. Uddenberg, P.-E. Almgren, and A. Nilsson, "Preference for Sex of the Child Among Pregnant Women," *Journal of Biosocial Science* 3 (1971): 267-80.

93. Dinitz et al., "Preferences for Male or Female Children?"

94. See Williamson, *Sons or Daughters*, for the most thorough, if slightly dated, review of this issue.

95. For examples of research on various European subpopulations, see Uddenberg et al., "Preference for Sex of the Child Among Pregnant Women"; G. Giurovich, "Sul Desiderio dei Coniugi di Avere Figli e di Avere Figli di un Dato Sesso" [On the Wish

of Married Couples to Have Children and to Have Children of a Specific Sex], in *Atti Della XV e XVI Riunione Scientifica (Roma: Aprile 1955-Giugno 1956)* (Rome: Società Italiana Di Stastica, 1956); C. Gini, "Esame Comparativo di Alcuni Risultati di Inchieste Italiane Straniere Sui Desiderio dei Genitori di Avere Figli Dell' uno o Piuttosto Dell' Altro Sesso" [Comparative Analysis of Some Results of Italian and Foreign Studies on Parents' Sex Preferences for their Children], in *Atti Della XV e XVI Riunione Scientifica (Roma: Aprile 1955-Giugno 1956)*, (Rome: Società Italiana Di Statistica, 1956), 319-32; J. Peel, "The Hull Family Survey. I. The Survey Couples, 1966," *Journal of Biosocial Science* 2 (1970): 45-70; R. Freedman and L.C. Coombs, "Preferences About Sex of Children," in *Cross-Cultural Comparisons: Data on Two Factors in Fertility Behavior: Report of a Project of the Subcommittee on Comparative Fertility Analysis of the International Union for the Scientific Study of Population* (New York: Population Council, 1974); R. Carr-Hill, M. Samphier, and B. Sauve, "Socio-Demographic Variations in the Sex Composition and Preferences of Aberdeen Families," *Journal of Biosocial Science* 14 (1982): 429-43; G. Dahlberg, "Do Parents Want Boys or Girls?" *Acta Genetica et Statistica Medica* 1 (1948): 163-67.

96. Markle, "Sex Ratio at Birth."

97. Dinitz et al., "Preferences for Male or Female Children?"

98. A.M. Leahy, "Some Characteristics of Adoptive Parents," *American Journal of Sociology* 38 (1933): 548-63; R. Brenner, *A Follow-Up Study of Adoptive Families* (New York: Child Adoption Research Committee, 1951); R. Michaels, "Casework Considerations in Rejecting the Adoption Application," in *Readings in Adoption*, ed. I.E. Smith (New York: Philosophical Library, 1963); E.A. Lawder et al., *A Study of Black Adoption Families: A Comparison of a Traditional and a Quasi-Adoption Program* (New York: Child Welfare League of America, 1971); B. Jaffee and D. Fanshel, *How They Fared in Adoption: A Follow-Up Study* (New York: Columbia University Press, 1970).

99. For example, see Jaffee and Fanshel, *How They Fared*; for similar data on Canadian adoptive parents, see H.D. Kirk, "Differential Sex Preference in Family Formation: A Serendipitous Datum Followed Up," *Canadian Review of Sociology and Anthropology* 1 (1964): 31-48.

100. See F. Arnold and E.C.Y. Kuo, "The Value of Daughters and Sons: A Comparative Study of the Gender Preferences of Parents," *Journal of Comparative Family Studies* 15 (1984): 299-318; Calway-Fagen et al., "The Relationship Between Attitudinal and Behavioral Measures"; Carr-Hill et al., "Socio-Demographic Variations"; P. Cutright, S. Belt, and J. Scanzoni, "Gender Preferences, Sex Predetermination, and Family Size in the United States," *Social Biology* 21 (1974): 242-48; Peterson and Peterson, "Preference for Sex of Offspring as a Measure of Change in Sex Attitudes"; C.F. Westoff and R.R. Rindfuss, "Sex Preselection in the United States: Some Implications," *Science* 184 (1974): 633-36; Williamson, *Sons or Daughters?*

101. G.E. Markle and C.B. Nam, "Sex Predetermination: Its Impact on Fertility," *Social Biology* 18 (1971): 73-83.

102. J.B. Ullman and L.S. Fidell, "Gender Selection and Society," in *Gender in Transition*, ed. J. Offerman-Zuckerberg (New York: Plenum Press, 1989).

103. M. Farr, "Dangerous Determination: Disturbing Trends in High Tech Sex Selection Won't Go Away by Ignoring the Problem," *This Magazine* 24 (April-May 1991): 10-15.

104. Adelman and Rosenzweig, "Parental Predetermination of the Sex of Offspring."

105. R.L. Matteson and G. Terranova, "Social Acceptance of New Techniques of Child Conception," *Journal of Social Psychology* 101 (1977): 225-29.

106. S.F. Hartley, "Attitudes Toward Reproductive Engineering: An Overview," *Journal of Family Issues* 2 (1981): 5-24.

107. Pebley and Westoff, "Women's Sex Preferences."

108. S.F. Hartley and L.M. Pietraczyk, "Preselecting the Sex of Offspring: Technologies, Attitudes and Implications," *Social Biology* 26 (1979): 232-46.

109. Fidell et al., "Some Social Implications."

110. Markle and Nam, "Sex Predetermination."

111. Gilroy and Steinbacher, "Preselection of Child's Sex."

112. Steinbacher and Gilroy, "Preference for Sex of Child."

113. Markle and Nam, "Sex Predetermination."

114. United States. National Commission for the Protection of Human Subjects of Biomedical and Behavioral Research, *Special Study: Implications of Advances in Biomedical and Behavioral Research* (Washington, DC: U.S. Department of Health, Education, and Welfare, 1978).

115. Rosenzweig and Adelman, "Parental Predetermination of the Sex of Offspring: The Attitudes of Young Married Couples with University Education," *Journal of Biosocial Science* 8 (1976): 335-46.

116. G. Largey, "Sex Control, Sex Preferences, and the Future of the Family," *Social Biology* 19 (1972): 379-92.

117. R. Dawkins, *The Selfish Gene* (Oxford: Oxford University Press, 1976).

118. Westoff and Rindfuss, "Sex Preselection in the United States."

119. Dawkins, *The Selfish Gene.*

120. Those commenting on the possible increase in male homosexuality, or on public perceptions of that possibility, include N.P. Chico and S.F. Hartley, "Widening Choices in Motherhood of the Future," *Psychology of Women Quarterly* 6 (1981): 12-25.

121. Zarutskie et al., "The Clinical Relevance."

122. A. Chahnazarian, "Determinants of the Sex Ratio at Birth," Ph.D. dissertation, Princeton University, 1986.

123. For an elaboration of this point, see L. Dulude, "Getting Old: Men in Couples and Women Alone," in *Women and Men: Interdisciplinary Readings on Gender*, ed. G.H. Nemiroff (Markham: Fitzhenry and Whiteside, 1987).

References

Adelman, S., and S. Rosenzweig. "Parental Predetermination of the Sex of Offspring. II. The Attitudes of Young Married Couples with High School and with College Education." *Journal of Biosocial Science* 10 (1978): 235-47.

Arnold, F., and E.C.Y. Kuo. "The Value of Daughters and Sons: A Comparative Study of the Gender Preferences of Parents." *Journal of Comparative Family Studies* 15 (1984): 299-318.

Barlow, P., and C.G. Vosa. "The Y Chromosome in Human Spermatozoa." *Nature* 226 (1970): 961-62.

Beatty, R.A. "F-Bodies as Y Chromosome Markers in Mature Human Sperm Heads: A Quantitative Approach." *Cytogenetics and Cell Genetics* 18 (1977): 33-49.

Beckett, T.A., R.H. Martin, and D.I. Hoar. "Assessment of the Sephadex Technique for Selection of X-Bearing Human Sperm by Analysis of Sperm Chromosomes, Deoxyribonucleic Acid and Y-Bodies." *Fertility and Sterility* 52 (1989): 829-35.

Beernink, F.J., and R.J. Ericsson. "Male Sex Preselection Through Sperm Isolation." *Fertility and Sterility* 38 (1982): 493-95.

Bennett, D., and E.A. Boyse. "Sex Ratio in Progeny of Mice Inseminated with Sperm Treated with H-Y Antiserum." *Nature* 246 (1973): 308-309.

Bennett, N.G. "Sex Selection of Children: An Overview." In *Sex Selection of Children*, ed. N.G. Bennett. New York: Academic Press, 1983.

Billings, E.L., et al. "Symptoms and Hormonal Changes Accompanying Ovulation." *Lancet* (5 February 1972): 282-84.

Bishop, D.W. "Biology: X and Y Spermatozoa." *Nature* 187 (1960): 255-56.

Brandriff, B.F., et al. "Chromosomal Abnormalities in Human Sperm: Comparisons Among Four Healthy Men." *Human Genetics* 66 (1984): 193-201.

—. "Sex Chromosome Ratios Determined by Karyotypic Analysis in Albumin-Isolated Human Sperm." *Fertility and Sterility* 46 (1986): 678-85.

Brenner, R. *A Follow-Up Study of Adoptive Families.* New York: Child Adoption Research Committee, 1951.

Broer, K.H., U. Dauber, and R. Kaiser. "Enrichment of X-Spermatozoa and *In Vitro* Penetration Through Cervical Mucus." *Andrologia* 9 (1977): 74-78.

Bumpass, L., and C. Westoff. *The Later Years of Childbearing.* Princeton: Princeton University Press, 1970.

Cabut, M. "De l'influence des apports nutritionnels en ions K⁺, Na⁺, Ca⁺⁺, Mg⁺⁺ sur la sex-ratio chez l'homme. Étude rétrospective chez 102 femmes n'ayant que des enfants du même sexe." M.D. dissertation, Université de Paris-Val de Marne, 1977.

Calway-Fagen, N., B.S. Wallston, and H. Gabel. "The Relationship Between Attitudinal and Behavioral Measures of Sex Preference." *Psychology of Women Quarterly* 4 (1979): 274-80.

Carr-Hill, R., M. Samphier, and B. Sauve. "Socio-Demographic Variations in the Sex Composition and Preferences of Aberdeen Families." *Journal of Biosocial Science* 14 (1982): 429-43.

Carson, S.A. "Sex Selection: The Ultimate in Family Planning." *Fertility and Sterility* 50 (1988): 16-19.

Chahnazarian, A. "Determinants of the Sex Ratio at Birth." Ph.D. dissertation, Princeton University, 1986.

Chaudhuri, J.P., and W.-B. Schill. "A Possibility of Unbiased Sex Preselection in Humans by Enrichment of X or Y Chromosome Bearing Spermatozoa." *Andrologia* 19 (1987): 157-60.

Chaudhuri, J.P., and R. Yanagimachi. "An Improved Method to Visualize Human Sperm Chromosomes Using Zona-Free Hamster Eggs." *Gamete Research* 10 (1984): 233-39.

Check, J.H., et al. "Male Sex Preselection: Swim-Up Technique and Insemination of Women After Ovulation Induction." *Archives of Andrology* 23 (1989): 165-66.

Chen, J., and T.R. Balakrishnan. "Do Gender Preferences Affect Fertility and Family Dissolution in Canada?" Discussion Paper 90-7. London: University of Western Ontario, Population Studies Centre, 1990.

Chico, N.P., and S.F. Hartley. "Widening Choices in Motherhood of the Future." *Psychology of Women Quarterly* 6 (1981): 12-25.

Coombs, C.H., L.C. Coombs, and G.H. McClelland. "Preference Scales for Number and Sex of Children." *Population Studies* 29 (1975): 273-98.

Corson, S.L., et al. "Sex Selection by Sperm Separation and Insemination." *Fertility and Sterility* 42 (1984): 756-60.

Cutright, P., S. Belt, and J. Scanzoni. "Gender Preferences, Sex Predetermination, and Family Size in the United States." *Social Biology* 21 (1974): 242-48.

Dahlberg, G. "Do Parents Want Boys or Girls?" *Acta Genetica et Statistica Medica* 1 (1948): 163-67.

Daniell, J.F., et al. "Initial Evaluation of a Convection Counter Streaming Galvanization Technique of Sex Separation of Human Spermatozoa." *Fertility and Sterility* 38 (1982): 233-37.

Dawkins, R. *The Selfish Gene*. Oxford: Oxford University Press, 1976.

Deininger, P.L., et al. "Base Sequence Studies of 300 Nucleotide Renatured Repeated Human DNA Clones." *Journal of Molecular Biology* 151 (1981): 17-33.

Diasio, R.B., and R.H. Glass. "Effects of pH on the Migration of X and Y Sperm." *Fertility and Sterility* 22 (1971): 303-305.

Dinitz, S., R.R. Dynes, and A.C. Clarke. "Preferences for Male or Female Children: Traditional or Affectional?" *Marriage and Family Living* 16 (May 1964): 128-30.

Dmowski, W.P., et al. "Use of Albumin Gradients for X and Y Sperm Separation and Clinical Experience with Male Sex Preselection." *Fertility and Sterility* 31 (1979): 52-57.

Downing, D.C., et al. "The Effect of Ion-Exchange Column Chromatography on Separation of X and Y Chromosome-Bearing Human Spermatozoa." *Fertility and Sterility* 27 (1976): 1187-90.

Dulude, L. "Getting Old: Men in Couples and Women Alone." In *Women and Men: Interdisciplinary Readings on Gender*, ed. G.H. Nemiroff. Markham: Fitzhenry and Whiteside, 1987.

Engelmann, U., E.-M. Parch, and W.-B. Schill. "Modern Techniques of Sperm Preparation — Do They Influence the Sex of Offspring?" *Andrologia* 21 (1989): 523-28.

Engelmann, U., et al. "Separation of Human X and Y Spermatozoa by Free-Flow Electrophoresis." *Gamete Research* 19 (1988): 151-60.

Ericsson, R.J., C.N. Langevin, and M. Nishino. "Isolation of Fractions Rich in Human Y Sperm." *Nature* 246 (1973): 421-24.

Evans, J.M., T.A. Douglas, and J.P. Renton. "An Attempt to Separate Fractions Rich in Human Y Sperm." *Nature* 253 (1975): 352-54.

Fancher, H.L. "The Relationship Between Occupational Status of Individuals and the Sex Ratio of Their Offspring." *Human Biology* 28 (1956): 316-22.

Farr, M. "Dangerous Determination: Disturbing Trends in High Tech Sex Selection Won't Go Away by Ignoring the Problem." *This Magazine* 24 (March-April 1991): 10-15.

Fidell, L., D. Hoffman, and P. Keith-Spiegel. "Some Social Implications of Sex-Choice Technology." *Psychology of Women Quarterly* 4 (1979): 32-42.

France, J.T., et al. "A Prospective Study of the Preselection of the Sex of Offspring by Timing Intercourse Relative to Ovulation." *Fertility and Sterility* 41 (1984): 894-900.

Freedman, D.S., R. Freedman, and P.K. Whelpton. "Size of Family and Preference for Children of Each Sex." *American Journal of Sociology* 66 (1960): 141-46.

Freedman, R., and L.C. Coombs. "Preferences About Sex of Children." In *Cross-Cultural Comparisons: Data on Two Factors in Fertility Behavior: Report of a Project of the Subcommittee on Comparative Fertility Analysis of the International Union for the Scientific Study of Population*. New York: Population Council, 1974.

Geier, M.R., J.L. Young, and D. Kessler. "Too Much or Too Little Science in Sex Selection Techniques?" *Fertility and Sterility* 53 (1990): 1111-14.

Gilroy, F., and R. Steinbacher. "Preselection of Child's Sex: Technological Utilization and Feminism." *Psychological Reports* 53 (1983): 671-76.

Gini, C. "Esame Comparativo di Alcuni Risultati di Inchieste Italiane e Straniere Sul Desiderio dei Genitori di Avere Figli Dell' uno o Piuttosto Dell' Altro Sesso" [Comparative Analysis of Some Results of Italian and Foreign Studies on Parents' Sex Preferences for Their Children]. In *Atti Della XV e XVI Riunione Scientifica (Roma: Aprile 1955-Giugno 1956)*. Rome: Società Italiana Di Statistica, 1956.

Giurovich, G. "Sul Desiderio dei Coniugi di Avere Figli e di Avere Figli di un Dato Sesso" [On the Wish of Married Couples to Have Children and to Have

Children of a Specific Sex]. In *Atti Della XV e XVI Riunione Scientifica (Roma: Aprile 1955-Giugno 1956)*. Rome: Società Italiana Di Statistica, 1956.

Gledhill, B.L. "Control of Mammalian Sex Ratio by Sexing Sperm." *Fertility and Sterility* 40 (1983): 572-74.

Guerrero, R. "Association of the Type and Time of Insemination Within the Menstrual Cycle with the Human Sex Ratio at Birth." *New England Journal of Medicine* 291 (1974): 1056-59.

Hammer, M., and J. McFerran. "Preference for Sex of Child: A Research Update." *Individual Psychology: Journal of Adlerian Theory, Research and Practice* 44 (1988): 481-91.

Harlap, S. "Gender of Infants Conceived on Different Days of the Menstrual Cycle." *New England Journal of Medicine* 300 (1979): 1445-48.

Hartley, R.E., F.P. Hardesty, and D.S. Gorfein. "Children's Perceptions and Expressions of Sex Preference." *Child Development* 33 (1962): 221-27.

Hartley, S.F. "Attitudes Toward Reproductive Engineering: An Overview." *Journal of Family Issues* 2 (1981): 5-24.

Hartley, S.F., and L.M. Pietraczyk. "Preselecting the Sex of Offspring: Technologies, Attitudes and Implications." *Social Biology* 26 (1979): 232-46.

Hilgers, T.W., and A.J. Bailey. "Natural Family Planning. II. Basal Body Temperature and Estimated Time of Ovulation." *Obstetrics and Gynecology* 55 (1980): 333-39.

Holmes, H.B. "Sex Preselection: Eugenics for Everyone?" In *Biomedical Ethics Reviews*, ed. J.M. Humber and R.F. Almeder. Clifton: Humana Press, 1985.

Jaffe, S.B., et al. "A Controlled Study for Gender Selection." *Fertility and Sterility* 56 (1991): 254-58.

Jaffee, B., and D. Fanshel. *How They Fared in Adoption: A Follow-Up Study*. New York: Columbia University Press, 1970.

James, W.H. "The Sex Ratio of Infants Born After Hormonal Induction of Ovulation." *British Journal of Obstetrics and Gynaecology* 92 (1985): 299-301.

Kirk, H.D. "Differential Sex Preference in Family Formation: A Serendipitous Datum Followed Up." *Canadian Review of Sociology and Anthropology* 1 (1964): 31-48.

Kleegman, S. "Can Sex Be Predetermined by the Physician?" In *Proceedings of the Fifth World Congress on Fertility and Sterility: 16-22 June 1966, Stockholm*, ed. B. Westin et al. Amsterdam: Excerpta Medica Foundation, 1967.

Labro, F., and F. Papa. *Boy or Girl? Choosing Your Child Through Diet*. London: Souvenir Press, 1984.

Largey, G. "Sex Control, Sex Preferences, and the Future of the Family." *Social Biology* 19 (1972): 379-92.

Lawder, E.A., et al. *A Study of Black Adoption Families: A Comparison of a Traditional and a Quasi-Adoption Program*. New York: Child Welfare League of America, 1971.

Leahy, A.M. "Some Characteristics of Adoptive Parents." *American Journal of Sociology* 38 (1933): 548-63.

Levin, R.J. "Human Sex Pre-Selection." In *Oxford Review of Reproductive Biology*, vol. 9, ed. J.R. Clarke. Oxford: Clarendon Press, 1987.

Lyster, W.R., and M.W.H. Bishop. "An Association Between Rainfall and Sex in Man." *Journal of Reproduction and Fertility* 10 (1965): 35-47.

Markle, G.E. "Sex Ratio at Birth: Values, Variance, and Some Determinants." *Demography* 11 (1974): 131-42.

Markle, G.E., and C.B. Nam. "Sex Predetermination: Its Impact on Fertility." *Social Biology* 18 (1971): 73-83.

Martin, R.H., et al. "The Chromosome Constitution of 1,000 Human Spermatozoa." *Human Genetics* 63 (4)(1983): 305-309.

Matteson, R.L., and G. Terranova. "Social Acceptance of New Techniques of Child Conception." *Journal of Social Psychology* 101 (1977): 225-29.

Michaels, R. "Casework Considerations in Rejecting the Adoption Application." In *Readings in Adoption*, ed. I.E. Smith. New York: Philosophical Library, 1963.

Norman, R. "Sex Differences in Preferences for Sex of Children: A Replication After 20 Years." *Journal of Psychology* 88 (1974): 229-39.

Oakley, A. "What Makes Girls Differ from Boys?" *New Society* 46 (21-28 December 1978): xii-xiv.

Pebley, A.R., and C.F. Westoff. "Women's Sex Preferences in the United States: 1970 to 1975." *Demography* 19 (1982): 177-89.

Peel, J. "The Hull Family Survey: I. The Survey Couples, 1966." *Journal of Biosocial Science* 2 (1970): 45-70.

Perez, A., et al. "Sex Ratio Associated with Natural Family Planning." *Fertility and Sterility* 43 (1985): 152-53.

Peterson, C.C., and J.L. Peterson. "Preference for Sex of Offspring as a Measure of Change in Sex Attitudes." *Psychology* 10 (2)(1973): 3-5.

Pharis, M.E., and M. Manosevitz. "Sexual Stereotyping of Infants: Implications for Social Work Practice." *Social Work Research and Abstracts* 20 (1)(1984): 7-12.

Quinlivan, W.L.G., et al. "Separation of Human X and Y Spermatozoa by Albumin Gradients and Sephadex Chromatography." *Fertility and Sterility* 37 (1982): 104-107.

Rent, C.S., and G.S. Rent. "More on Offspring-Sex Preference: A Comment on Nancy E. Williamson's 'Sex Preference, Sex Control, and the Status of Women.'" *Signs: Journal of Women in Culture and Society* 3 (1977): 505-15.

Roberts, A.M. "Gravitational Separation of X and Y Spermatozoa." *Nature* 238 (1972): 223-25.

Roberts, A.M., and H. Goodall. "Y Chromosome Visibility in Quinacrine-Stained Human Spermatozoa." *Nature* 262 (1976): 493-94.

Rorvik, D.M., and L.B. Shettles. *Your Baby's Sex: Now You Can Choose.* New York: Bantam Books, 1971.

Rosenzweig, S., and S. Adelman. "Parental Predetermination of the Sex of Offspring: The Attitudes of Young Married Couples with University Education." *Journal of Biosocial Science* 8 (1976): 335-46.

Ross, A., J.A. Robinson, and H.J. Evans. "Failure to Confirm Separation of X- and Y-Bearing Human Sperm Using BSA Gradients." *Nature* 253 (1975): 354-55.

Rothschild, V. "Biology: X and Y Spermatozoa." *Nature* 187 (1960): 253-54.

Rotter, G.S., and N.G. Rotter. "Preferred Family Constellations: A Pilot Study." *Social Biology* 19 (1972): 401-404.

Rudak, E., P.A. Jacobs, and R. Yanagimachi. "Direct Analysis of the Chromosome Constitution of Human Spermatozoa." *Nature* 274 (1978): 911-13.

Sampson, J.H., et al. "Gender After Artificial Induction of Ovulation and Artificial Insemination." *Fertility and Sterility* 40 (1983): 481-84.

Sarkar, S. "Human Sperm Swimming in Flow." *Differentiation* 27 (1984): 126-32.

—. "Motility, Expression of Surface Antigen, and X and Y Human Sperm Separation in *In Vitro* Fertilization Medium." *Fertility and Sterility* 42 (1984): 899-905.

Shettles, L.B. "Factors Influencing Sex Ratios." *International Journal of Gynecology and Obstetrics* 8 (1970): 643-47.

—. "Human Spermatozoan Types." *Gynaecologia* 152 (1961): 153-62.

—. "Separation of X and Y Spermatozoa." *Journal of Urology* 116 (1976): 462-64.

Shishito, S., M. Shirai, and K. Sasaki. "Galvanic Separation of X and Y Bearing Human Spermatozoa." *International Journal of Fertility* 20 (1975): 13-16.

Simcock, B.W. "Sons and Daughters — A Sex Preselection Study." *Medical Journal of Australia* (13 May 1985): 541-42.

Stark, E. "The Sexes: Boys 1, Girls 1." *Psychology Today* 19 (August 1985): 18.

Steeno, O., A. Adimoelja, and J. Steeno. "Separation of X- and Y-Bearing Human Spermatozoa with the Sephadex Gel-Filtration Method." *Andrologia* 7 (1975): 95-97.

Steinbacher, R., and F.D. Gilroy. "Preference for Sex of Child Among Primiparous Women." *Journal of Psychology* 119 (1985): 541-47.

Stolkowski, J., and J. Choukroun. "Preconception Selection of Sex in Man." *Israel Journal of Medical Sciences* 17 (1981): 1061-67.

Stolkowski, J., and J. Lorrain. "Preconceptional Selection of Fetal Sex." *International Journal of Gynecology and Obstetrics* 18 (1980): 440-43.

Thomas, M. "The Impact of Gender Preselection on Gender Maldistribution." In *Feminist Research: Prospect and Retrospect,* ed. P. Tancred-Sheriff. Montreal and Kingston: McGill-Queen's University Press, 1988.

Thomsen, J.L., and E. Niebuhr. "The Frequency of False-Positive and False-Negative Results in the Detection of Y-Chromosome in Interphase Nuclei." *Human Genetics* 73 (1986): 27-30.

Uddenberg, N., P.-E. Almgren, and A. Nilsson. "Preference for Sex of the Child Among Pregnant Women." *Journal of Biosocial Science* 3 (1971): 267-80.

Ueda, K., and R. Yanagimachi. "Sperm Chromosome Analysis as a New System to Test Human X- and Y-Sperm Separation." *Gamete Research* 17 (1987): 221-28.

Ullman, J.B., and L.S. Fidell. "Gender Selection and Society." In *Gender in Transition*, ed. J. Offerman-Zuckerberg. New York: Plenum Press, 1989.

United States. National Commission for the Protection of Human Subjects of Biomedical and Behavioral Research. *Special Study: Implications of Advances in Biomedical and Behavioral Research.* Washington, DC: U.S. Department of Health, Education, and Welfare, 1978.

Van Duijn, C. "Nuclear Structure of Human Spermatozoa." *Nature* 188 (1960): 916-18.

Vear, C.S. "Preselective Sex Determination." *Medical Journal of Australia* 2 (19 November 1977): 700-702.

West, J.D., K.M. West, and R.J. Aitken. "Detection of Y-Bearing Spermatozoa by DNA-DNA In Situ Hybridisation." *Molecular Reproduction and Development* 1 (1989): 201-207.

Westoff, C.F., and R.R. Rindfuss. "Sex Preselection in the United States: Some Implications." *Science* 184 (1974): 633-36.

Williamson, N.E. "Sex Preferences, Sex Control, and the Status of Women." *Signs: Journal of Women in Culture and Society* 1 (1976): 847-62.

—. *Sons or Daughters: A Cross-Cultural Survey of Parental Preferences.* Beverly Hills: Sage Publications, 1976.

Zaneveld, L.J.D., et al. "Scanning Electron Microscopy of Mammalian Spermatozoa." *Journal of Reproductive Medicine* 6 (4)(1971): 147-51.

Zarutskie, P.W., et al. "The Clinical Relevance of Sex Selection Techniques." *Fertility and Sterility* 52 (1989): 891-905.

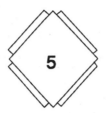

5

Bibliography on Preferences for the Sex of One's Children, and Attitudes Concerning Sex Preselection

Martin Thomas

Executive Summary

This bibliography includes two substantive categories of publications: those dealing with preferences for the sex of one's children and those referring to any social scientific or ethical aspect of sex preselection.

Sex preselection refers to sex selection approximately at the time of conception, and does not subsume selection by fetal sex determination and selective abortion. Publications whose focus is on abortion for sex selection are included only if they deal primarily or extensively with parental preference for the sex of their children.

Social scientific aspects of sex preselection include both attitudes concerning preselection and public knowledge of preselection.

Publications dealing with the technical aspects of sex selection are not included in this bibliography; however, some are cited in a companion research report on sex preference and sex selection in this volume.

The author intends to maintain an updated bibliography on this topic as a resource for scholars, and earnestly solicits both corrections to the current version and the identification of other relevant publications, preferably with annotations, for inclusion in subsequent versions.

This paper was completed for the Royal Commission on New Reproductive Technologies in May 1992.

Bibliography

Abdulla, A.S., M.A.F. All-Rubeaj, and E. Gray. "Desired Family Size and Sex of Children in Libya." *Journal of Heredity* 75 (1984): 76-78.

Adelman, S. "Parental Choice of Offspring Sex: An Investigation of the Effects of Information, Education, and Family Size on Sex-Choice Attitudes, with Special Reference to the Idiodynamic Bases of Antenatal Sex Preferences." Ph.D. dissertation, Washington University, 1977.

Adelman, S., and S. Rosenzweig. "Parental Predetermination of the Sex of Offspring. II. The Attitudes of Young Married Couples with High School and with College Education." *Journal of Biosocial Science* 10 (1978): 235-47.

Adimoelja, A., et al. "The Separation of X- and Y-Spermatozoa with Regard to the Possible Clinical Application by Means of Artificial Insemination." *Andrologia* 9 (1977): 289-92.

Ahmed, K., ed. *Nutrition Survey of Rural Bangladesh 1975-76.* Dacca: University of Dacca, Institute of Nutrition and Food Science, 1977.

Ahmed, N.R. "Family Size and Sex Preferences Among Women in Rural Bangladesh." *Studies in Family Planning* 12 (1981): 100-109.

Aly, H., and M. Sheilds. "Son Preference and Contraception in Egypt." *Economic Development and Cultural Change* 39 (1991): 353-70.

Arditti, R. "Reducing Women to Matter." *Women's Studies International Forum* 8 (1985): 577-82.

Arnold, F. "The Effect of Sex Preference on Fertility: A Reply to Bairagi." *Demography* 24 (1987): 139-42.

—. "Measuring the Effect of Sex Preference on Fertility: The Case of Korea." *Demography* 22 (1985): 280-88.

Arnold, F., and E.C.Y. Kuo. "The Value of Daughters and Sons: A Comparative Study of the Gender Preferences of Parents." *Journal of Comparative Family Studies* 15 (1984): 299-318.

Arnold, F., and L. Zhaoxiang. "Sex Preference, Fertility and Family Planning in China." *Population and Development Review* 12 (1986): 221-46.

Arnold, F., et al. *The Value of Children: A Cross-National Study.* Vol. 1, *Introduction and Comparative Analysis.* Honolulu: East-West Population Institute, East-West Center, 1975.

Asimov, I. "Choosing an Unborn Child's Sex." *American Way* 11 (9 February 1978): 9-10.

"Babies to Order." *American Demographics* 9 (July 1987): 23.

"The Baby Scientists vs. Mother Nature." *Toronto Star* (21 September 1987): A18.

"Baby Shopping: Sex Selection." *Vogue* (May 1989): 255.

Bairagi, R. "A Comment on Fred Arnold's 'Measuring the Effect of Sex Preference on Fertility.' " *Demography* 24 (1987): 137-38.

Bairagi, R., and R.L. Langsten. "Preference for Sex of Children and Its Implications for Fertility in Rural Bangladesh." Paper presented at the Annual Meeting of the Population Association of America, San Francisco, April 1986.

Balikci, A. *The Netsilik Eskimo.* Garden City: Natural History Press, 1970.

Bardhan, P. "Little Girls and Death in India." *Economic and Political Weekly* 17 (4 September 1982): 1448-50.

Barkat, K. "The Value of Children in Village Barkait." Paper presented at the Seminar on Fertility, Which Way Is It Going?, Cox's Bazaar, Bangladesh, 21-23 December 1976.

Baruch, E.H., A.F. D'Adamo, Jr., and J. Seager, eds. *Embryos, Ethics, and Women's Rights: Exploring the New Reproductive Technologies.* New York: Harrington Park Press, 1988.

Bayles, M.D. *Reproductive Ethics.* Englewood Cliffs: Prentice-Hall, 1984.

Beaujot, R. "Attitudes Among Tunisians Toward Family Formation." *International Family Planning Perspectives* 14 (June 1988): 54-61.

Bennett, N.G. "Sex Selection of Children: An Overview." In *Sex Selection of Children,* ed. N.G. Bennett. New York: Academic Press, 1983.

Bennett, N.G., and A. Mason. "Decision Making and Sex Selection with Biased Technologies." Paper presented at the Annual Meeting of the Population Association of America, Atlanta, April 1978.

—. "Decision Making and Sex Selection with Biased Technologies." In *Sex Selection of Children,* ed. N.G. Bennett. New York: Academic Press, 1983.

Ben-Porath, Y. *Do Sex Preferences Really Matter?* Santa Monica: Rand Corporation, 1975.

Ben-Porath, Y., and F. Welch. *Chance, Child Traits, and Choice of Family Size.* Santa Monica: Rand Corporation, 1975.

—. "Do Sex Preferences Really Matter?" *Quarterly Journal of Economics* 90 (1976): 285-309.

—. "On Sex Preferences and Family Size." *Research in Population Economics* 2 (1980): 387-99.

Berelson, B., and R. Freedman. "A Study in Fertility Control." *Scientific American* 210 (May 1964): 29-37.

Berg, K. "Ethical Problems Arising from Research Progress in Medical Genetics." In *Research Ethics*, ed. K. Berg and K.E. Tranøy. New York: Alan R. Liss, 1983.

Bhatia, J.C. "Ideal Number and Sex Preference of Children in India." *Journal of Family Welfare* 24 (4)(1978): 3-16.

Bhattacharya, B.C. *Guide to Pre-Arranging the Sex of Offspring.* Ralson: Action Press, 1977.

Birke, L., S. Himmelweit, and G. Vines. *Tomorrow's Child.* London: Virago Press, 1990.

"Birth Test Said to Help Indians Abort Females." *Washington Post* (25 August 1982): A24.

Blank, R. *The Political Implications of Human Genetic Technology.* Boulder: Westview Press, 1981.

Bloom, D.E., and G. Grenier. "The Economics of Sex Preference and Sex Selection." In *Sex Selection of Children,* ed. N.G. Bennett. New York: Academic Press, 1983.

Bollen, G. *Bijdrage Tot De Methode Der Paarsgewijze Vergelijking: Een Onderzoek naar de voorkeur voor bepaalde Familiesamenstellingen* [Contribution to the Method of Paired Comparisons. An Experiment on Preference for Families]. Leuven: University of Leuven, 1962.

Boserup, E. *Woman's Role in Economic Development.* London: Allen and Unwin, 1970.

"Boy or Girl." *Economist* 316 (28 July 1990): 16.

Brandewie, E.H. "Family Size and Kinship Pressures in the Philippines." *Philippines Quarterly of Culture and Society* 1 (1)(1973): 6-18.

Braun, R.A. "From the Stone Age to Mechanized Paradise." *Bryn Mawr Now* 2 (April 1975): 8-9.

Brefkenridge, J. "Clinic Improves Chances of Choosing Child's Sex." *Globe and Mail* (23 September 1987): A1-A2.

Brenner, R. *A Follow-Up Study of Adoptive Families.* New York: Child Adoption Research Committee, 1951.

Brittain, A.W., W.T. Morrill, and J.A. Kurland. "Parental Choice and Infant Mortality in a West Indian Population." *Human Biology* 60 (1988): 679-92.

Brodribb, S. *Reproductive Technologies, Masculine Dominance and the Canadian State.* Toronto: Centre for Women's Studies in Education, 1984.

Brown, J. "Sex Selection: The Ultimate Sexist Act." *Kinesis* 19 (October 1990): 7.

Bulatao, R.A. "Values and Disvalues of Children in Successive Childbearing Decisions." *Demography* 18 (1981): 1-25.

Bulatao, R.A., and F. Arnold. "Roots of the Preference for Sons or Daughters: Comparisons of Wives and Husbands in Seven Countries." Paper presented at the Annual Meeting of the Population Association of America, Boston, 28-30 March 1985.

Bumpass, L., and C. Westoff. *The Later Years of Childbearing.* Princeton: Princeton University Press, 1970.

Burling, R. *Rengsangrii: Family and Kinship in a Garo Village.* Philadelphia: University of Pennsylvania Press, 1963.

Cahill, L. "A Hard Look at the Implications of Artificial Birth." *Globe and Mail* (10 August 1985): E16.

Callan, V.J. *The Value of Children to Australian, Greek and Italian Parents in Sydney.* Report 60-C. Honolulu: East-West Center, 1980.

Callan, V.J., and P.-K. Kee. "Sons or Daughters? Cross-Cultural Comparisons of the Sex Preferences of Australian, Greek, Italian, Malay, Chinese and Indian Parents in Australia and Malaysia." *Population and Environment* 4 (Summer 1981): 97-108.

Calway-Fagen, N., B.S. Wallston, and H. Gabel. "The Relationship Between Attitudinal and Behavioral Measures of Sex Preference." *Psychology of Women Quarterly* 4 (1979): 274-80.

Campbell, C. "What Happens When We Get the Manchild Pill?" *Psychology Today* 10 (August 1976): 86-91.

Campbell, E.K. "Sex Preferences for Offspring Among Men in the Western Area of Sierra Leone." *Journal of Biosocial Science* 23 (1991): 337-42.

"Can You Choose Your Child's Sex? Maybe." *Verve* 2 (August-September 1986): 71.

Carr-Hill, R., M. Samphier, and B. Sauve. "Socio-Demographic Variations in the Sex Composition and Preferences of Aberdeen Families." *Journal of Biosocial Science* 14 (1982): 429-43.

Carson, S.A. "Sex Selection: The Ultimate in Family Planning." *Fertility and Sterility* 50 (1988): 16-19.

Carter, C.O. "Eugenic Implications of New Techniques." In *Developments in Human Reproduction and Their Eugenic, Ethical Implications*, ed. C.O. Carter. New York: Academic Press, 1983.

Cassen, R.H. *India: Population, Economy and Society.* London: Macmillan, 1978.

—. "Population and Development: A Survey." *World Development* 4 (1976): 785-830.

Cha, J.-H. "Alternative Approaches to Measurement of Son Preference." Paper presented at the Conference on the Measurement of Preferences for Number and Sex of Children, East-West Center, Honolulu, 2-5 June 1975.

Chahnazarian, A. "Determinants of the Sex Ratio at Birth." Ph.D. dissertation, Princeton University, 1986.

Chaudhury, R.H. *Social Aspects of Fertility: With Special References to Developing Countries.* Mayapuri: Vikas, 1982.

—. "Socio-Cultural Factors Affecting Practice of Contraception in a Metropolitan Urban Area of Bangladesh." In *Fertility in Bangladesh: Which Way Is It Going?*, ed. M. Hossain, M.A.R. Khan, and L.C. Chen (Seminar on Fertility in Bangladesh 1976: Cox's Bazaar, Bangladesh), 1979.

—. "Some Aspects of Seasonal Dimensions to Rural Poverty in Bangladesh." Paper presented to the Conference on Seasonal Dimensions to Rural Poverty, Institute of Development Studies, University of Sussex, 3-6 July 1978.

Chen, J., and T.R. Balakrishnan. "Do Gender Preferences Affect Fertility and Family Dissolution in Canada?" Discussion Paper 90-7. London: University of Western Ontario, Population Studies Centre, 1990.

Chen, P.-C., and A. Kols. *Population and Birth Planning in the People's Republic of China.* Report J25. Baltimore: Johns Hopkins University, Population Information Program, 1982.

Cherfas, J., and J. Gribbin. *The Redundant Male: Is Sex Irrelevant in the Modern World?* London: Bodley Head, 1984.

Chico, N.P. "Confronting the Dilemmas of Reproductive Choice: The Process of Sex Preselection." Ph.D. dissertation, University of California, San Francisco, 1989.

Chico, N.P., and S.F. Hartley. "Widening Choices in Motherhood of the Future." *Psychology of Women Quarterly* 6 (1981): 12-25.

"China's She-Baby Cull." *Economist* 287 (16-22 April 1983): 36.

Chitre, K.T., R.N. Saxena, and H.N. Ranganathan. "Motivation for Vasectomy." *Journal of Family Welfare* 11 (1)(1964): 36-49.

Cho, L.-J., F. Arnold, and T.H. Kwon. *The Determinants of Fertility in the Republic of Korea.* Washington, DC: National Academy Press, 1982.

Cho, N.H., et al. *Effects of Economic Factors on Fertility Behavior.* Seoul: Korean Institute for Family Planning, 1977.

"Choosing the Baby's Sex." *British Medical Journal* 280 (1980): 272-73.

Chung, B.M., J.-H. Cha, and S.J. Lee. *A Study on Boy Preference and Family Planning in Korea.* Seoul: Korean Institute for Research in the Behavioral Sciences, 1974.

Cillov, H. "Attitudes on Family Planning in Turkey." Paper presented at the Meeting of the International Union for the Scientific Study of Population, Sydney, Australia, 1967.

Clare, J.E. "Preference Regarding the Sex of Children and Its Relation to Size of Family." Master's thesis, Columbia University, 1951.

Clare, J.E., and C.V. Kiser. "Social and Psychological Factors Affecting Fertility: Preference for Children of Given Sex in Relation to Fertility." *Milbank Memorial Fund Quarterly* (1951): 440-92.

Clark, M. "Choosing Your Child's Sex." *Newsweek* (30 May 1983): 102.

Cleland, J., J. Verrall, and M. Vaessen. "Preferences for the Sex of Children and Their Influence on Reproductive Behaviour." *World Fertility Survey Comparative Studies No. 27.* Voorburg: International Statistical Institute, 1983.

Cohn, V. "Fetuses Aborted to Prevent Child of 'Wrong' Sex." *Washington Post* (6 September 1979): A1, A5.

Cole, S.G. "Baby Design Dilemma: High-Tech Sex Selection Is a Step Backward to Greater Gender Barriers, Say Detractors of This New Reproductive Tampering." *Now* (29 October-4 November 1987): 9-10.

Connors, S. "Scientist Licensed to Work on 'Pre-Embryos.'" *New Scientist* 108 (21 November 1985): 21.

Coombs, C.H., L.C. Coombs, and G.H. McClelland. "Preference Scales for Number and Sex of Children." *Population Studies* 29 (1975): 273-98.

Coombs, L.C. *Are Cross-Cultural Preference Comparisons Possible? A Measurement Theoretic Approach.* IUSSP Papers 5. Liege: International Union for the Scientific Study of Population, 1976.

—. "Comparative Fertility Analysis: A Project of the International Union for the Scientific Study of Population." Paper presented at the Annual Meeting of the Population Association of America, University of Michigan, Population Studies Center, Ann Arbor, April 1973.

—. "IUSSP Preference Scale Study." Paper presented at the Conference on the Measurement of Preferences for Number and Sex of Children, East-West Center, Honolulu, 2-5 June 1975.

—. *The Measurement of Family Composition Preferences.* United Nations document POP/SPAFB/99. Bangkok: United Nations. Economic and Social Commission for Asia and the Pacific, 1974. In *Report and Papers of the Expert Group Meeting on Social and Psychological Aspects of Fertility Behaviour.* Asian Population Studies No. 21.

—. "The Measurement of Family Size Preferences and Subsequent Fertility." *Demography* 11 (1974): 587-611.

—. "Preferences for Sex of Children Among U.S. Couples." *Family Planning Perspectives* 9 (1977): 259-65.

—. "Prospective Fertility and Underlying Preferences: A Longitudinal Study in Taiwan." *Population Studies* 33 (1979): 447-55.

—. "Underlying Family-Size Preferences and Reproductive Behavior." *Studies in Family Planning* 10 (1979): 25-36.

Coombs, L.C., and C.H. Coombs. "Measurement of Family Composition Preferences." Paper presented at the Annual Meeting of the Population Association of America, New York, April 1974.

Coombs, L.C., and R. Freedman. "Some Roots of Preference: Roles, Activities and Familial Values." *Demography* 16 (1979): 359-76.

Coombs, L.C., and T.-H. Sun. "Familial Values in Developing Society: A Decade of Change in Taiwan." *Social Forces* 59 (1981): 1229-55.

—. "Family Composition Preferences in a Developing Culture: The Case of Taiwan, 1973." *Population Studies* 32 (1978): 43-64.

Copeland, J., and M. Hager. "Couples Playing Doctor — and God." *Newsweek* (6 October 1986): 43.

Corea, G. *The Mother Machine: Reproductive Technologies from Artificial Insemination to Artificial Wombs.* New York: Harper and Row, 1986.

Corea, G., and S. Ince. "Report of a Survey of IVF Clinics in the US." In *Made to Order: The Myth of Reproductive and Genetic Progress*, ed. P. Spallone and D.L. Steinberg. New York: Pergamon Press, 1987.

Corea, G., et al. "Prologue." In *Made to Order: The Myth of Reproductive and Genetic Progress*, ed. P. Spallone and D.L. Steinberg. New York: Pergamon Press, 1987.

Cornacchia, C. "New Franchises Offer You a Designer Baby; Picky Parents Could Disturb Mother Nature." *Montreal Gazette* (12 March 1988): A1, A4.

Crawford, T.J., and R. Boyer. "Salient Consequences, Cultural Values, and Childbearing Intentions." *Journal of Applied Social Psychology* 15 (1985): 16-30.

Crew, F.A.E. *Sex-Determination.* 3d ed. London: Methuen, 1954.

Culpepper, E.E. "Sex Preselection: Discussion Moderator's Remarks." In *The Custom-Made Child? Women-Centered Perspectives*, ed. H.B. Holmes, B.B. Hoskins, and M. Gross. Clifton: Humana Press, 1981.

Cusine, D.J. *New Reproductive Techniques: A Legal Perspective.* Aldershot: Gower, 1988.

Cutright, P., S. Belt, and J. Scanzoni. "Gender Preferences, Sex Predetermination, and Family Size in the United States." *Social Biology* 21 (1974): 242-48.

Dada, V. *Choose the Sex of Your Baby: A Psychological Approach.* New York: Vantage Press, 1983.

D'Adamo, A.F., Jr. "Reproductive Technologies: The Two Sides of the Glass Jar." In *Embryos, Ethics and Women's Rights: Exploring the New Reproductive Technologies*, ed. E.H. Baruch, A.F. D'Adamo, Jr., and J. Seager. New York: Harrington Park Press, 1988.

Dahlberg, G. "Do Parents Want Boys or Girls?" *Acta Genetica et Statistica Medica* 1 (1948): 163-67.

Daniell, J.F. "Sex-Selection Procedures." *Journal of Reproductive Medicine* 28 (1983): 235-37.

Das, N. "The Sex of Previous Children and Subsequent Fertility Intention in India." *Canadian Studies in Population* 13 (1)(1986): 19-36.

—. "Sex Preference and Fertility Behavior: A Study of Recent Indian Data." *Demography* 24 (1987): 517-30.

—. "Sex Preference Pattern and Its Stability in India: 1970 to 1980." *Demography India* 13 (1984): 108-12.

Datin, N.L.A.B., T.B. Ann, and T.N. Peng. "Preferences for Number and Sex of Children in the Rural Areas of Peninsular Malaysia." *Southeast Asian Journal of Social Science* 12 (2)(1984): 18-35.

Dawes, R.M. "Sexual Heterogeneity of Children as a Determinant of American Family Size." *ORI Research Bulletin* 10 (8)(1970): 1-7.

Dawkins, R. *The Selfish Gene*. Oxford: Oxford University Press, 1976.

Dela Paz, D.R. "Preferences for Number and Sex of Children in the Philippines." Paper presented at the Conference on the Measurement of Preferences for Number and Sex of Children, East-West Center, Honolulu, 2-5 June 1975.

DeTray, D. *Son Preference in Pakistan: An Analysis of Intentions Versus Behavior*. Report P-6504. Santa Monica: Rand Corporation, 1980.

Dietz, T. "Normative and Microeconomic Models of Voluntary Childlessness." *Sociological Spectrum* 4 (1984): 209-28.

Dinitz, S., R.R. Dynes, and A.C. Clarke. "Preferences for Male or Female Children: Traditional or Affectional?" *Marriage and Family Living* 16 (May 1964): 128-30.

Dixon, R.D., and D.E. Levy. "Sex of Children: A Community Analysis of Preferences and Predetermination Attitudes." *Sociological Quarterly* 26 (1985): 251-71.

Donchin, A. "The Growing Feminist Debate over the New Reproductive Technologies." *Hypatia* 4 (3)(1989): 136-49.

Dove, G.A., and C. Blow. "Boy or Girl Parental Choice?" *British Medical Journal* (1 December 1979): 1399-1400.

Dunlop, M. "Toronto Centre Lets You Pick Sex of Baby." *Toronto Star* (1 September 1987): A2.

Dunnell, K. *Family Formation 1976: A Survey Carried out on Behalf of Population Statistics Division 1 of the Office of Population Censuses and Surveys of a Sample of Women (Both Single and Ever Married) Aged 16-49 in Great Britain.* London: HMSO, 1976.

Edward, R.G. "Fertilization of Human Eggs *In Vitro*: Morals, Ethics and the Law." *Quarterly Review of Biology* 49 (1974): 3-26.

Ehrlich, P.R. *The Population Bomb.* New York: Ballantine Books, 1971.

El-Badry, M.A. "Higher Female than Male Mortality in Some Countries of South Asia: A Digest." *Journal of the American Statistical Association* 64 (1969): 1234-44.

Elder, G.H., Jr., and C.E. Bowerman. "Family Structure and Child-Rearing Patterns: The Effect of Family Size and Sex Composition." *American Sociological Review* 28 (1963): 891-905.

Elshtain, J.B. "Technology as Destiny." *Progressive* 53 (June 1989): 19-23.

Erba, P. "I desideri dei genitori riguardo ai loro figli" [Parents' Wishes with Regards to Their Children]. In *Atti Della XV e XVI Riunione Scientifica (Roma: Aprile 1955-Giugno 1956).* Rome: Società Italiana Di Statistica, 1956.

Etzioni, A. *Genetic Fix: The Next Technological Revolution.* New York: Harper and Row, 1975.

—. "Sex Control, Science and Society." *Science* 161 (1968): 1107-12.

Evans, J. "Legal Aspects of Prenatal Sex Selection." In *Sex Selection of Children,* ed. N.G. Bennett. New York: Academic Press, 1983.

Evans, M.I., et al. "Attitudes on the Ethics of Abortion, Sex Selection, and Selective Pregnancy Termination Among Health Care Professionals, Ethicists, and Clergy Likely to Encounter Such Situations." *American Journal of Obstetrics and Gynecology* 164 (1991): 1092-99.

Fancher, H.L. "The Relationship Between Occupational Status of Individuals and the Sex Ratio of Their Offspring." *Human Biology* 28 (1956): 316-22.

Farber, B., and L.S. Blackman. "Marital Role Tensions and Number and Sex of Children." *American Sociological Review* 21 (1956): 596-601.

Farr, M. "Dangerous Determination: Disturbing Trends in High Tech Sex Selection Won't Go Away by Ignoring the Problem." *This Magazine* 24 (March-April 1991): 10-15.

Fawcett, J.T. "The Value and Cost of Children: Converging Theory and Research." In *The Economic and Social Supports for High Fertility: Proceedings of the Conference Held in Canberra 16-18 November 1976,* ed. L.T. Ruzicka. Canberra: Australian National University, Department of Demography, 1977.

—. "Value of Children." In *International Encyclopedia of Population*, ed. J.A. Ross. New York: Free Press, 1982.

Fawcett, J.T., et al. *Papers of the East-West Population Institute, No. 32.* Honolulu: East-West Center, 1974.

Feil, R.N., G.P. Largey, and M. Miller. "Attitudes Toward Abortion as a Means of Sex Selection." *Journal of Psychology* 116 (1984): 269-72.

Fidell, L., D. Hoffman, and P. Keith-Spiegel. "Some Social Implications of Sex-Choice Technology." *Psychology of Women Quarterly* 4 (1979): 32-42.

Findley, S.E., R.G. Potter, and T.W. Findley. "Alternative Strategies of Fetal Sex Diagnoses and Sex Preselection." *Social Biology* 31 (1984): 120-39.

Finnell, R.B. "Daughters or Sons?" *Natural History* 4 (1988): 63-83.

Flanagan, J.C. "A Study of Factors Determining Family Size in a Selected Professional Group." *Genetic Psychology Monograph* 25 (1942): 3-99.

Fletcher, J. *The Ethics of Genetic Control: Ending Reproductive Roulette.* Buffalo: Prometheus Books, 1988.

Fletcher, J.C. "Ethics and Amniocentesis for Fetal Sex Identification." *New England Journal of Medicine* 301 (1979): 550-53.

—. "Ethics and Public Policy: Should Sex Choice Be Discouraged?" In *Sex Selection of Children*, ed. N.G. Bennett. New York: Academic Press, 1983.

—. "Is Sex Selection Ethical?" In *Research Ethics*, ed. K. Berg and K.E Tranøy. New York: Alan R. Liss, 1983.

Fletcher, J.C., and D.C. Wertz. "Ethics, Law and Medical Genetics: After the Human Genome Is Mapped." *Emory Law Journal* 39 (1990): 747-809.

Frankel, M.S. "Sex Preselection." *Science* 185 (1974): 1109.

Fraser, F.C., and C. Pressor. "Attitudes of Counselors in Relation to Prenatal Sex-Determination Simply for Choice of Sex." In *Genetic Counseling*, ed. H.A. Lubs and F. De la Cruz. New York: Raven Press, 1977.

Freedman, D.S., R. Freedman, and P.K. Whelpton. "Size of Family and Preference for Children of Each Sex." *American Journal of Sociology* 66 (1960): 141-46.

Freedman, R., and L.C. Coombs. *Cross-Cultural Comparisons: Data on Two Factors in Fertility Behavior: Report of a Project of the Subcommittee on Comparative Fertility Analysis of the International Union for the Scientific Study of Population.* New York: Population Council, 1974.

—. "Preferences About Sex of Children." In *Cross-Cultural Comparisons: Data on Two Factors in Fertility Behavior: Report of a Project of the Subcommittee on Comparative Fertility Analysis of the International*

Union for the Scientific Study of Population. New York: Population Council, 1974.

Freedman, R., et al. "Trends in Fertility, Family Size Preferences, and Practice of Family Planning: Taiwan, 1965-1973." *Studies in Family Planning* 5 (1974): 270-88.

Frias Bautista, M.L. "Historical Influences on Gender Preference in the Philippines." *Journal of Comparative Family Studies* 19 (1988): 143-53.

Fribourg, S. "Morality of Induced Abortion and Freedom of Choice." *American Journal of Obstetrics and Gynecology* 157 (1987): 215.

Fried, E.S., S.L. Hofferth, and J.R. Udry. "Parity-Specific and Two-Sex Utility Models of Reproductive Intentions." *Demography* 17 (1980): 1-11.

Fruman, L. "Choosing Your Baby's Sex — New Controversy for Parents." *Toronto Star* (30 January 1987): B1, B6.

Gallin, B. *Hsin-Hsing, Taiwan: A Chinese Village in Change.* Berkeley: University of California Press, 1966.

Galton, L. "Decisions, Decisions, Decisions." *New York Times Magazine* (30 June 1974): 22, 23, 26, 27.

Gearhart, S. "The Future — If There Is One — Is Female." In *Reweaving the Web of Life: Feminism and Nonviolence*, ed. P. McAllister. Philadelphia: New Society Publishers, 1982.

Geier, M.R., J.L. Young, and D. Kessler. "Too Much or Too Little Science in Sex Selection Techniques?" *Fertility and Sterility* 53 (1990): 1111-14.

"Gender Choice a Gross Deception." *FDA Consumer* 21 (April 1987): 2.

"Gender Kits — Caveat Emptor." *U.S. News and World Report* 102 (9 February 1987): 12.

Gille, H., and R.H. Pardoko. "A Family Life Study in East Java: Preliminary Findings." In *Family Planning and Population Programs: A Review of World Developments.* ed. B. Berelson et al. Chicago: University of Chicago Press, 1966.

Gilroy, F., and R. Steinbacher. "Preselection of Child's Sex: Technological Utilization and Feminism." *Psychological Reports* 53 (1983): 671-76.

Gini, C. "Combinations and Sequences of Sexes in Human Families and Mammal Litters." *Acta Genetica et Statistica Medica* 2 (1951): 220-44.

—. "Esame Comparativo di Alcuni Risultati di Inchieste Italiane e Straniere Sul Desiderio dei Genitori di Avere Figli Dell' uno o Piuttosto Dell' Altro Sesso" [Comparative Analysis of Some Results of Italian and Foreign Studies on Parents' Sex Preferences for Their Children]. In *Atti Della XV e XVI Riunione Scientifica (Roma: Aprile 1955-Giugno 1956).* Rome: Società Italiana Di Statistica, 1956.

Giurovich, G. "Sul Desiderio dei Coniugi di Avere Figli e di Avere Figli di un Dato Sesso" [On the Wish of Married Couples to Have Children and to Have Children of a Specific Sex]. In *Atti Della XV e XVI Riunione Scientifica (Roma: Aprile 1955-Giugno 1956)*. Rome: Società Italiana Di Statistica, 1956.

Glass, R.H. "Sex Preselection." *Obstetrics and Gynecology* 49 (1977): 122-26.

Glass, R.H., and R.J. Ericsson. *Getting Pregnant in the 1980s: New Advances in Infertility Treatment and Sex Preselection.* Berkeley: University of California Press, 1982.

Gledhill, B.L. "Control of Mammalian Sex Ratio by Sexing Sperm." *Fertility and Sterility* 40 (1983): 572-74.

—. "Gender Preselection: Historical, Technical, and Ethical Perspectives." *Seminars in Reproductive Endocrinology* 6 (1988): 385-95.

Glover, J., et al. *Fertility and the Family: The Glover Report on Reproductive Technologies to the European Commission.* London: Fourth Estate, 1989.

Goh, T.N. "Quantitative Analysis of Some Decision Rules for Family Planning in an Oriental Society." *Interfaces* 11 (April 1981): 31-37.

Goldfarb, C.S. "The Folklore of Pregnancy." *Psychological Reports* 62 (1988): 891-900.

Goodale, J.C. *Tiwi Wives: A Study of the Women of Melville Island, North Australia.* Seattle: University of Washington Press, 1971.

Gooderham, M. "Parents Consult Gender Timepiece: Makers Claim Watch Can Help Produce Child of Desired Sex." *Globe and Mail* (6 April 1991): A1, A2.

Goodman, L.A. "Some Possible Effects of Birth Control on the Human Sex Ratio." *Annals of Human Genetics* 25 (1961): 75-81.

Goody, J.R., et al. "Implicit Sex Preferences: A Comparative Study." *Journal of Biosocial Science* 13 (4)(October 1981): 455-66.

—. "On the Absence of Implicit Sex-Preference in Ghana." *Journal of Biosocial Science* 13 (1981): 87-96.

Gordon, M.J. "The Control of Sex." *Scientific American* 199 (November 1958): 87-88, 90, 92, 94.

Goshen-Gottstein, E.R. *Marriage and First Pregnancy: Cultural Influence on Attitudes of Israeli Women.* London: Tavistock, 1966.

Gould, C.C., ed. *Beyond Domination: New Perspectives on Women and Philosophy.* Totowa: Rowman and Allanheld, 1983.

Gould, R.A. "The Wealth Quest Among the Tolowa Indians of Northwestern California." *Proceedings of the American Philosophical Society* 110 (1966): 67-89.

Gray, E. "Influence of Sex of First Two Children on Family Size." *Journal of Heredity* 63 (1972): 91-92.

Gray, E., and M. Morrison. "Influence of Combinations of Sexes of Children on Family Size." *Journal of Heredity* 65 (1974): 169-74.

Gray, E., V.K. Hurt, and S. Oyewole. "Desired Family Size and Sex of Children in Nigeria." *Journal of Heredity* 74 (1983): 204-206.

Gribnau, F.W.J. "Selecting the Sex of One's Children." *Lancet* (15 June 1974): 228-29.

Grobstein, C. *From Chance to Purpose*. Reading: Addison-Wesley, 1981.

Grossman, E. "The Obsolescent Mother: A Scenario." *Atlantic Monthly* 227 (1971): 39-50.

Growe, S. "Debate Urged on Artificial Reproduction." *Toronto Star* (29 March 1988), B2.

Guerrero, R. "Timing Intercourse Can Alter Sex Ratio, but There's a Catch." *Family Planning Perspectives* 7 (March-April 1975): 58.

Gulati, S.C. *Some Reflections on Son Preference and Its Influence on Additional Desired Fertility*. Delhi: Institute of Economic Growth, 1987.

Guthrie, G.M., and P.J. Jacobs. *Child Rearing and Personality Development in the Philippines*. University Park: Pennsylvania State University Press, 1966.

Guttentag, M., and P.F. Secord. *Too Many Women? The Sex Ratio Question*. Beverly Hills: Sage Publications, 1983.

Hafez, E.S.E. *Assisted Human Reproductive Technology*. New York: Hemisphere Publishing Corporation, 1991.

Ham, P.C. "Report on a Study on the Korean Preference for Male Children." Yonsei University, Social Science Research Institute, Division of Demography, Center for Population and Family Planning, 1971.

Hammer, M., and J. McFerran. "Preference for Sex of Child: A Research Update." *Individual Psychology: Journal of Adlerian Theory, Research and Practice* 44 (1988): 481-91.

Han, S.-H., and S.-B. Lee. "An Analysis for Factors Affecting Parity Progression — Longitudinal Approach." *Journal of Family Planning Studies* (Kajok kyehoek nonjip) 4 (November 1977): 55-69.

Hanmer, J. "Reproductive Technology: The Future for Women?" In *Machina Ex Dea: Feminist Perspectives on Technology*, ed. J. Rothschild. Elmsford: Pergamon Press, 1983.

—. "Sex Predetermination, Artificial Insemination and Maintenance of Male-Dominated Culture." In *Women, Health and Reproduction*, ed. H. Roberts. Boston: Routledge and Kegan Paul, 1981.

—. "A Womb of One's Own." In *Test-Tube Women: What Future for Motherhood?* ed. R. Arditti, R.D. Klein, and S. Minden. London: Pandora Press, 1984.

Hanmer, J., and P. Allen. "Reproductive Engineering: The Final Solution?" In *Alice Through the Microscope: The Power of Science over Women's Lives*, ed. L. Birke et al. London: Virago, 1980.

Hardee-Cleaveland, K. "Desired Family Size and Sex Preference in Rural China: Evidence from Fujian Province." Ph.D. dissertation, Cornell University, 1988.

Harper, M.J.K. *Birth Control Technologies: Prospects by the Year 2000.* Austin: University of Texas Press, 1983.

Harper, M.R. "Parental Preference with Respect to the Sex of Children." Master's thesis, Sociology, University of Chicago, December 1936.

Harrison, B.G. "Ladies Last: Will Women Lose the Sex-Selection Sweepstakes?" *Mademoiselle* (October 1984): 244.

Hart, C.W.M., and A.R. Pilling. *The Tiwi of North Australia.* New York: Holt, 1960.

Hartley, R.E. "Children's Perceptions of Sex Preference in Four Culture Groups." *Journal of Marriage and the Family* 31 (1969): 380-87.

Hartley, R.E., F.P. Hardesty, and D.S. Gorfein. "Children's Perceptions and Expressions of Sex Preference." *Child Development* 33 (1962): 221-27.

Hartley, S.F. "Attitudes Toward Reproductive Engineering: An Overview." *Journal of Family Issues* 2 (1981): 5-24.

Hartley, S.F., and L.M. Pietraczyk. "Preselecting the Sex of Offspring: Technologies, Attitudes and Implications." *Social Biology* 26 (1979): 232-46.

Hassan, S.S. "Religion Versus Child Mortality as a Cause of Differential Fertility." Paper presented at the Annual Meeting of the Population Association of America, Cincinnati, April 1967.

Hawley, A.H., and V. Prachuabmoh. "Family Growth and Family Planning in a Rural District of Thailand." In *Family Planning and Population Programs: A Review of World Developments*, ed. B. Berelson et al. Chicago: University of Chicago Press, 1966.

Heer, D.M., and H.-Y. Wu. "The Separate Effects of Individual Child Loss, Perception of Child Survival and Community Mortality Level upon Fertility and Family-Planning in Rural Taiwan with Comparison Data from Urban Morocco." In *Seminar on Infant Mortality in Relation to the Level of Fertility, 6-12 May 1975, Bangkok, Thailand.* Paris: Committee for International Coordination of National Research in Demography, 1975.

Heer, D.M., et al. *Child Mortality, Son Preference, and Fertility: A Report with Particular Attention to the Kentucky Pretest.* Cambridge: Harvard University, School of Public Health, 1969.

Hewitt, J. "Preconceptional Sex Selection." *British Journal of Hospital Medicine* 37 (1987): 149, 151-52, 154-55.

Hill, E.C. "Your Morality or Mine? An Inquiry into the Ethics of Human Reproduction." *American Journal of Obstetrics and Gynecology* 154 (1986): 1173-80.

Hill, R., M.J. Stycos, and K.W. Back. *The Family and Population Control: A Puerto Rican Experiment in Social Change.* New Haven: College and University Press, 1959.

Hoffman, L.W. "Social Change, the Family and Sex Differences." Minneapolis: National Council on Family Relations, 1976.

—. "Working Paper on Measurement of Preference for Number and Sex of Children." Paper presented at the Conference on the Measurement of Preferences for Number and Sex of Children, East-West Center, Honolulu, 2-5 June 1975.

Holmes, H.B. "Book Review of *Gendercide*, by M.A. Warren, 1955." *Bioethics* 1 (1987): 100-109.

—. "Sex Preselection: Eugenics for Everyone?" In *Biomedical Ethics Reviews*, ed. J.M. Humber and R.F. Almeder. Clifton: Humana Press, 1985.

Holmes, H.B., and B.B. Hoskins. "Prenatal and Preconception Sex Choice Technologies: A Path to Femicide?" In *Man-Made Women: How New Reproductive Technologies Affect Women*, ed. G. Corea et al. Bloomington: Indiana University Press, 1987.

Holmes, H.B., B.B. Hoskins, and M. Gross, eds. *The Custom-Made Child? Women-Centered Perspectives.* Clifton: Humana Press, 1981.

Homans, H., ed. *The Sexual Politics of Reproduction.* Brookfield: Gower, 1985.

Hong, S., et al. *Population Status Report.* Seoul: Korea Development Institute, 1978.

Hoskins, B.B., and H.B. Holmes. "Technology and Prenatal Femicide." In *Test-Tube Women: What Future for Motherhood?* ed. R. Arditti, R.D. Klein, and S. Minden. London: Pandora Press, 1984.

—. "When Not to Choose: A Case Study." *Journal of Medical Humanities and Bioethics* 6 (1985): 28-37.

Houska, W. "The Characteristics of Son Preference in an Urban Scheduled Caste Community." *Eastern Anthropologist* 34 (January-March 1981): 27-35.

Hubbard, R. "Personal Courage Is Not Enough: Some Hazards of Childbearing in the 1980s." In *Test-Tube Women: What Future for Motherhood?* ed. R. Arditti, R.D. Klein, and S. Minden. London: Pandora Press, 1984.

Hubbard, R., and W. Sandford. "New Reproductive Technologies." In *The New Our Bodies, Ourselves: A Book by and for Women.* 2d ed. New York: Simon and Schuster, 1984.

India. Ministry of Health and Family Welfare. Operation Research Group. *Survey of Family Planning Practices in India.* Baroda: 1970-1971.

Inkeles, A., and D.H. Smith. *Becoming Modern: Individual Change in Six Developing Countries.* Cambridge: Harvard University Press, 1974.

Jaffee, B., and D. Fanshel. *How They Fared in Adoption: A Follow-Up Study.* New York: Columbia University Press, 1970.

James, W.H. "The Human Sex Ratio. Part 1. A Review of the Literature." *Human Biology* 59 (1987): 721-52.

—. "The Human Sex Ratio. Part 2. A Hypothesis and a Program of Research." *Human Biology* 59 (1987): 873-900.

—. "Timing of Fertilization and Sex Ratio of Offspring — A Review." *Annals of Human Biology* 3 (1976): 549-56.

—. "Timing of Fertilization and the Sex Ratio of Offspring." In *Sex Selection of Children,* ed. N.G. Bennett. New York: Academic Press, 1983.

Jeambrun, P. "The Preconception Selection of Sex by Means of Diet." *Servir* 38 (3)(1989): 179-82.

Johnson, B. "Move Over, Mother Nature! A New Diet May Help Moms Select Their Babies' Sex." *People* (23 August 1982): 48-51.

Johnston, K. "Sex of New Embryos Known." *Nature* 327 (1987): 547.

Jones, G.W. "Economic and Social Support for High Fertility Conceptual Framework." In *The Economic and Social Supports for High Fertility: Proceedings of the Conference Held in Canberra 16-18 November 1976,* ed. L.T. Ruzicka. Canberra: Australian National University, Department of Demography, 1977.

Jones, R.J. "Sex Predetermination and the Sex Ratio at Birth." *Social Biology* 20 (1973): 203-11.

Kagitcibasi, C. *The Changing Value of Children in Turkey.* Report 60-E. Honolulu: East-West Population Institute, 1982.

Kapadia, K.M. *Marriage and Family in India.* 3d ed. London: Oxford University Press, 1966.

Karlin, S., and S. Lessard. *Theoretical Studies on Sex Ratio Evolution.* Princeton: Princeton University Press, 1986.

Karp, L.E. "The Arguable Propriety of Preconceptual Sex Determination." *American Journal of Medical Genetics* 6 (1980): 185-87.

Katagiri, T. "A Report on the Family Planning Program in the People's Republic of China." *Studies in Family Planning* 4 (1973): 216-18.

Kazazian, H. "Prenatal Diagnosis for Sex Choice: A Medical View." *Hastings Center Report* 10 (February 1980): 17-18.

KCTS, T.V. Seattle. *Hard Choice: Boy or Girl — Should the Choice Be Ours? (Telecast, United States Public Broadcasting Services).* Kent: PTV Publications, January 1981.

Kee, P.-K. *Measuring Parental Sex Preferences: Some Methodological Issues.* Working Paper 20. Honolulu: East-West Population Institute, 1981.

Kenna, K. "Couples Wanting Only Boys Flock to MD for Gender Test." *Toronto Star* (10 December 1990): B1, B3.

Kent, M.M., and A. Larson. *Family Size Preferences: Evidence from the World Fertility Surveys.* Report 4. Washington, DC: Population Reference Bureau, 1982.

Kerin, J. "Sex Preselection: A Scientific Appraisal in 1982." *International Review of Natural Family Planning* 7 (1)(1983): 69-72.

Keyfitz, N. "Foreword." In *Sex Selection of Children,* ed. N.G. Bennett. New York: Academic Press, 1983.

—. *Introduction to the Mathematics of Population.* Rev. ed. Reading: Addison-Wesley, 1977.

Khan, M.A., and I. Sirageldin. "Son Preference and the Demand for Additional Children in Pakistan." *Demography* 14 (1977): 481-95.

Khatamee, M.A., et al. "Sex Preselection in New York City: Who Chooses Which Sex and Why." *International Journal of Fertility* 34 (1989): 353-54.

Khatri, A., and B. Siddiqui. "'A Boy or a Girl?' Preferences of Parents for Sex of Offspring as Perceived by East Indian and American Children: A Cross-Cultural Study." *Journal of Marriage and the Family* 31 (1969): 388-92.

Killien, M.G. "Birth Planning Values and Intentions of Professional Couples." Ph.D. dissertation, University of Washington, 1982.

Kim, N.-I., and B.M. Choi. "Preferences for Number and Sex of Children and Contraceptive Use in Korea." *World Fertility Survey: Scientific Reports* 22 (June 1981): 1-29.

Kirk, H.D. "Differential Sex Preference in Family Formation: A Serendipitous Datum Followed Up." *Canadian Review of Sociology and Anthropology* 1 (1964): 31-48.

Kishwar, M. "The Continuing Deficit of Women in India and the Impact of Amniocentesis." In *Man-Made Women: How New Reproductive Technologies Affect Women*, ed. G. Corea et al. Bloomington: Indiana University Press, 1987.

Klinger, A. "The Longitudinal Study of Marriages Contracted in 1974 in Hungary." Paper presented at the Conference on the Measurement of Preferences for Number and Sex of Children, East-West Center, Honolulu, 2-5 June 1975.

Knodel, J., and S. De Vos. "Preferences for the Sex of Offspring and Demographic Behaviour in Eighteenth- and Nineteenth-Century Germany: An Examination of Evidence from Village Genealogies." *Journal of Family History* 5 (1980): 145-66.

Knodel, J., and P. Pitaktepsombati. "Thailand: Fertility and Family Planning Among Rural and Urban Women." *Studies in Family Planning* 4 (1973): 229-55.

Knodel, J., and V. Prachuabmoh. "Preferences for Sex of Children in Thailand: A Comparison of Husbands' and Wives' Attitudes." *Studies in Family Planning* 7 (1976): 137-43.

Kobrin, F.E., and R.G. Potter, Jr. "Sex Selection Through Amniocentesis and Selective Abortion." In *Sex Selection of Children*, ed. N.G. Bennett. New York: Academic Press, 1983.

Koo, S.Y. *A Study of Fertility and Labor Force Participation of Married Women in Korea*. Honolulu: University of Hawaii, 1979.

The Korean National Fertility Survey: 1974: First Country Report. Seoul: National Bureau of Statistics of the Economic Planning Board, Korean Institute for Family Planning, 1977.

Kornitzer, M. *Adoption and Family Life*. London: Putnam, 1968.

Kovacs, G.T., and K. Waldron. "Sex Preselection — A Review." *Australian Family Physician* 16 (1987): 608-10, 13.

Krigier, L.M. "Medical Technology Helps Couples Select Sex of Baby." *Winnipeg Free Press* (30 July 1986), 33.

Krishnamoorthy, S. "Effects of Sex Preference and Mortality on Family Size." *Demography India* 3 (1)(1974): 120-32.

Krishnan, V. "Preferences for Sex of Children: A Multivariate Analysis." *Journal of Biosocial Science* 19 (1987): 367-76.

Krober, A.L. *People of the Philippines*. Westport: Greenwood Press, 1974.

Kumar, A. *Preference for Sons: A Study for Developing Communication Strategy.* Uttar Pradesh: Lucknow Population Centre, India Population Project, 1977.

Kumar, D. "Male Utopias or Nightmares." *Economic and Political Weekly* 18 (15 January 1983): 61-64.

—. "Should One Be Free to Choose the Sex of One's Child?" In *Ethics, Reproduction and Genetic Control,* ed. R.F. Chadwick. London: Routledge, 1990.

Kwon, T.H., and H.Y. Lee. "Preference for Number and Sex of Children in a Korean Town." *Bulletin of the Population and Development Studies Center* 5 (1976): 1-13.

Labro, F., and F. Papa. *Boy or Girl? Choosing Your Child Through Diet.* London: Souvenir Press, 1984.

Lahiri, S. *Preference for Sons and Ideal Family in Urban India.* Bombay: International Institute for Population Studies, 1973.

—. "Preference for Sons and Ideal Family in Urban India." *Indian Journal of Social Work* 34 (1974): 323-36.

—. "Sex Consciousness Among Child-Desiring Husbands in Relation to Family Gender." *Journal of Population Research* 4 (1)(1977): 29-42.

—. "Sex Preference in Relation to Desire for Additional Children in Urban India." *Demography India* 4 (1)(1975): 86-107.

Langendoen, S., and W. Proctor. *The Preconception Gender Diet: Diet A = Boy, Diet B = Girl.* New York: M. Evans, 1982.

Lappé, M., and P. Steinfels. "Choosing the Sex of Our Children: A Dream Come True or ...?" *Hastings Center Report* 4 (February 1974): 1-4.

Largey, G. "Reproductive Technologies: I. Sex Selection." In *Encyclopedia of Bioethics,* ed. W. Reich. New York: Free Press, 1978.

—. "Sex Control, Sex Preferences, and the Future of the Family." *Social Biology* 19 (1972): 379-92.

—. "Sociological Aspects of Sex Pre-Selection: A Study of the Acceptance of a Medical Innovation." Ph.D. dissertation, State University of New York, Buffalo, 1972.

Lawder, E.A., et al. *A Study of Black Adoption Families: A Comparison of a Traditional and a Quasi-Adoption Program.* New York: Child Welfare League of America, 1971.

Leahy, A.M. "Some Characteristics of Adoptive Parents." *American Journal of Sociology* 38 (1933): 548-63.

Leifer, M. *Psychological Effects of Motherhood: A Study of First Pregnancy.* New York: Praeger, 1980.

Lewis, R. "Your Next Child Will Be a: Boy...Girl." *Health* 19 (January 1987): 58-62.

Lightbourne, R.E. *Fertility Preferences in Guyana, Jamaica, and Trinidad and Tobago, from World Fertility Survey, 1975-77: A Multiple Indicator Approach.* WFS Scientific Reports 68. Voorburg: International Statistical Institute, 1984.

Lloyd, M., O. Lloyd, and W. Lyster. "Slugs and Snails Against Sugar and Spice. Changes in the Ratios of Boys and Girls Might Have Profound Consequences." *British Medical Journal* (24-31 December 1988): 1627-28.

Lockridge, F.L. *Adopting a Child.* New York: Greenberg, 1947.

Lorrain, J., and R. Gagnon. "Sélection préconceptionnelle du sexe." *L'Union médicale du Canada* 104 (1975): 800-803.

Luce, C.B. "Next: Pills to Make Most Babies Male." *Washington Star* (8 July 1978): C1, C4.

—. "Only Women Have Babies." *National Review* (7 July 1978): 824-27.

McClelland, G.H. "Determining the Impact of Sex Preferences on Fertility: A Consideration of Parity Progression Ratio, Dominance, and Stopping Rule Measures." *Demography* 16 (1979): 377-88.

—. "Measuring Sex Preferences and Their Effects on Fertility." In *Sex Selection of Children,* ed. N.G. Bennett. New York: Academic Press, 1983.

—. "Theoretical and Methodological Implications of the Influence of Sex Preferences on the Fertility Attitude-Behavior Relationship." *Journal of Population* 2 (1979): 224-34.

McClelland, G.H., and B.H. Hackenberg. "Subjective Probabilities for Sex of Next Child: U.S. College Students and Philippine Villagers." *Journal of Population* 1 (1978): 132-47.

McClelland, G.H., C.H. Coombs, and L.C. Coombs. "Measurement and Analysis of Family-Composition Preferences." In *Population Psychology: Research and Educational Issues,* ed. S.H. Newman and V.D. Thompson. Washington, DC: U.S. Government Printing Office, 1976.

McClulloch, M. *Peoples of Sierra Leone.* London: International African Institute, 1964.

McCormack, T. "When Is Biology Destiny?" In *The Future of Human Reproduction,* ed. C. Overall. Toronto: Women's Press, 1989.

McDonald, J. "Sex Predetermination: Demographic Effects." *Mathematical Bioscience* 17 (1973): 137-46.

Magarick, R.H., and R.T. Burkman, eds. *Reproductive Health Education and Technology: Issues and Future Directions.* Baltimore: Johns Hopkins

University Program for International Education in Gynecology and Obstetrics, 1988.

Mahoney, J. "The Ethics of Sex Selection." In *Medicine, Medical Ethics and the Value of Life*, ed. P. Byrne. Chichester: John Wiley and Sons, 1990.

Mamdani, M. *The Myth of Population Control: Family, Caste, and Class in an Indian Village*. New York: Monthly Review Press, 1972.

Markle, G.E. "An Analysis of Attitudes and Issues Concerning the Future Prospect of Sex Determination." Master's thesis, Department of Sociology, Florida State University, 1969.

—. "The Potential Impact of Sex Predetermination on Fertility." Ph.D. dissertation, Florida State University, 1973.

—. "Sex Ratio at Birth: Values, Variance, and Some Determinants." *Demography* 11 (1974): 131-42.

Markle, G.E., and C.B. Nam. "The Impact of Sex Predetermination on Fertility." Paper presented at the Annual Meeting of the Population Association of America, Atlanta, April 1970.

—. "Sex Predetermination: Its Impact on Fertility." *Social Biology* 18 (1971): 73-83.

—. "Sex Predetermination: Its Impact on Fertility." *Social Biology* 29 (1982): 168-79.

Markle, G.E., and R.F. Wait. *The Development of Family Size and Sex Composition Norms Among U.S. Children*. Honolulu: East-West Center, 1976.

Mason, A., and N.G. Bennett. "Sex Selection with Biased Technologies and Its Effect on the Population Sex Ratio." *Demography* 14 (1977): 285-96.

Mason, K.O., and A.M. Taj. *Gender Differences in Reproductive Goals in Developing Countries*. Research Report 87-105. Ann Arbor: University of Michigan, Population Studies Center, 1987.

Matheson, G. "What's Wrong with Choosing Your Baby's Sex?" *Globe and Mail* (3 December 1990): A15.

Matteson, R.L., and G. Terranova. "Social Acceptance of New Techniques of Child Conception." *Journal of Social Psychology* 101 (1977): 225-29.

May, D.A., and D.M. Heer. "Son Survivorship Motivation and Family Size in India: A Computer Simulation." *Population Studies* 22 (1968): 199-210.

Mazzeo, J.A. "Technology, Power and the State." In *Embryos, Ethics, and Women's Rights: Exploring the New Reproductive Technologies*, ed. E.H. Baruch, A.F. D'Adamo, Jr., and J. Seager. New York: Harrington Park Press, 1988.

Mead, M. *Sex and Temperament in Three Primitive Societies*. New York: Morrow, 1935.

Meier, R. "Sex Determination and Other Innovations." In *Population in Perspective*, ed. L.B. Young. Toronto: Oxford University Press, 1968.

Michaels, R. "Casework Considerations in Rejecting the Adoption Application." In *Readings in Adoption*, ed. I.E. Smith. New York: Philosophical Library, 1963.

Michel, A. "The Preference for the Sex of the Children." In *The Modernization of North African Families in the Paris Area*. The Hague: Mouton, 1974.

Michelmore, S. *Sexual Reproduction*. New York: Doubleday, 1964. As cited in *Population in Perspective*, ed. L.B. Young. New York: Oxford University Press, 1968.

Miller, B.D. "Daughter Neglect, Women's Work and Marriage: Pakistan and Bangladesh Compared." *Medical Anthropology* 8 (1984): 109-26.

—. *The Endangered Sex: Neglect of Female Children in Rural India*. Ithaca: Cornell University Press, 1981.

—. *Prenatal and Postnatal Sex-Selection in India: The Patriarchal Context, Ethical Questions and Public Policy*. East Lansing: Michigan State University, 1985.

—. *Son Preference, Daughter Neglect, and Juvenile Sex Ratios: Pakistan and Bangladesh Compared*. Ann Arbor: Michigan State University, Women in International Development, 1983.

Miller, W. "Reproduction, Technology, and the Behavioral Sciences." *Science* 183 (1974): 149.

Minkler, M. "Fertility and Female Labour Force Participation in India: A Survey of Workers in Old Delhi Area." *Journal of Family Welfare* 17 (1)(1970): 31-43.

Minturn, L., and J.T. Hitchcock. "The Rājputs of Khalapur, India." In *Six Cultures: Studies of Child Rearing*, ed. B.B. Whiting. New York: John Wiley and Sons, 1963.

Mitra, S. "Preferences Regarding the Sex of Children and Their Effects on Family Size Under Varying Conditions." *Indian Journal of Statistics* (Series B) 32 (June 1970): 55-62.

Mittenthal, S. "Amniocentesis on the Increase." *New York Times* (22 August 1984), C1, C10.

Mode, C.J. "A Study of the Impact of Age of Marriage, Sex Preference, Abortion, Contraception, and Sterilization on Population Growth in Korea by Computer Simulation." Paper presented at the Annual Meeting of the Population Association of America, Seattle, April 1975.

Moore, D.H., II, and B.L. Gledhill. "How Large Should My Study Be so that I Can Detect an Altered Sex Ratio?" *Fertility and Sterility* 50 (1988): 21-25.

Morgan, K.P. "Of Woman Born? How Old-Fashioned! — New Reproductive Technologies and Women's Oppression." In *The Future of Human Reproduction*, ed. C. Overall. Toronto: Women's Press, 1989.

Morsa, J. "The Tunisia Survey: A Preliminary Analysis." In *Family Planning and Population Programs: A Review of World Developments*, ed. B. Berelson et al. Chicago: University of Chicago Press, 1966.

Motulsky, A.G. "Brave New World." *Science* 185 (1974): 653-63.

Muthiah, A., et al. "Comments on 'The Mania for Sons: An Analysis of Social Values in South Asia' [by A. Ramanamma and U. Bambawale]." *Social Science and Medicine* 16 (1982): 879-85.

Myers, G.C., and J.D. Roberts. "A Technique of Measuring Preferential Family Size and Composition." *Eugenics Quarterly* 15 (3)(1968): 164-72.

Nag, M., B. White, and R.C. Peet. "An Anthropological Approach to the Study of the Economic Value of Children in Java and Nepal." *Current Anthropology* 19 (1978): 293-306.

Nair, N.K., and L.P. Chow. "Fertility Intentions and Behavior: Some Findings from Taiwan." *Studies in Family Planning* 11 (1980): 255-63.

Namboodirim, N.K. "Sequential Fertility Decision Making and the Life Course." In *Determinants of Fertility in Developing Countries*, ed. R.A. Bulatao et al. New York: Academic Press, 1983.

Nemeth, R.J. "Son Preference and Its Effect on Korean Lactation Practices: A Social Epidemiological Study." Paper presented at the Annual Meeting of the Population Association of America, Washington, DC, March 1981.

Nentwig, M.R. "Technical Aspects of Sex Preselection." In *The Custom-Made Child? Women-Centered Perspectives*, ed. H.B. Holmes, B.B. Hoskins, and M. Gross. Clifton: Humana Press, 1981.

Nimkoff, M. "Technology, Biology, and the Changing Family." *American Journal of Sociology* 57 (July 1951): 20-26.

—. "Will Parents Pick Sex of Child?" *Science Digest* 30 (5)(1951): 65-68.

Norman, R. "Sex Differences in Preferences for Sex of Children: A Replication After 20 Years." *Journal of Psychology* 88 (1974): 229-39.

Oakley, A. *Becoming a Mother*. New York: Schocken Books, 1980.

—. "From Walking Wombs to Test-Tube Babies." In *Reproductive Technologies: Gender, Motherhood and Medicine*, ed. M. Stanworth. Minneapolis: University of Minnesota Press, 1987.

—. "What Makes Girls Differ from Boys?" *New Society* 46 (21-28 December 1978): xii-xiv.

Okore, A.O. "The Ibos of Arochukwu in Imo State, Nigeria." In *The Persistence of High Fertility*, ed. J.C. Caldwell. Canberra: Australian National University, 1977.

Orubuloye, O. "Values and Costs of Daughters and Sons to Yoruba Mothers and Fathers." In *Sex Roles, Population and Development in West Africa: Policy-Related Studies on Work and Demographic Issues*, ed. C. Oppong. Portsmouth: Heinemann, 1987.

Osman, M., and T. Yamashita. "A Model for Evaluating the Effect of Son or Daughter Preference on Population Size." *Journal of Heredity* 78 (1987): 377-82.

Overall, C. *Ethics and Human Reproduction: A Feminist Analysis*. Boston: Unwin Hyman, 1987.

—, ed. *The Future of Human Reproduction*. Toronto: Women's Press, 1989.

Panigrahi, L. *British Social Policy and Female Infanticide in India*. New Delhi: Munshiam Manoharlal, 1972.

Papp, A. "A Matter of Gender." *Healthsharing* 12 (Spring 1991): 12.

Pappert, A. "Can Feminism Survive Test-Tube Reproduction?" *Toronto Star* (10 October 1989): A20.

—. "Defining Limits for Test-Tube Technologies." *Toronto Star* (12 October 1989): A30.

—. "New Techniques of Reproductive Technology." *Toronto Star* (7 October 1989): A16.

Park, C.B. "The Fourth Korean Child: The Effect of Son Preference on Subsequent Fertility." *Journal of Biosocial Science* 10 (1978): 95-106.

—. "Preference for Sons, Family Size, and Sex Ratio: An Empirical Study in Korea." *Demography* 20 (1983): 333-52.

Patel, V. "Sex-Determination and Sex-Preselection Tests in India: Modern Techniques for Femicide." *Bulletin of Concerned Asian Scholars* 21 (January-March 1989): 2-11.

Pathak, K.B. "On a Model for Studying Variation in the Family Size Under Different Sex Preferences." *Biometrics* 29 (1973): 589-95.

Pathak, K.B., and P.C. Saxena. "On the Time Required for Attaining the Desired Size and Sex Composition of the Family." *Canadian Studies in Population* 6 (1979): 101-10.

Pebley, A.R., and C.F. Westoff. "Women's Sex Preferences in the United States: 1970 to 1975." *Demography* 19 (1982): 177-89.

Pebley, A.R., H. Delgado, and E. Brineman. "Family Sex Composition Preferences Among Guatemalan Men and Women." *Journal of Marriage and the Family* 42 (1980): 437-47.

Peel, J. "The Hull Family Survey: I. The Survey Couples, 1966." *Journal of Biosocial Science* 2 (1970): 45-70.

Peterson, C.C., and J.L. Peterson. "Preference for Sex of Offspring as a Measure of Change in Sex Attitudes." *Psychology* 10 (2)(1973): 3-5.

Pharis, M.E., and M. Manosevitz. "Sexual Stereotyping of Infants: Implications for Social Work Practice." *Social Work Research and Abstracts* 20 (1)(1984): 7-12.

Poffenberger, T. "Age of Wives and Number of Living Children of a Sample of Men Who Had the Vasectomy in Meerut District, U.P." *Journal of Family Welfare* 13 (4)(1967): 48-51.

Poffenberger, T., and S. Poffenberger. "The Social Psychology of Fertility Behavior in a Village in India." In *Psychological Perspectives on Population*, ed. J.T. Fawcett. New York: Basic Books, 1973.

Pogrebin, L.C. *Growing Up Free: Raising Your Child in the 80's*. Toronto: Bantam, 1981.

Pohlman, E. "Some Effects of Being Able to Control Sex of Offspring." *Eugenics Quarterly* 14 (1967): 274-81.

"Poll: Most Wouldn't Choose Baby's Sex." *Montreal Gazette* (20 November 1986): E18.

Postgate, J. "Bat's Chance in Hell." *New Scientist* 58 (5 April 1973): 12-14, 16.

Potts, M., and P. Selman. *Society and Fertility*. Plymouth: Macdonald and Evans, 1979.

Powledge, T.M. "Prenatal Diagnosis: New Techniques, New Questions." *Hastings Center Report* 9 (June 1979): 16-17.

—. "Reproductive Technologies and the Bottom Line." In *Embryos, Ethics and Women's Rights: Exploring the New Reproductive Technologies*, ed. E.H. Baruch, A.F. D'Adamo, Jr., and J. Seager. New York: Harrington Park Press, 1988.

—. "Toward a Moral Policy for Sex Choice." In *Sex Selection of Children*, ed. N.G. Bennett. New York: Academic Press, 1983.

—. "Unnatural Selection: On Choosing Children's Sex." In *The Custom-Made Child? Women-Centered Perspectives*, ed. H.B. Holmes, B.B. Hoskins, and M. Gross. Clifton: Humana Press, 1981.

Prachuabmoh, V., and J. Knodel. *Preferences for Sex of Children in Thailand: Results from the Second Round of a National Survey*. Report

23. Bangkok: Chulalongkorn University, Institute of Population Studies, 1977.

Prachuabmoh, V., J. Knodel, and O. Alers. "Preference for Sons, Desire for Additional Children, and Family Planning in Thailand." *Journal of Marriage and the Family* 36 (1974): 601-14.

Prothro, E. *Child-Rearing in the Lebanon.* Cambridge: Harvard University Press, 1961.

Rainwater, L. *Family Design: Marital Sexuality, Family Size, and Contraception.* Chicago: Aldine, 1965.

Ramanamma, A., and U. Bambawale. "The Mania for Sons: An Analysis of Social Values in South Asia." *Social Science and Medicine* 14 (May 1980): 107-10.

Rao, P.V.V., and N.V. Rao. "Alternatives in Intimacy, Marriage, and Family Lifestyles." *Alternative Lifestyles* 3 (1980): 485-98.

—. "Family Size and Sex Preference of Children: A Biracial Comparison." *Adolescence* 16 (1981): 385-401.

Rao, R. "Sex Selection Continues in Maharastra." *Nature* 341 (1990): 497.

Rao, R., and E. Ebbert. "Move to Ban Sex Determination." *Nature* 331 (11 February 1988): 467.

Raymond, J. "Sex Preselection: A Response." In *The Custom-Made Child? Women-Centered Perspectives*, ed. H.B. Holmes, B.B. Hoskins, and M. Gross. Clifton: Humana Press, 1981.

Reinhart, W. *Sex Preselection — Not Yet Practical.* Population Report Series I (2). Washington, DC: George Washington University Medical Center, May 1975.

Rent, C.S., and G.S. Rent. "More on Offspring-Sex Preference: A Comment on Nancy E. Williamson's 'Sex Preference, Sex Control, and the Status of Women.'" *Signs: Journal of Women in Culture and Society* 3 (1977): 505-15.

Repetto, R. "Son Preference and Fertility Behavior in Developing Countries." *Studies in Family Planning* 3 (4)(1972): 70-76.

Repetto, R., et al. *Economic Development, Population Policy, and Demographic Transition in the Republic of Korea.* Cambridge: Harvard University Press, 1981.

Rice, S.A., and M.M. Willey. "College Men and Birth Rate: A Note on the Present Day Undergraduate Mores Relating to Family Size." *Journal of Heredity* 17 (1926): 11-12.

Robbins, H. "A Note on Gambling Systems and Birth Statistics." *American Mathematical Monthly* 59 (1952): 685-86.

Rodgers, J.L. "Effects of Sex Preselection on Family Planning." Master's thesis, University of North Carolina, May 1979.

Rogerson, P.A. "The Effects of Sex Preselection on the Sex Ratio of Families." *Journal of Heredity* 82 (1991): 239-43.

Roggencamp, V. "Abortion of a Special Kind: Male Sex Selection in India." In *Test-Tube Women: What Future for Motherhood?* ed. R. Arditti, R.D. Klein, and S. Minden. London: Pandora Press, 1984.

Rorvik, D.M., and L.B. Shettles. *Choose Your Baby's Sex: The One Sex-Selection Method That Works.* New York: Dodd, Mead, 1977.

—. "How to Choose Your Baby's Sex." *Look* (21 April 1970): 88-98.

Rose, H. "Victorian Values in the Test-Tube: The Politics of Reproductive Science and Technology." In *Reproductive Technologies: Gender, Motherhood and Medicine,* ed. M. Stanworth. Minneapolis: University of Minnesota Press, 1987.

Rosenzweig, S., and S. Adelman. "Parental Predetermination of the Sex of Offspring: The Attitudes of Young Married Couples with University Education." *Journal of Biosocial Science* 8 (1976): 335-46.

Rosner, F. "Ancient Descriptions of Hemophilia and Preconception Gender Selection." *JAMA* 252 (1984): 900.

—. "The Biblical and Talmudic Secret for Choosing One's Baby's Sex." *Israel Journal of Medical Sciences* 15 (1979): 784-87.

Rothman, B.K. *The Tentative Pregnancy: Prenatal Diagnosis and the Future of Motherhood.* New York: Penguin, 1987.

Rotter, G.S., and N.G. Rotter. "Preferred Family Constellations: A Pilot Study." *Social Biology* 19 (1972): 401-404.

Rowland, R. "Motherhood, Patriarchal Power, Alienation and the Issue of 'Choice' in Sex Preselection." In *Man-Made Women: How New Reproductive Technologies Affect Women,* ed. G. Corea et al. Bloomington: Indiana University Press, 1987.

—. "Of Women Born, but for How Long? The Relationship of Women to the New Reproductive Technologies and the Issue of Choice." In *Made to Order: The Myth of Reproductive and Genetic Progress,* ed. P. Spallone and D.L. Steinberg. New York: Pergamon Press, 1987.

—. "Reproductive Technologies: The Final Solution to the Woman Question?" In *Test-Tube Women: What Future for Motherhood?* ed. R. Arditti, R.D. Klein, and S. Minden. London: Pandora, 1984.

Rubin, J.Z., F.J. Provenzano, and Z. Luria. "The Eye of the Beholder: Parents' Views on Sex of Newborns." *American Journal of Orthopsychiatry* 44 (1974): 512-19.

Rubin, L.R. "It's Getting Easier to Choose Your Baby's Sex." *Saturday Evening Post* (October 1988), 58-59.

Ruegsegger, V.C., and R. Jewelewicz. "Gender Preselection: Facts and Myths." *Fertility and Sterility* 49 (1988): 937-40.

Rukanuddin, A.R. "The Effect of Sex Preference and Infant and Child Mortality on Fertility Behavior of Couples in Pakistan." Ph.D. dissertation, Johns Hopkins University, 1975.

Sadler, C. "The Right to Keep Mum." *Nursing Times* 87 (24-30 July 1991): 16-17.

Sarma, D.V.N., and A.K. Jain. "Preference About Sex of Children and Use of Contraception Among Women Wanting No More Children in India." *Demography India* 3 (1)(1974): 81-104.

Schaaf, C.H. "One Daughter, One Son." *Populi* 3 (4)(1976): 38-43.

Schulz, B., and R. Schulz. "Family Size Preferences and Sex Composition." *Sociological Symposium* 8 (1972): 73-82.

Sears, R.R., E.E. Maccoby, and H. Levin. *Patterns of Child Rearing.* Evanston: Row, Peterson, 1957.

"Selecting the Sex of Your Infant." *Science News* 115 (3 March 1979): 135.

Sell, R.R., K.J. Roghmann, and R.A. Doherty. "Attitudes Toward Abortion and Prenatal Diagnosis of Fetal Abnormalities: Implications for Educational Programs." *Social Biology* 25 (1978): 288-301.

Serow, W.J., and V.J. Evans. "Demographic Effects of Prenatal Sex Selection." *Population Index* 36 (1970): 319.

"Sex Determination." *Science* 126 (1957): 1059.

"Sex Selection Worries Japanese." *Vancouver Sun* (1 November 1986): B6.

Sheps, M.C. "Effects on Family Size and Sex Ratio of Preferences Regarding the Sex of Children." *Population Studies* 17 (1)(1963): 66-72.

Shettles, L.B. "Conception and Birth Sex Ratios: A Review." *Obstetrics and Gynecology* 18 (1961): 122-30.

—. "Factors Influencing Sex Ratios." *International Journal of Gynecology and Obstetrics* 8 (1970): 643-47.

Shettles, L.B., and D. Shettles. *How to Choose the Sex of Your Baby: A Complete Update on the Method Best Supported by the Scientific Evidence.* New York: Doubleday, 1984.

Simcock, B.W. "Sons and Daughters — A Sex Preselection Study." *Medical Journal of Australia* (13 May 1985): 541-42.

Singer, P. *The Expanding Circle: Ethics and Sociobiology.* New York: Farrar, Straus and Giroux, 1981.

Singer, P., and D. Wells. *Making Babies: The New Science and Ethics of Conception.* New York: Scribner, 1985.

Sloane, D., and C.F. Lee. "Sex of Previous Children and Intentions for Further Births in the United States, 1965-1976." *Demography* 20 (1983): 353-67.

Sloman, S.S. "Emotional Problems in 'Planned for' Children." *American Journal of Orthopsychiatry* 18 (1948): 523-28.

Smith, D.P. "Generating Functions for Partial Sex Control Problems." *Demography* 11 (1974): 683-89.

—. "Sex Selection." In *International Encyclopedia of Population,* ed. J.A. Ross. New York: Free Press, 1982.

Snitow, A. "The Paradox of Birth Technology. Exploring the Good, the Bad, and the Scary." *Ms.* (December 1986): 42ff.

Sorenson, J. "From Social Movement to Clinical Medicine: The Role of Law and the Medical Profession in Regulating Applied Human Genetics." In *National Symposium on Genetics and the Law,* ed. A. Milunsky and G. Annas. New York: Plenum Press, 1976.

South, S.J. "Sex Ratios and Women's Roles: A Cross-National Analysis." *American Journal of Sociology* 93 (1988): 1096-1115.

Spallone, P. *Beyond Conception: The New Politics of Reproduction.* Houndmills: Macmillan Education, 1989.

Spallone, P., and D.L. Steinberg, eds. *Made to Order: The Myth of Reproductive and Genetic Progress.* New York: Pergamon Press, 1987.

Stark, E. "The Sexes: Boys 1, Girls 1." *Psychology Today* 19 (August 1985): 18.

Steinbacher, R. "Futuristic Implications of Sex Preselection." In *The Custom-Made Child? Women-Centered Perspectives,* ed. H.B. Holmes, B.B. Hoskins, and M. Gross. Clifton: Humana Press, 1981.

—. "Preselection of Sex: The Social Consequences of Choice." *The Sciences* 20 (April 1980): 6-9, 28.

—. "Sex Preselection: From Here to Fraternity." In *Beyond Domination: New Perspectives on Women and Philosophy,* ed. C. Gould. Totowa: Rowman and Allanheld, 1983.

Steinbacher, R., and F.D. Gilroy. "Preference for Sex of Child Among Primiparous Women." *Journal of Psychology* 119 (1985): 541-47.

—. "Sex Selection Technology: A Prediction of Its Use and Effect." *Journal of Psychology* 124 (1990): 283-88.

Steinbacher, R., and H.B. Holmes. "Sex Choice: Survival and Sisterhood." In *Man-Made Women: How New Reproductive Technologies Affect*

Women, ed. G. Corea et al. Bloomington: Indiana University Press, 1987.

Stenchever, M.A. "An Abuse of Prenatal Diagnosis." *JAMA* 221 (1972): 408.

Stephens, J.D. "Editorial." *Lancet* (23 March 1991): 739.

—. "Morality of Induced Abortion and Freedom of Choice." *American Journal of Obstetrics and Gynecology* 158 (1988): 218.

Stinner, W.F. "Sons, Daughters or Both? An Analysis of Family Sex Composition Preferences in the Philippines." *Demography* 12 (1975): 67-79.

Stinner, W.F., and P.D. Mader. "Son Preference Among Filipino Muslims: A Causal Analysis." *Social Biology* 22 (1975): 181-88.

Stolkowski, J., and J. Choukroun. "Preconception Selection of Sex in Man." *Israel Journal of Medical Sciences* 17 (1981): 1061-67.

Strunk, M. "The Quarter's Poll: Children." *Public Opinion Quarterly* 11 (1947-1948): 641.

Stycos, J.M. *Family and Fertility in Puerto Rico: A Study of the Lower Income Group.* New York: Columbia University Press, 1955.

Sufian, A.J.M., and N.E. Johnson. "Son Preference and Child Replacement in Bangladesh: A New Look at the Child Survival Hypothesis." *Journal of Biosocial Science* 21 (1989): 207-16.

Sun, T.H. "Measurement of Preference for Number and Sex of Children in Taiwan: An Application of Coombs' Preference Scales." Paper presented at the Conference on the Measurement of Preferences for Number and Sex of Children, East-West Center, Honolulu, 2-5 June 1975.

Suzuki, D. *Genetics: The Clash Between New Genetics and Human Values.* Cambridge: Harvard University Press, 1989.

Swinbanks, D. "Japanese Gynaecology: Gender Selection Sparks Row." *Nature* 321 (1986): 720.

Taeuber, I.B., and L.A. Orleans. "Mainland China." In *Family Planning and Population Programs: A Review of World Developments*, ed. B. Berelson et al. Chicago: University of Chicago Press, 1966.

Talwar, P.P. "Effect of Desired Sex Composition in Families on the Birthrate." *Journal of Biosocial Science* 7 (1975): 133-39.

Teachman, J.D., and P.T. Schollaert. "Gender of Children and Birth Timing." *Demography* 26 (1989): 411-23.

Thobani, S. "More than Sexist." *Healthsharing* 12 (Spring 1991): 10-11, 13.

Thomas, M. "The Impact of Gender Preselection on Gender Maldistribution." In *Feminist Research: Prospect and Retrospect*, ed. P. Tancred-Sheriff. Montreal and Kingston: McGill-Queen's University Press, 1988.

Thomas, M.H. "Sex Pattern and Size of Family." *British Medical Journal* (7 April 1951): 733-34.

Trexler, R.C. "Infanticide in Florence: New Sources and First Results." *History of Childhood Quarterly* 1 (Summer 1973): 102.

Tsui, A.O., and D.J. Bogue. *A Work Plan for a Family Planning Analysis of World Fertility Survey Data.* Chicago: University of Chicago, Community and Family Study Center, 1978.

Turner, J., and A. Simmons. "Family Size Attitudes: A Comparison of Measures." Paper presented at the Conference on the Measurement of Preferences for Number and Sex of Children, East-West Center, Honolulu, 2-5 June 1975.

Uddenberg, N., P.-E. Almgren, and A. Nilsson. "Preference for Sex of the Child Among Pregnant Women." *Journal of Biosocial Science* 3 (1971): 267-80.

Ullman, J.B., and L.S. Fidell. "Gender Selection and Society." In *Gender in Transition,* ed. J. Offerman-Zuckerberg. New York: Plenum Press, 1989.

Underwood, N. "Choosing Baby's Gender." *Maclean's* (9 November 1987): 66.

United Nations. Department of International Economic and Social Affairs. *Selected Factors Affecting Fertility and Fertility Preferences in Developing Countries.* New York: United Nations, 1981.

United States. National Commission for the Protection of Human Subjects of Biomedical and Behavioral Research. *Special Study: Implications of Advances in Biomedical and Behavioral Research.* Washington, DC: U.S. Department of Health, Education, and Welfare, 1978.

United States. President's Commission for the Study of Ethical Problems in Medicine and Biomedical and Behavioral Research. *Screening and Counseling for Genetic Conditions: A Report on the Ethical, Social and Legal Implications of Genetic Screening, Counseling and Education Programs.* Washington, DC: U.S. Government Printing Office, 1983.

Verny, T., and J. Kelly. *The Secret Life of the Unborn Child.* Toronto: Collins, 1981.

Virshup, A. "Perfect People: The Promise and the Peril of Genetic Testing." *New York* (27 July 1987): 26-34.

Vreland, N. *Area Handbook for the Philippines.* 3d ed. Washington, DC: U.S. Government Printing Office, 1984.

Waheed, M. "Effect on Family Size of Varying Sex Preference Rules." *Journal of Family Welfare* 19 (March 1973): 35-41.

Waller, J.H. "Sex of Children and Ultimate Family Size by Time and Class." *Social Biology* 23 (1976): 210-25.

Wallis, C. "Can Science Pick a Child's Sex." *Time* (27 August 1984): 59.

Walter, S.D. "The Transitional Effect on the Sex Ratio at Birth of a Sex Predetermination Program." *Social Biology* 21 (1974): 340-52.

Warnock, M. *A Question of Life: The Warnock Report on Human Fertilisation and Embryology.* Oxford: Basil Blackwell, 1985.

Warren, M.A. *Gendercide: The Implications of Sex Selection.* Totowa: Rowman and Allanheld, 1985.

Weatherbee, C. "Toward Preselected Sex." *Science News* 94 (1968): 119-20.

Weiler, H. "Sex Ratio and Birth Control." *American Journal of Sociology* 65 (1959): 298-99.

Welch, F. *Sex of Children, Prior Uncertainty and Subsequent Fertility Behavior.* Santa Monica: Rand, 1974.

Wells, D., and P. Singer. *The Reproductive Revolution: New Ways of Making Babies.* New York: Oxford University Press, 1984.

Wells, R. *Human Sex Determination: An Historical Review and Synthesis.* Tharwa: Riverlea Press, 1990.

Wertz, D.C., and J.C. Fletcher. "Attitudes of Genetic Counselors: A Multinational Survey." *American Journal of Human Genetics* 42 (1988): 592-600.

—. "Ethical Decision Making in Medical Genetics: Women as Patients and Practitioners in Eighteen Nations." In *Healing Technology: Feminist Perspectives*, ed. K.S. Ratcliff et al. Ann Arbor: University of Michigan Press, 1989.

—. "Ethical Issues in Prenatal Diagnosis." *Pediatric Annals* 18 (1989): 739-49.

—. "Ethical Problems in Prenatal Diagnosis: A Cross-Cultural Survey of Medical Geneticists in 18 Nations." *Prenatal Diagnosis* 9 (1989): 145-57.

—. "Ethics and Medical Genetics in the United States: A National Survey." *American Journal of Medical Genetics* 29 (1988): 815-27.

—. "Fatal Knowledge? Prenatal Diagnosis and Sex Selection." *Hastings Center Report* 19 (May-June 1989): 21-27.

—. "Moral Reasoning Among Medical Geneticists in Eighteen Nations." *Theoretical Medicine* 10 (1989): 123-38.

Wertz, D.C., J.C. Fletcher, and J.J. Mulvihill. "Medical Geneticists Confront Ethical Dilemmas: Cross-Cultural Comparisons Among 18 Nations." *American Journal of Human Genetics* 46 (1990): 1200-1213.

Wessels, P.H., M.D. Trumpelmann, and A.P. Oosthuizen. "Sex Selection as Done by the Infertility Clinic, Universitas Hospital, Bloemfontein." *South African Medical Journal* 77 (4)(1990): 196-98.

Westoff, C.F. *Family Growth in Metropolitan America.* Princeton: Princeton University Press, 1961.

—. "The Social-Psychological Structure of Fertility." In *International Population Conference at Vienna 1959.* Vienna: Working Committee of the Conference, 1959.

—. *The Third Child: A Study in the Prediction of Fertility.* Princeton: Princeton University Press, 1963.

Westoff, C.F., and R.R. Rindfuss. "Sex Preselection in the United States: Some Implications." *Science* 184 (1974): 633-36.

Whelan, E.M. *Boy or Girl?: How to Help Choose the Sex of Your Baby.* Indianapolis: Bobbs-Merrill, 1984.

—. *Boy or Girl?: The Sex Selection Technique That Makes All Others Obsolete.* Indianapolis: Bobbs-Merrill, 1977.

Whelpton, P.K., A.A. Campbell, and J.E. Patterson. *Fertility and Family Planning in the United States.* Princeton: Princeton University Press, 1966.

Widmer, K.R., G.H. McClelland, and C.A. Nickerson. "Determining the Impact of Sex Preferences on Fertility: A Demonstration Study." *Demography* 18 (1981): 27-37.

Wiegle, T.C. "The Biotechnology of Sex Preselection: Social Issues in a Public Policy Context." *Policy Studies Review* 4 (1985): 445-60.

Williams, L.S. *But What Will They Mean for Women? Feminist Concerns About the New Reproductive Technologies.* Ottawa: Canadian Research Institute for the Advancement of Women, 1986.

Williamson, N.E. "Boys or Girls? Parents' Preferences and Sex Control." *Population Bulletin* 33 (January 1978): 3-35.

—. "Future Life Histories: A Method of Measuring Family Size and Sex Preferences." Paper presented at the Conference on the Measurement of Preferences for Number and Sex of Children, East-West Center, Honolulu, 2-5 June 1975.

—. "Parental Sex Preference and Sex Selection." In *Sex Selection of Children,* ed. N.G. Bennett. New York: Academic Press, 1983.

—. "Preference for Sons Around the World." Ph.D. dissertation, Harvard University, 1973.

—. "Problems of Measuring Son Preference." Paper presented at the Annual Meeting of the Population Association of America, New York, April 1974.

—. "A Reply to Rent and Rent's 'More on Offspring-Sex Preference.' " *Signs: Journal of Women in Culture and Society* 3 (1977): 513-15.

—. "Sex Preferences, Sex Control, and the Status of Women." *Signs: Journal of Women in Culture and Society* 1 (1976): 847-62.

—. *Sons or Daughters: A Cross-Cultural Survey of Parental Preferences.* Beverly Hills: Sage Publications, 1976.

Williamson, N.E., T. Lean, and D. Vengadasalam. "Evaluation of an Unsuccessful Sex Preselection Clinic in Singapore." *Journal of Biosocial Science* 10 (1978): 375-88.

Williamson, N.E., S.L. Putnam, and H.R. Wurthmann. *Future Autobiographies: Expectations of Marriage, Children, and Careers.* Honolulu: East-West Center, 1975.

Winston, S. "Birth Control and the Sex-Ratio at Birth." *American Journal of Sociology* 38 (1932): 225-31.

—. "The Influence of Social Factors upon the Sex-Ratio at Birth." *American Journal of Sociology* 37 (1931): 1-21.

—. "Some Factors Related to Differential Sex-Ratios at Birth." *Human Biology* 4 (1932): 272-79.

Winters, B. "Engineered Conception: The New Parenthood." In *The Technological Woman: Interfacing with Tomorrow*, ed. J. Zimmerman. New York: Praeger, 1983.

Wolf, M. *Women and Family in Rural Taiwan.* New York: Appleton-Stanford University Press, 1972.

Wood, C.H. "Ethnic Status and Sex Composition as Factors Mediating Income Effects on Fertility." Ph.D. dissertation, University of Texas, 1975.

Woods, F.J., and A.C. Lancaster. "Cultural Factors in Negro Adoptive Parenthood." *Social Work* 7 (October 1962): 14-21.

Wynne, E.M. *Would You Like to Have a Boy or Girl First? Now You May Choose.* New York: House of Great Creations, 1986.

Wyon, J.B., and J.E. Gordon. *The Khanna Study: Population Problems in the Rural Punjab.* Cambridge: Harvard University Press, 1971.

Xie, Y. "Measuring Regional Variation in Sex Preference in China: A Cautionary Note." *Social Science Research* 18 (1989): 291-305.

Yaukey, D. *Fertility Differences in a Modernizing Country: A Survey of Lebanese Couples.* Princeton: Princeton University Press, 1961.

Yi, H.-T. *Causes of Son Preference in Korea: A Socio-Demographic Analysis: A Research Report to W.H.O.* Geneva: World Health Organization, 1982.

Young, C.M. "Family Building Differences Between Same Sex and Mixed Sex Families in Australia." *Australian Journal of Statistics* 19 (August 1977): 83-95.

"Ys & Wherefores." *Economist* 316 (28 July 1990): 68.

Acknowledgments

The bulk of the work in organizing this bibliography was done by Natalie Wallach, who served as primary research assistant on this project. She both reviewed a large number of the publications, to determine their relevance, and entered almost all of the bibliographic data in a computerized bibliographic system.

There are so many librarians at various institutions who made valuable discoveries for me, both small and large, which otherwise might not have been made. I thank them collectively, but offer special thanks to those at the York University Libraries and at the Library of Congress.

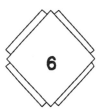

6

Attitudes of Genetic Counsellors with Respect to Prenatal Diagnosis of Sex for Non-Medical Reasons

Z.G. Miller and F.C. Fraser

Executive Summary

This paper reports the authors' survey of the attitudes about prenatal sex selection for non-medical reasons of Canadian genetic counsellors associated with centres providing prenatal diagnosis. It found very few (2%) genetic counsellors approved personally of testing simply for preference of one sex. The survey also tested the hypothesis that genetic counsellors' responses to such a request for prenatal diagnosis are influenced by the way in which the question is put — that is, whether or not they are given the reasons and circumstances behind a couple's request for this service.

The survey asked if respondents approved of such requests, and, if not, whether they would refer the couple to their own centre or, if their centre was not willing to do the test, to a centre that would. The data are reported by sex and professional discipline of two groups — those who were given the circumstances for the request and those who were not. The authors conclude there is no suggestion of a trend toward increasing approval by genetic counsellors in Canada with respect to

This paper was completed for the Royal Commission on New Reproductive Technologies in April 1992.

prenatal sex selection for non-medical reasons. There is a difference in willingness to refer for testing if detailed circumstances are outlined.

Introduction

Prenatal sex selection for non-medical reasons was among the concerns about genetics and the new reproductive technologies frequently expressed in the public hearings of the Royal Commission on New Reproductive Technologies. It is also well represented in the literature on the ethics of prenatal diagnosis (Corea 1986; Hoskins and Holmes 1989; Overall 1987; Powledge and Fletcher 1979; Warren 1985; Wertz and Fletcher 1989). It therefore seemed of interest to survey attitudes on this topic of Canadian genetic counsellors associated with centres providing prenatal diagnosis.

We repeated an approach that was used 15 years ago to survey North American genetic counsellors about this issue. The previous survey showed that the counsellor's response was influenced by the nature of the situation in which the request for prenatal diagnosis simply for choice of sex was made (Fraser and Pressor 1977). In that survey one group was asked, "Would you recommend amniocentesis to allow parents to choose the sex of their unborn child?" A second group was supplied with some cogent reasons why the couple wanted prenatal diagnosis and was asked the same question. As predicted, the percentage of "Yes" responses was higher in the second group than in the first (28% vs. 15%; p < 0.05).

Materials and Methods

The names of genetic counsellors associated with Canadian genetics centres providing prenatal diagnosis were obtained from directories of the Canadian College of Medical Genetic Counsellors, the Canadian Association of Genetic Counsellors, and the American Society of Human Genetics. These were randomly divided into two groups. As in the previous survey (Fraser and Pressor 1977), those in group A were sent a questionnaire that referred simply to a couple who wanted prenatal diagnosis of sex for non-medical reasons; group B's questionnaire described the reasons behind the couple's request. The reasons given were: "A pregnant immigrant woman, from a culture where son preference is strong, requests prenatal diagnosis to determine the sex of the fetus. She already has three daughters and her husband has told her he will send her back to her own country without her children if she has another daughter." This statement was modified somewhat from that of the previous survey in an attempt to make it more relevant to the present social climate.

Both groups were asked whether they would refer such a couple for prenatal diagnosis, but we went further than the previous survey by trying to distinguish between the respondent's personal approval and whether he or she would refer the couple regardless of personal view. Question 1 asked, "Would you personally approve [of the couple's request]?" The "yes" responses are shown in Table 1. Question 2 asked, "Would you nevertheless recommend to your centre that the test be done?" (Table 2). Question 2 should be equivalent to the "Would you recommend amniocentesis?" question of the previous survey.

We also added a question asking whether, if the respondent knew his or her centre would not do the test for this reason, the respondent would refer the couple to a centre that did. Table 3, therefore, represents all those who would refer the couple to a centre where the test was done.

Data were also obtained on the respondent's age, gender, religious affiliation, and academic status (M.D., Ph.D., R.N., or M.Sc.). Those with both M.D. and Ph.D. were arbitrarily counted as M.D.s for purposes of analysis. Statistical analysis was limited to Chi square tests; the material was not considered suitable for more sophisticated methods.

Results

Of 249 questionnaires sent to respondents, 80% were completed and returned.* The data are summarized in Tables 1 to 3. Very few (2%) genetic counsellors personally approved of prenatal diagnosis simply for choice of sex when no reasons were given. However, as predicted, the percentage of those who approved of the couple's request was higher (14%) when detailed reasons were given for the couple wanting a child of a particular sex ($p < 0.01$ — see Table 1, line 1). The responses to the question of whether they would nevertheless refer the couple for testing showed that 20% would if no reason was given, and 26% would if the circumstances were outlined (Table 2, line 1). The difference is not statistically significant. In the two groups' responses to the question of whether they would refer to another centre (Table 3, line 1), the effect of providing detailed reasons for wanting the test is maintained (55% vs. 41%; $p < 0.05$).

---

* We thank those who replied for their kind cooperation.

Table 1. **"Yes" Responses to Question 1 in Two Groups of Respondents Queried About Prenatal Diagnosis Simply for Choice of Sex**

Respondents	Group A*		Group B**	
	% "Yes"	n	% "Yes"	n
All respondents	2	97	14	103
M.D.s and Ph.D.s	3	61	14	70
R.N.s and M.Sc.s	0	36	12	33
All females	2	65	12	60
All males	3	32	16	43
M.D./Ph.D. females	3	29	11	28
M.D./Ph.D. males	3	32	17	42

Note: The percentages are accurate, but to simplify the table we have not shown minor variations in n due to a few "not sure" or "no" answers.

* Question 1 (administered to group A): Would you personally approve of a request for prenatal diagnosis to allow parents to know the sex of the fetus, on the assumption the fetus would be aborted if it were not of the preferred sex?

** Question 2 (administered to group B): A pregnant immigrant woman from a culture where son preference is strong requests prenatal diagnosis to determine the sex of the fetus. She already has three daughters and her husband has told her he will send her back to her own country without her children if she has another daughter. Would you personally approve of a request for prenatal diagnosis to allow this couple to know the sex of the fetus, on the assumption that the fetus would be aborted if it were a girl?

Table 2. "Yes" Responses to Question 2 in Two Groups of Respondents Queried About Prenatal Diagnosis Simply for Choice of Sex

Respondents	Group A		Group B	
	% "Yes"	n	% "Yes"	n
All respondents	20	97	26	103
M.D.s and Ph.D.s	18	61	21	70
R.N.s and M.Sc.s	24	36	38	33
All females	27	65	30	60
All males	6	32	21	43
M.D./Ph.D. females	31	29	21	28
M.D./Ph.D. males	6	32	21	42

Note: The percentages are accurate, but to simplify the table we have not shown minor variations in n due to a few "not sure" or "no" answers.

Question 2 (administered to groups A and B): Would you nevertheless recommend to your centre that the test be done (assuming that you knew your centre would not categorically deny the request)?

Table 3. "Yes" Responses to Question 3 in Two Groups of Respondents Queried About Prenatal Diagnosis Simply for Choice of Sex

Respondents	Group A		Group B	
	% "Yes"	n	% "Yes"	n
All respondents	41	97	55	103
M.D.s and Ph.D.s	31	61	44	70
R.N.s and M.Sc.s	58	36	79	33
All females	51	65	60	60
All males	22	32	44	43
M.D./Ph.D. females	41	29	39	28
M.D./Ph.D. males	22	32	48	42

Note: The percentages are accurate, but to simplify the table we have not shown minor variations in n due to a few "not sure" or "no" answers.

Question 3 (administered to groups A and B): If you knew your centre would deny the request, would you refer the couple to a centre that you know would do the test?

M.D.s and Ph.D.s were very similar in their responses, as were R.N.s and M.Sc.s. Women seem to be somewhat more permissive than men in the circumstances outlined, as indicated by Question 2 — 27% vs. 6% in sample A (p < 0.05) and 30% vs. 21% in sample B (not significant) (Table 2, lines 4 and 5). There is a similar, though not significant, trend for R.N.s and M.Sc.s to be more permissive than M.D.s and Ph.D.s in sample B (38% vs. 21% — see Table 2, lines 2 and 3), which might be explained, at least in part, by the fact that the former group is almost exclusively female as compared to 44% of the latter group. Although these trends are suggestive, they are not highly significant, and not much weight should be placed on them.

There were no appreciable differences relating to religion, age, or family status of the respondents, and these data are therefore not presented.

Discussion

These data show that very few genetic counsellors (2%) approve of prenatal testing for sex preference if no reasons are given. They also support the hypothesis that the response to the request for prenatal diagnosis simply for choice of sex is influenced by the way in which the question is put, confirming the suggestion put forward by Fraser and Pressor (1977).

They also reveal the quandary in which counsellors sometimes find themselves: they may not approve of the reason for a request, but feel a responsibility to respect the tenet that couples should be free to make their own reproductive choices (Powledge and Fletcher 1979). In group A, where no reasons were given, although only 2% approved personally, 20% were nevertheless willing to refer for the test, and 41% would refer to another centre for the test. In group B, where the couple's reasons were given, although only 14% of respondents personally approved of the procedure for the stated purpose, 26% would refer the couple for prenatal diagnosis nevertheless and 55% would refer the couple elsewhere if they knew that their own centre would not accept the request. The figures indicating that only 41% of group A and 55% of group B would be willing to refer elsewhere are lower than might be expected given the consensus that physicians who feel a requested procedure is against their moral principles are obliged to refer the couple if it is available elsewhere. However, the existence of Canadian guidelines that say that sex preference is not an indication for prenatal diagnosis may act in the opposite direction.

It is also interesting that in previous surveys female counsellors tended to be more permissive than males (Wertz and Fletcher 1989) and that M.Sc.-level counsellors tended to be more permissive than M.D. and

Ph.D. counsellors (ibid.; Pencarinha et al. 1992). This suggests that the differences noted in our survey may be real.

With regard to trends over time in attitudes about this topic, in the previous survey no Canadian respondents would refer a couple for prenatal diagnosis simply for sex; however, the sample was very small. In a questionnaire study by Sorenson (1976), which corresponded most closely to our group A Question 2, only 1% of respondents said they would endorse the procedure, as compared to 20% in our study, suggesting an increase in tolerance of the practice since that time.

Wertz and Fletcher (1989), in a 1985 survey of genetic counsellors in many countries, included a question on the use of prenatal diagnosis solely for selecting the sex of the child. It is interesting that this question caused the respondents the greatest ethical conflict of all those in the questionnaire. The question presented social reasons underlying the request, and is most comparable to our group B, Question 2. In the Wertz and Fletcher study, the proportion of U.S. respondents who would refer the couple to their own centre was 34%, and the proportion of Canadian respondents who would refer the couple to their own centre was 30%, compared to 26% in our survey. The proportion who would refer to their own centre or elsewhere was 47%, compared to 55% in our survey, a striking similarity. Incidentally, there was wide variation among the countries. Most countries were less permissive than the United States and Canada — 7 of 17 had 10% or fewer "Yes" responses. Only 1 was more permissive (Hungary, 60%). A detailed discussion of the societal implications of prenatal diagnosis of sex will be found in the report by D. Wertz (Wertz 1993).

Conclusion

There is no suggestion of a trend over the past seven years toward increasing approval by genetic counsellors in Canada of prenatal diagnosis simply for sex determination. However, the data demonstrate a sharp divisiveness among genetic counsellors: there are those who support the collective view of society (except for certain cultures) that the sex of an unborn child is not sufficient grounds for abortion, while others support the individual right to freedom of choice. Will society decide that the collective view prevails, and regulate — or legislate — against prenatal diagnosis simply for choice of sex? Or will society recognize the right of couples to make choices based on what they are, or are not, prepared to live with?

Bibliography

Corea, G. 1986. *The Mother Machine: Reproductive Technologies from Artificial Insemination to Artificial Wombs.* New York: Harper and Row.

Fraser, F.C., and C. Pressor. 1977. "Attitudes of Counsellors in Relation to Prenatal Sex-Determination Simply for Choice of Sex." In *Genetic Counseling*, ed. H.A. Lubs and F. de la Cruz. New York: Raven Press.

Hoskins, B.B., and H.B. Holmes. 1989. "Technology and Prenatal Femicide." In *Test-Tube Women: What Future for Motherhood?* ed. R. Arditti, R.D. Klein, and S. Minden. London: Pandora Press.

Overall, C. 1987. *Ethics and Human Reproduction: A Feminist Analysis.* Boston: Unwin Hyman.

Pencarinha, D.F., et al. 1992. "Ethical Issues in Genetic Counseling: A Comparison of M.S. Counselor and Medical Geneticist Perspectives." *Journal of Genetic Counseling* 1: 19-30.

Powledge, T.M., and J. Fletcher. 1979. "Guidelines for the Ethical, Social and Legal Issues in Prenatal Diagnosis." *New England Journal of Medicine* 300: 168-72.

Sorenson, J.R. 1976. "From Social Movement to Clinical Medicine — The Role of Law and the Medical Profession in Regulating Applied Human Genetics." In *Genetics and the Law*, ed. A. Milunsky and G.J. Annas. New York: Plenum Press.

Warren, M.A. 1985. *Gendercide: The Implications of Sex Selection.* Totowa: Rowman and Allanheld.

Wertz, D.C. 1993. "Prenatal Diagnosis and Society." In *New Reproductive Technologies: Ethical Aspects*, vol. 1 of the research studies of the Royal Commission on New Reproductive Technologies. Ottawa: Minister of Supply and Services Canada.

Wertz, D.C., and J.C. Fletcher. 1989. "Fatal Knowledge? Prenatal Diagnosis and Sex Selection." *Hastings Center Report* 19 (May-June): 21-27.

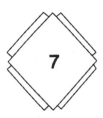

7

Preimplantation Diagnosis

F. Clarke Fraser

Executive Summary

Through preimplantation diagnosis, genetic disorders can be detected in the conceptus before it implants in the uterine wall.

The conceptus is recovered through the techniques of *in vitro* fertilization or uterine lavage, and one or several cells are removed. Techniques are available for measuring enzymes, making specific chromosomes visible, and detecting DNA mutations.

Problems exist with all of these methods of diagnosis. Because of the difficulties, preimplantation diagnosis is likely to remain limited to a small proportion of women at high risk for having offspring with genetic disorders.

Ethical questions are similar to those for conventional prenatal diagnosis and *in vitro* fertilization, and in addition involve consideration of the limitations of the procedure.

Origins of Preimplantation Diagnosis

Preimplantation diagnosis refers to the diagnosis of genetic disorders in the very early conceptus before it implants in the uterine wall. Its origins were threefold. First was the discovery that the conceptus (the

This paper was completed for the Royal Commission on New Reproductive Technologies in February 1991.

entity resulting from the joining of egg and sperm) could be biopsied; that is, if a few cells were removed at, say, the 8- or 16-cell stage, the remaining cells would reorganize themselves and continue normal development as if nothing had happened. This phenomenon had long been familiar to biologists working in Amphibia, who had been probing the nature of differentiation by separating the cells of the early embryo after one, two, or more divisions to see how long each of the individual cells kept the ability to develop into a normal embryo, or how late in development one could remove one or more cells from the embryo without interfering with its normal development. More recently, it was found that the mouse embryo could also develop normally after removal of a few cells — at, for example, the 8-cell stage. A British reproductive mouse geneticist, Anne McLaren, suggested that this would make it possible to biopsy the early human conceptus for diagnostic purposes (McLaren 1987), but not, of course, until there were diagnostic techniques that could be applied to one or a very few cells.

The second origin arose very soon after, when an American biochemist discovered an ingenious technique for "amplifying" a very small amount of DNA to achieve quantities large enough for sequencing or genetic diagnostic testing. This was the polymerase chain reaction, a technique that not only made preimplantation diagnosis possible but revolutionized molecular genetics (Mullis 1990). The discoverer had been working on the construction of DNA segments of specified sequence — *probes* — when he had his seminal idea. He was not involved with prenatal diagnosis.

The third origin was *in vitro* fertilization (IVF), which made available the very early embryo for biopsy.

The Techniques of Preimplantation Diagnosis

Recovery of Conceptus for Testing

In one method of preimplantation diagnosis, eggs are recovered by ultrasound (guided laparoscopic retrieval), and then the techniques of assisted human reproduction — IVF and related methods — are used to bring about fertilization. These techniques have been extensively reviewed elsewhere (Jones and Schrader 1988), and have been found to be costly, stressful, and inefficient. When used for preimplantation diagnosis, the success rates of these techniques are somewhat better than those for infertile women, with "take-home-baby" rates of up to 35 percent rather than 10-20 percent. There is not much optimism for further improvement.

Another method of recovering a conceptus for diagnosis is uterine lavage. The egg is ovulated and fertilized in the normal way and then the conceptus is flushed out of the uterus for examination. This avoids the stress of ovarian stimulation and laparoscopy and is less expensive (around $500 rather than $5 000). The disadvantages are that only one conceptus is obtained per menstrual cycle (and only in about 40 percent of cycles); only about one in four of these are in the blastocyst stage, suitable for biopsy; and only about 12 percent of replaced concepti implant successfully.

Early Biopsy of Conceptus

Much exploratory work is going on to establish optimal methods for the culture and biopsy of the early conceptus (Edwards and Hollands 1988; Handyside et al. 1989). Biopsy techniques include removal of the polar body, aspiration of one or more cells from the conceptus at the 4- to 16-cell stage, excising a few cells at the blastocyst stage (when it is a hollow sphere), or, later still, removing cells from the trophoblast, the tissue that will form the membranes around the embryo itself. The last method has the advantages of providing more cells for diagnosis and not invading the embryo itself, but so far the implantation rate is poor at this later stage. There are no large bodies of comparative data, but the best results so far seem to be obtained by aspirating one or two cells at around the 8-cell stage; this is successful perhaps half of the time. About 35 percent of replaced concepti successfully implant. With this method, if the biopsy is done at 8:00 a.m., the diagnosis can be available by 5:00 p.m. the same day.

With respect to the first technique (removal of the polar body), the first polar body — which is extruded from the egg after the first meiotic (reduction) division — is examined. It contains a haploid set of chromosomes and the egg contains the other set. Thus, for any genes for which the mother is heterozygous, the genotype of the egg can be inferred from that of the polar body (see below).

Diagnostic Techniques

To be useful for preimplantation diagnosis, the techniques for genetic diagnosis must be sensitive enough for use on single cells. There are now such techniques for measuring enzymes (for the diagnosis of inborn errors of metabolism), for visualizing specific chromosomes (in situ hybridization), and for detecting mutations in the DNA.

Enzyme Measurement

Enzyme determinations in single cells are at the limits of technical resolution. For example, in a mouse model of the Lesch-Nyhan syndrome of severe mental retardation and self-mutilation, the deficiency of the responsible enzyme, HPRT, can be detected in single cells. However, the enzyme is not present in the human egg and there is much variation, from embryo to embryo, in the stage at which it appears. For these and other reasons, the early diagnosis of inborn errors of metabolism by this approach does not hold much promise of success in the foreseeable future.

Detection of Chromosomal Disorders

Fluorescent probes are now available that bind to specific chromosomes (*in situ* hybridization), causing them to light up under the microscope and making it possible to detect extra or missing chromosomes (aneuploidy). The probes work in non-dividing cells, so a trisomic cell would have three dots of a particular colour instead of the usual two. There are probes for chromosomes 21, 18, 13, X, and Y — those that result in viable aneuploidies. These probes will be useful for rapid screening of fetal cells obtained by chorionic villus sampling or amniocentesis, but their use in preimplantation diagnosis will be very limited. They could be used to determine the sex of the early embryo, to back up the results of DNA analysis where there is a risk of a severe X-linked disorder, or in the rare case where the mother has a translocation involving one of these chromosomes. They would not be suitable for screening for aneuploidies because of the great effort and cost of obtaining the conceptus for biopsy. Neither would they be useful for polar body analysis, since there are false negatives, and several cells must be examined to ensure accuracy.

DNA Analysis

Biopsy of Conceptus

The technique of polymerase chain reaction (PCR) can amplify the DNA from a single cell (though two is better) to provide enough material for genetic testing. This means preimplantation diagnosis can be done for any genetic disorder resulting from an alteration in the DNA, in which the nature of the alteration is known. The number of such disorders is increasing rapidly, and it is expected that for every disorder that shows regular Mendelian segregation (caused by alteration in a single gene), the responsible gene will be mapped and its DNA alteration identified within the next five years.

There are still some problems, however. Amplification is successful in only about 80 percent of cells, and the technique is so sensitive that there is always a risk of contamination by foreign DNA. Data on sensitivity and specificity are being collected but are still sparse. Much of the exploratory work of testing very early embryos and checking the result by retesting them after further growth in culture has been done using DNA probes for genes in the X and Y chromosomes to diagnose the sex of the embryo. This approach is now beginning to be put into practice in the case of severe X-linked disorders in which the male is at high risk and the specific DNA alteration is not known. It is also being explored with selected disorders that can be identified in the DNA, such as cystic fibrosis, haemophilia A, and the fragile X syndrome of mental retardation.

Polar Body Analysis

PCR can also be used to examine the DNA of the polar body (Verlinsky et al. 1990). When the egg undergoes reduction division (meiosis), its two sets of chromosomes separate from one another, and one set is expelled from the egg in a small cell called the polar body.   If the female is heterozygous for a deleterious gene — for example, the sickle cell gene (Ss) — the polar body will get either the S or the s gene, and the egg the converse. Thus, the genotype of the egg can be inferred from that of the polar body.

However, there are problems with this technique. One problem arises because the fertilized egg (with its polar body) results from IVF or is recovered by uterine lavage, which has a limited success rate. In addition, removal of the polar body from the fertilized egg and PCR amplification are not always successful. A second and more fundamental problem is due to a normal genetic phenomenon, crossing-over, which is an exchange between homologous chromosomes during meiosis. Without crossing-over, the egg from a heterozygous woman will contain two copies of the chromosome, carrying either SS or ss, which separate at the second meiotic division. But if crossing-over occurs, both egg and polar body will be heterozygous (Ss) and the genotype of the egg cannot be inferred. Thus, only 25 percent of the tested eggs will be implantable. A third problem is that the transferred conceptus may not implant; therefore, this approach has had very limited success. This might improve if uterine lavage became simple and effective, but the prospects of this happening are not promising.

Results

Because of the difficulties mentioned above, progress over the first five years has been slow. At the 8th International Congress of Human Genetics in October 1991, two centres reported on their results. One had been testing eggs from females carrying severe X-linked disorders, using PCR and DNA probes to diagnose sex, and replacing only female embryos. Of 22 embryos diagnosed as female, 10 implanted. Of these, 7 reached the fetal heart stage. Of these, 6 were female. The misdiagnosis of the male resulted from failure of amplification (Handyside 1991). The other centre reported five pregnancies in which the embryo was predicted not to have cystic fibrosis; one had it (Verlinsky et al. 1991). Thus, the sensitivity of the method is not satisfactory, and preimplantation diagnosis pregnancies will have to be monitored by traditional methods of prenatal diagnosis for some time to come.

Use of preimplantation diagnosis is likely to be limited to mainly two groups of women. The first group consists of women known to be at high risk for having children with genetic or chromosomal disorders, who are so strongly opposed to abortion and so desirous of having children that they are willing to undergo the stresses and frustrations of IVF or uterine lavage rather than have prenatal diagnosis by chorionic villus sampling or early amniocentesis. (This would presumably not include older women for whom the risk of a chromosome problem is not high enough to justify the difficulty and expense of the preimplantation diagnosis procedure.) The second group consists of women known to be at high risk for genetic disorder in their children, who have experienced prenatal diagnosis and abortion for genetic reasons and find the loss of a wanted child so painful that they are not willing to face the experience again.

It seems clear, then, that preimplantation diagnosis will never supplant, or even compete with, other methods of prenatal diagnosis. This is because it will involve only a small proportion (about 3 percent) of women at high risk for having offspring with severe genetic disorders who are, in turn, only a small proportion of women currently referred for prenatal diagnosis.

Ethical Aspects

Ethical questions relating to preimplantation diagnosis are very much the same as those for conventional prenatal diagnosis (Modell 1990), IVF, and related techniques (Roy 1984). The main difference, from an ethical point of view, is the fact that preimplantation diagnosis is done before the embryonic axis (an imaginary line from the head end to the tail end of an embryo) is laid down, at which point there is some reason to believe that the embryo acquires individuality. Some would argue that being able to identify and discard embryos with genetic disorders before this point removes, or at least lessens, the moral objections that attend later stages.

Another ethical question raised by preimplantation diagnosis and certain other new technologies is whether it is justifiable to expend resources on a costly, stressful, and inefficient procedure, which benefits only a very small number of individuals, when there are so many other demands on health care dollars. It may be argued that research and development must continue in order to lower costs and improve efficiency. But if little progress is being made, and prospects for improvement are slim, is it appropriate to continue to provide support? Other questions arise: By what process, by what authority, and by whom would a decision to withdraw support be made?

Conclusion

Preimplantation diagnosis is a difficult, expensive, and inefficient means of diagnosing genetic disorders prenatally. The survival rate for concepti undergoing the procedure is approximately 20 percent, compared to over 99 percent for regular prenatal diagnosis. The cost-effectiveness ratio is very high indeed, but may go down somewhat as techniques improve. Risks and effectiveness are not yet well documented. Nevertheless, for a small number of women who are at high risk of having children with a particular genetic disorder, and who find the prospect of abortion intolerable, preimplantation diagnosis has promise of providing a means to have offspring free of that disorder.

Bibliography

Edwards, R.G., and P. Hollands. 1988. "New Advances in Human Embryology: Implications of the Preimplantation Diagnosis of Genetic Disease." *Human Reproduction* 3: 549-56.

Handyside, A.H. 1991. "Preimplantation Diagnosis: The First Five Years." *American Journal of Human Genetics* 49 (Suppl.): 24.

Handyside, A.H., et al. 1989. "Biopsy of Human Preimplantation Embryos and Sexing by DNA Amplification." *Lancet* (18 February): 347-49.

Jones, H.W., Jr., and C. Schrader, eds. 1988. "*In Vitro* Fertilization and Other Assisted Reproduction." *Annals of the New York Academy of Sciences* 541.

McLaren, A. 1987. "Can We Diagnose Genetic Disease in Pre-Embryos?" *New Scientist* (10 December): 42-47.

Modell, B. 1990. "The Ethics of Prenatal Diagnosis and Genetic Counselling." *World Health Forum* 11: 179-86.

Mullis, K.B. 1990. "The Unusual Origin of the Polymerase Chain Reaction." *Scientific American* 262 (April): 56-61, 64-65.

Roy, D. 1984. "Research and the IVF Human Embryo — Ethical Issues and Positions." In *Moral Priorities in Medical Research: The Second Hannah Conference*, ed. J.M. Nicholas. Toronto: Hannah Institute for the History of Medicine.

Verlinsky, Y., et al. 1990. "Analysis of the First Polar Body: Preconception Genetic Diagnosis." *Human Reproduction* 5: 826-29.

—. 1991. "Reliability of Preconception and Preimplantation Genetic Diagnosis." *American Journal of Human Genetics* 49 (Suppl.): 22.

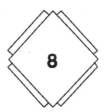

8

Somatic and Germ Line Gene Therapy:
Current Status and Prospects

Lynn Prior

Executive Summary

Human gene therapy involves the introduction of genetic material into humans for the purpose of correcting a genetic disorder. This document looks at the current status of, and research into, gene therapy.

Clinical trials of somatic cell gene therapy are currently under way, using the method of gene insertion. With current techniques, only diseases caused by recessive mutations in a single gene could be corrected by gene therapy; however, research is being done into techniques that may be used to treat dominant mutations and acquired diseases such as cancer and acquired immunodeficiency syndrome (AIDS). In addition, new approaches to somatic cell gene therapy have made seemingly inaccessible tissues, such as brain tissue, candidates for therapy. Current research into somatic cell gene therapy in Canada is discussed.

Somatic cell gene therapy does not present any unique ethical or legal problems but instead raises issues that apply to all new human therapeutic treatments.

Gene alteration for enhancement of "superior" traits in normal people would, if it were possible, present serious ethical concerns

This paper was completed for the Royal Commission on New Reproductive Technologies in December 1991 and released in March 1992.

because the procedure would not be used for the treatment of disease. Ethical analyses suggest that gene therapy should be reserved only for the treatment of serious disorders for which no equally effective alternative therapy exists.

Germ line gene therapy is not yet technically possible in humans, nor is it being considered for human therapeutic use. There is, however, a need for continued discussion of the ethical issues involved because it may become technically possible in the future.

Introduction

The prospect of using directed genetic alteration to treat serious inherited disorders is an exciting one that is just beginning to become a reality. It raises the hopes of patients and their families, but also the fears of those who perceive it as tampering with the secrets of life, or at least creating unknown hazards. This paper will discuss what directed gene alteration can do, what it cannot do, and why, and will review briefly the ethical issues raised by this new technology. It will begin with a description of the biological basis for directed gene alteration.

A gene is a particular region of deoxyribonucleic acid (DNA) in which a sequence of nucleotide base pairs codes for the amino acid sequence of a protein. Long stretches of DNA containing many genes constitute a chromosome. The DNA, which is in the nucleus of a cell, transmits its code to the cytoplasm by the synthesis (transcription) of a ribonucleic acid (RNA) molecule containing a base pair sequence complementary to that of its DNA. This RNA code provides the template on which the amino acids of the resulting protein are assembled (translation). A change in the base pair sequence of a gene can result in a change in the structure and function of the corresponding protein, and may result in a genetic disorder. Over 3 000 human genetic diseases have been identified. More than 5 percent of the population have diseases with important genetic components.[1]

Recent advances in molecular biology have allowed the identification of specific genes responsible for particular genetic diseases; this has created the potential to correct the molecular defect that caused the disease. Human gene therapy may be defined as "the deliberate administration of genetic material into a human patient with the intent of correcting a specific genetic defect."[2] More specifically, a genetic defect resulting from an alteration in the DNA of a specific gene is to be corrected by inserting a normal DNA sequence for that gene into the cells of the patient.

The application of gene therapy to human beings has potential in three areas: somatic cell gene insertion, gene alteration for enhancement of particular qualities, and germ line gene insertion. Somatic cell gene therapy involves the introduction of the corrective DNA into the somatic cells (the non-reproductive cells) of the patient; thus, the alteration is not inherited. Germ line gene therapy refers to the introduction of the corrective DNA into the germ cells (the reproductive cells), and the resulting genetic change can be passed on to subsequent generations. Enhancement genetics involves the insertion of a gene to enhance a known characteristic of a person, such as placing an additional growth hormone gene into a normal child, or to improve "desirable" human traits, such as personality or intelligence. The feasibility and ethical implications of each of these areas will be discussed.

Somatic Cell Gene Therapy

Strategies for Gene Therapy

There are three strategies for gene therapy: gene replacement, gene modification, and gene insertion. Only one of these (gene insertion) is currently feasible.

Gene replacement involves the specific excision of part of the mutant gene sequence from the chromosome and its replacement with the normal form of the gene. Currently, this is not technically feasible.

Gene modification entails the specific correction of a gene mutation in the cell without previous removal of the mutant gene. This has been demonstrated in mice by gene targeting,[3] which involves the introduction of a piece of DNA with the "correct" sequence into the cell in such a way that it is substituted for the "defective" DNA and incorporated into the genome of the cell during cell division. This approach may be applicable to human gene therapy in the future.

Gene insertion involves the introduction of a normal version of a gene somewhere in the chromosomes of an affected cell. In many cases, the genetic function may be restored by the addition of genetic sequences into non-specific sites of the genome without removal or correction of the non-functional mutant gene. Once expressed, the inserted genes produce sufficient quantities of the missing product to overcome the defect. Several techniques have been developed to insert DNA into human cells, including the use of viruses, microinjection, physical and chemical treatments, and membrane fusion. Such methods involve removing cells from the patient, treating them in culture, and returning the treated cells to the patient.

Viral Vectors

Viruses are small packages of genetic information that enter (infect) cells and insert their information into the infected cell. Viruses are useful as carriers (vectors) of DNA into cells for gene therapy because they enter with high efficiency, are easy to manipulate in the laboratory, and can affect many cells. When they are used as vectors for DNA, many safeguards are built in to guard against their "escape." Nevertheless, there is concern about their safety (see Safety).

Retroviruses

The most promising vector for inserting DNA into cells is the retrovirus. The genetic code of the retrovirus is composed of RNA, rather than DNA. It is called a "retro" virus because it can synthesize DNA from RNA, rather than the other way around. When the retrovirus infects the cell, its genetic information is transcribed into a double strand of DNA. This DNA, called a provirus, integrates into the genome of the host cell. An intact retrovirus contains all of the enzymatic machinery required for the integration of its genetic material into the target cell genome. To form a retroviral vector, the viral protein coding sequences are deleted and substituted with a complementary RNA copy of the normal gene to be used for therapy. To enter the target cells, the vector sequences must be packaged into virions — virus particles with an external protein — which can be accomplished only if the deleted viral gene products are supplied. These products are obtained by the use of packaging cell lines, called helper cells, that assemble the viral RNA into virions. The virions can then infect the target cells where the genetic information will become incorporated into the host genome. Thus, a DNA copy of the therapeutic gene is incorporated into the genome of the host cell.

Although retroviral vectors are capable of infecting a broad class of cell types, cell division and DNA synthesis are required for the provirus to integrate into the host genome. This restricts the use of retroviral vectors to dividing cells.

Herpes Simplex Virus

Retroviruses cannot work in the nervous system because neurons do not divide. However, the herpes simplex virus infects neurons, where it remains latent, but yet expresses foreign genes incorporated into the viral DNA. Use of the herpes simplex virus would be advantageous to gene therapy because its large genome would increase the capacity of vectors to carry large foreign sequences. In addition, certain strains of the virus can enter the peripheral nervous system and travel to the central nervous system, which may provide access to the brain.

What triggers the herpes simplex virus to become active is not yet understood; however, once it does, it reproduces and destroys the infected neuron. Various versions of the replication-defective virus are being developed that can express the infected genes but never reproduce.[4] This method may allow the possibility of introducing genes into previously inaccessible tissues.

Adenovirus

To treat genetic diseases involving the lungs, the therapeutic gene can be delivered directly to the lung epithelial cells *in vivo* by tracheal instillation. However, lung epithelial cells do not divide very rapidly, and most of the cells are fully differentiated. Thus, retroviruses are not suitable vectors for gene transfer into such cells. The use of a recombinant adenovirus vector has been suggested.[5] The adenovirus, which is normally found in the lungs, does not require host-cell division for gene expression, rarely recombines to form pathogenic strains, and is not associated with human malignancies. Once adenoviral vectors have been shown to be safe, they may be useful in the treatment of genetic lung diseases such as alpha$_1$-antitrypsin deficiency and cystic fibrosis.

Microinjection

Microinjection involves injection of a solution of DNA directly into cells. This technique is highly reliable because a high proportion of cells that receive the genes express them, but it is limited by the number of cells that can be directly injected. Only hundreds or thousands of cells can be injected compared to the billions of cells that can be treated using viruses or chemical treatments. In addition, microinjection often results in cell death.

It has been reported that, after the injection of a solution of DNA and water directly into mouse muscle tissue, some of the genes were incorporated into the muscle cells and the proteins expressed.[6] However, the level of chromosomal integration was low, and most of the injected DNA remained non-integrated. If the efficiency of the technique can be improved, this procedure, known as gene therapeutics, may prove useful to treat muscular diseases caused by an absent or defective protein, since muscle cells are unusually large and have many nuclei. An example of such a disease is Duchenne-type muscular dystrophy in which the protein dystrophin is defective.

Chemical and Physical Treatments

The cell membrane of a host cell can be made more permeable by treatment with chemicals such as calcium phosphate or by small electric charges (electroporation), so that the DNA can enter the cells. This method has the advantage of not requiring a vector; however, the treatment is relatively uncontrolled and unpredictable. DNA is incorporated into a small proportion of treated cells, and often multiple copies of the gene, in tandem, are inserted. For Canadian research in this area see the section entitled Research in Canada.

Membrane Fusion

Membrane fusion involves putting DNA inside membranes (liposomes) that can then be fused with the outer membrane of target cells, allowing the contents of the liposome to empty into the cells. This method is relatively simple and can be used to treat many cells; however, it is unreliable and non-specific in its delivery of DNA to cells. It may prove useful if membranes can be constructed that target specific cells with highly reliable delivery, which might be accomplished by the use of antibodies on the liposome surface to direct the liposome to the desired target cell.[7]

Combined Gene Transfer-Implantation

A novel approach for treating genetic brain disorders involves the combination of *in vitro* gene transfer with cell grafting into specific regions of the mammalian brain. Gene therapy is used to introduce the missing gene into fibroblasts. The genetically modified cells, which are then able to produce and secrete therapeutically useful metabolites, would be grafted into the brain of the patient to supply the missing product.[8] This approach has been applied to rat models for two major human neurologic disorders: Parkinson's disease[9] and Alzheimer's disease.[10] In both cases, the genetic modification of fibroblasts *in vitro*, followed by the grafting of the modified cells into the brain, led to a decrease in the degeneration of neurons.

Limitations of Gene Therapy

With the current technology, the range of genetic disorders that are potential candidates for gene therapy is limited. Chromosomal disorders or diseases caused by more than one gene, environmental factors, or both, cannot be treated. Chromosomal disorders involve the absence or duplication of fragments of chromosomes or entire chromosomes: for example, Down syndrome (trisomy 21). Since no techniques are available to insert or remove sufficient DNA to correct such large defects, gene therapy for chromosomal disorders is not possible. Multifactorial disorders are determined by a combination of genetic predisposition and interaction with the environment; some examples are cardiovascular disease and some types of cancer. The genetic components are not understood sufficiently to merit serious contemplation of any genetic intervention in most, if any. However, treatment of one form of cancer is being explored by the insertion of a gene that produces a substance that kills tumour cells. In addition, research is being done into treating acquired diseases, such as AIDS, by gene therapy. With the large amount of research being done into new techniques for gene therapy, the applications will probably expand rapidly.

For single-gene disorders, only diseases that are inherited as recessive mutations, such as adenosine deaminase (ADA) deficiency (an immune defect) and phenylketonuria (a type of mental retardation), are currently potential candidates for gene therapy. In dominant disorders, such as Huntington disease (a progressive dementia of adult onset), having just one copy of the gene leads to expression of the disease. Thus, simple gene insertion of the normal gene would not be sufficient; either gene surgery or gene modification to remove or replace the defective gene would be necessary. The technique of targeting a transferred gene to a specific site on a chromosome is being developed by several laboratories. One group[11] has demonstrated the targeted transfer of the β-globin gene in mice by a technique called "homologous recombination." This involves the use of a vector to introduce into cells the new gene that carries nucleotide sequences identical to those of the DNA at the chromosomal site where the gene is to be integrated. The shared nucleotide sequences guide the vector to the desired chromosomal location where the exchange of DNA is to occur. However, the technique has limited success because of the low frequency of cells that integrate the transferred gene and the small fraction of these cells in which targeted integration occurs. Research efforts to improve the frequency of targeted gene transfer involve insertion of a selectable marker along with the therapeutic gene, followed by selection of the cells that receive the transferred gene in the correct genomic location from those that do not.[12] Until the efficiency of targeting is greatly improved, gene therapy will not be feasible for dominant disorders.

Another limitation to gene therapy is that the target organ for the gene product must be accessible. The clinical consequences of a disorder must be due either to effects occurring in a single accessible tissue such as blood, bone marrow, or liver, or to changes in protein or metabolites that circulate freely in the blood. Several gene disorders affect relatively inaccessible tissues such as the brain (e.g., Tay-Sachs disease) or bone; new techniques such as genetically engineered fibroblasts are being developed to treat such disorders, as mentioned above.

If a gene disorder produces irreversible malformation or damage from toxic metabolites, gene therapy would need to be performed before the damage occurs. In many cases, this would mean treating the fetus. For example, in Tay-Sachs disease, degenerative changes of the central nervous system occur early in fetal development. Successful gene transfer has been performed in fetal lambs[13] and will probably be possible in human fetuses *in utero* in the future. The altered genes could be delivered into the affected fetus by perinatal umbilical cord catheterization under ultrasound guidance. This method permits therapy only in the mid-to-late second trimester of pregnancy, after the organs have formed. No viable approaches to fetal gene therapy exist for the first trimester; thus, the diseases that cause damage at such an early stage of development would not yet be candidates for gene therapy.

For most clinical applications of gene therapy, the expression of the introduced gene will need to be regulated appropriately. Inappropriate timing or magnitude of gene expression will make disease correction difficult or dangerous. Much still needs to be learned about transcriptional and translational control before gene therapy can be used for disorders in which genes are highly regulated, such as the thalassaemia group of anaemias.

The current technology limits the use of gene therapy to single-gene recessive disorders in an accessible tissue for which little regulation of expression of the gene product is required, and some types of cancer. Only a few diseases are in this category. However, current research may lead to the development of new techniques for treating more disorders.

Ethical Issues

The ethical problems raised by somatic cell gene therapy are not unique, and are raised by other methods of therapy. The most probable applications of gene therapy closely resemble well-accepted medical interventions, such as organ transplantation (without the complication of graft rejection). They provide promising approaches to correct certain well-understood genetic diseases caused by a single defective or missing protein in a person.   The same issues are raised that apply to all human therapeutic experimentation or new medical treatment.

The ethical issues raised by human therapeutic experimentation are benefit and risk assessment (including an analysis of the potential safety and effectiveness of the therapy and the presence of alternative treatments), selection of candidates, informed consent, confidentiality, review boards, and allocation of resources.

Benefit and Risk Assessment

A comparison of the potential benefits and types of harm of gene therapy must be made for each potential disorder.   Therapy should be undertaken only if the foreseeable benefits of the therapy outweigh the potential risks. The severity of the disease and the presence of any existing therapies must be considered.   Until the safety and efficiency of gene therapy are shown, gene therapy should be considered only for severe diseases that have no effective alternative therapy.

Safety

Some concerns have been raised regarding the safety of gene therapy for both the individual and society. These include immediate fears about the safety of retroviral vectors, and concerns about the long-term impact on the human gene pool and the possible inadvertent transfer of inserted genes from somatic cells to the germ cells. Therefore, before any gene therapy is attempted on humans, the evidence for the safety of each proposal, based on *in vitro* and animal studies, should be evaluated.

a. *In Vitro* and Animal Studies

The safety of gene therapy should be based on animal trials designed to study the short- and long-term impacts of the therapy. Ideally, trials should be conducted on small animals and on primates. If no animal model exists, the therapy should be assessed on the basis of tissue culture and indirect animal experiments. Before gene therapy is attempted in humans, technical and animal data must be provided showing that every possible precaution has been taken to minimize risks. This would include demonstrating the correction of disease, observing treated laboratory animals to determine the risk of infection and cancer, and studying offspring with respect to the possible transfer of inserted genes to the germ cells. Extensive studies of this kind have been done at the U.S. National Institutes of Health (NIH) and elsewhere.[14]

b. Safety of Retroviral Vectors

The use of retroviral vectors to introduce functional genes into humans presents several possible types of harm: the induction of harmful mutations in the patient; the induction of cancer in the patient; and the exposure of the patient and people in close contact with the patient to infectious viruses resulting from the therapy.

It is not yet possible to control how and where the inserted DNA integrates into the host cell. This random integration could occur in or near an essential cellular gene, inactivating the gene and killing the infected cell. It has been suggested that random retroviral integrations into pronuclei of mice induce mutations at an overall frequency of about 5 percent.[15] The percentage would probably be lower in diploid cells because some mutations would be recessive. However, death of an infected cell will not harm the patient and will merely decrease the efficiency of treatment.

Second, random integration of inserted genes could result in activation of a proto-oncogene or inactivation of a tumour suppressor gene, which could increase the probability of subsequent development of cancer in the patient. The probability of such an occurrence depends on the number of cells infected, the number of retroviral integrations per cell, the number of proto-oncogenes activated, the number of tumour suppressor genes inactivated, and the efficiency with which sequences in the retroviral vector can activate proto-oncogenes or inactivate tumour suppressor genes. The insertional activation of one proto-oncogene by a wild-type retrovirus is not sufficient for the induction of cancer. Furthermore, the increased probability of developing cancer may be extremely small, as the frequency with which gene transfer results in a deleterious mutation or predisposition to cancer appears to be quite low.[16] The human genome contains only a very small number of proto-oncogenes compared to its total number of genes, so the probability is low that a provirus will insert into the chromosome next to a proto-oncogene. However, even if the increased risk of cancer is measurable, it may not be a barrier to gene therapy for life-threatening conditions. A higher probability of developing cancer occurs after undergoing other therapies for life-threatening conditions, such as kidney transplantation or radiotherapy or chemotherapy for cancer in children.

Also, the elements of the viral genome may interfere with the proper expression of the inserted human gene. Mutations in retroviruses occur at a high rate due to genetic variation during replication of the vector.[17] Such mutations could inactivate the vector or the gene it carries, which is not dangerous to the patient but decreases the efficiency of the therapy.

There is concern that once retroviruses enter the target cells, they may recombine to form an infectious agent. The infectious viral vector could then cause disease in the patient and could be transmitted inadvertently to people in contact with the patient. A retrovirus competent to replicate could be formed by recombination of the retroviral vector with genomes of helper cells, infected cells, or other viruses. The probability of recombination depends on the amount of sequence homology between the vector and other genomes. Because the retroviral vector contains less than 10 percent of the genome of a replication-competent retrovirus, to form an infectious viral vector the other sequences would have to come from a replication-competent helper cell or from an endogenous retrovirus. The proper design of vectors and delivery systems may be able to remove most of the potential foreseen risks. Retroviral vectors have been constructed to produce the safest possible retroviral vector system — the retroviral vector-helper cell system. The system involves a retroviral vector containing the minimal number of retrovirus sequences required for transcription, packaging, and reverse transcription of the vector RNA, and for integration of the vector DNA. This vector is produced by a helper cell that has no sequence homology with the vector; thus, the homologous recombination between the vector and the helper cell is not possible. This greatly decreases the chance of recombination between the vector and helper cell sequences to form a replication-competent retrovirus; it could occur only by non-homologous recombination. No infectious endogenous viral sequences are known in the human genome; however, the sequence of the human genome is not known sufficiently to establish that these sequences do not exist.

If a replication-competent retrovirus was formed, it would probably contain the gene inserted for gene therapy. Since the size of the retrovirus has a package limit, the recombinant would probably be too large to be packaged successfully in the genome with all of the viral protein coding sequences; it would probably contain only some of the vector control sequences required and would not be replication-competent.

Also relevant is that murine amphotropic retroviruses, which are most commonly used as retroviral vectors, are not pathogenic in primates.[18] Since both the formation of replication-competent virus and the induction of disease are unlikely together, the probability is extremely low that disease will be induced by a replication-competent retrovirus formed by recombination with the vector. In addition, retroviruses usually are not transmitted easily. Thus, it is very unlikely that replication-competent retroviruses, formed by recombination, would have any observable biological effect. No replication-competent retroviruses in patients of the first human gene transfer experiments have been detected.[19]

c. Impact on the Human Gene Pool

If people with rare lethal genetic disorders are treated successfully, they may have children, thus passing on their abnormal genes. The result would be an increase in the number of abnormal genes in the human gene pool. However, because only recessive, single-gene defects will be treated initially, the impact on the human gene pool will be extremely small. For recessive genetic disorders, an overwhelming proportion of the relevant genes exist only in one dose in carriers; affected individuals are quite rare. A small increase in the number of carriers will have little effect on the total number of mutant genes in the human population. The successful treatment of X-linked diseases would increase the gene frequency somewhat more.

Any medical treatment of genetic disorders might have some impact on the human gene pool. For example, the pool is being altered by current traditional methods of treatment for genetic disease, such as haemophilia or phenylketonuria, which allow affected individuals to mature and have children. Because somatic cell gene therapy does not alter the germ line, its effect on the distribution of genes in the population is no greater than that which has already resulted from the introduction of other therapies for inherited disease.

d. Transfer of Genetic Information from Somatic to Germ Cells

The possibility of insertion of the retroviral vector into the germ line of the patient is remote because the vector is crippled and infection is to be performed outside the body with the helper virus-free stocks. There is no opportunity for a free infectious virus to be transmitted. If an inserted gene is inadvertently transferred to germ line cells, the offspring of the person could be affected by some unintended mutations. The long-term consequences are unknown, but the impact is likely to be small. Only the children of a few people who have been treated could contribute to the gene pool. This addition would be trivial compared to the total number of mutations that are constantly occurring. In addition, the risk of inadvertently affecting the germ line is not unique to gene therapy; other medical practices such as chemotherapy and radiation therapy also carry this risk.

e. *In Vitro* Versus *In Vivo* Therapy

Gene therapy can be performed by removing cells from the body, genetically altering the cells *in vitro*, and then restoring the cells to the patient. This provides a built-in safety factor. If a mishap occurs in the gene-transfer process, such as a lethal mutation in the treated cells, the attempt can be stopped with no harm done to the patient. Also, *in vitro* therapy decreases the chance of altering the germ line and lowers the probability of unintentionally affecting other tissues that need not be treated. So far, only bone marrow and skin cells (fibroblasts) can be so manipulated.

Efficiency of Gene Therapy

For gene therapy to be effective, the gene must be delivered to the targeted tissue, must express a sufficient amount of product, and must remain in the cells long enough to have an effect.

The product of the inserted gene must be expressed sufficiently at the proper time and in the proper amount. If the gene requires precise regulation of expression, it is a poor candidate for gene therapy because the current understanding of gene regulation is insufficient to ensure precise control. Also, the gene must be inserted into enough cells to produce enough product to have a significant effect. If insufficient gene product is produced by genetically modified cells, the genetic disorder may be only partially corrected so that the lethal genetic disease is converted to one that allows the patient to survive but causes great suffering.

The inserted gene must be stable and continue to make product for a long time. Ideally, gene therapy should involve either non-dividing cells or cycling stem cells to perpetuate a genetic correction. If only differentiated, replicating cells are infected, the newly introduced gene function will be lost as the cells mature and die; the disease will reappear, and the gene therapy will have to be repeated.

Alternative Treatments

Gene therapy is acceptable only if it offers the best prospect of success among all potential treatments for a given patient. Factors to be considered include the expected efficacy, anticipated cost, and the magnitude and type of risks.

Selection of Candidates

Candidate Genetic Diseases

For a disease to be a candidate for gene therapy, the anticipated benefits of the therapy must outweigh the possible types of harm. Only serious genetic disorders (severely debilitating or lethal diseases) that have no effective conventional treatments should be considered at this time. If somatic cell gene therapy proves to be effective and safe in fatal diseases, and if its use appeared to be safer and more efficient than that of other therapies, it could be considered for less burdensome diseases. Any increased probability of later cancer or other untoward events would have to be evaluated against the benefits of the gene therapy.

Candidate Research Subjects

Theoretically, cancer could be induced by gene therapy; therefore, only patients with serious conditions should be candidates at first. The centres working on new methods are likely to be few, and there will possibly be more people affected than can be treated. Therefore, it will be important to establish equitable criteria for selecting research subjects. The Recombinant DNA Advisory Committee (RAC) Subcommittee on Human Gene Therapy[20] (see Regulation of Gene Therapy) indicated that investigators must describe recruitment procedures and patient eligibility requirements. In the first gene therapy clinical protocol,[21] patients were chosen from among the fewer than 20 children worldwide who have severe combined immunodeficiency due to ADA deficiency. Only patients without a sibling-matched bone marrow transplant as an alternative treatment were considered. Children with human immunodeficiency virus (HIV) infection were excluded. For special considerations relating to the fact that most, if not all, candidates for directed gene alteration will be children, see Gene Therapy Involving Children.

Principles of Consent

Informed Decision Making

The Medical Research Council of Canada (MRC) Guidelines[22] declared that involvement in research of a human subject should be informed and voluntary. The subject should be informed fully about the therapy and should make the decision about whether to participate with no pressure. Prospective subjects must receive enough information about the proposed therapy and their role in it, in an easily understood form, to enable them to decide whether or not to participate. The MRC Guidelines suggested that the prospective subject might be told

(a) the reasons for the study;

(b) research techniques which will involve the prospective subject, such as randomization [or not] of treatments;

(c) the reason why the prospective subject is being invited to take part;

(d) the reasonably anticipated benefits and consequences of the study;

(e) the reasonably anticipated benefits and consequences of the study for the prospective subject and society (if none, this should be stated);

(f) the foreseeable risks, including discomforts and inconveniences, to the prospective subject;

(g) the foreseeable risks of the study itself;

(h) complete details regarding confidentiality of prospective subjects;

(i) the expected time commitment for subjects;

(j) the intent to conduct a follow-up study ... and the retention of data;

(k) the rules for stopping the study and withdrawing the subject; and

(l) the right of the subject to withdraw from the study at any time and without penalty.

Additional information requirements must be met for potential research subjects who are also patients ... Information would include

(a) the patient's prognosis without intervention;

(b) alternative interventions available;

(c) experimental aspects of interventions proposed;

(d) interventions to be unavailable to a patient who becomes a subject, for the sake of the research;

(e) an estimate of the likely success and failure of all the interventions which may be offered and withheld;

(f) an estimate of the risks and possible adverse effects of interventions offered; and

(g) a clear distinction between procedures in the research protocol and those that would be part of usual patient care.

The level of disclosure should be proportionate to the likelihood and the scale of possible harm, but even the remote possibility of injury should be disclosed.

Several problems arise with respect to informed consent for gene therapy, as for other treatments. First, because gene therapy is irreversible, revocable consent may not be meaningful. Also, by withdrawing, the patient will lose the benefit of follow-up and early recognition of any harm that might manifest itself later. In addition, for assessment of the potential harm of the therapy to third parties in contact with the subject, the subject must adhere to long-term monitoring aspects of the protocol. If the subject no longer wishes to participate, withdrawal will deny any future subjects the benefit of the information resulting from long-term monitoring of the patient for harmful effects. If there is possible harm to others, public policy might overcome the individual's right to withdraw from monitoring.

Free Consent

Individual freedom of choice must be allowed when obtaining the consent of the patient. Undue influence must not be used, and the person should be allowed sufficient time to consider the information given.

The law presumes that any agreement between a weaker and a stronger party, from which the stronger party gains an unusual advantage, is suspect. Such a relationship exists when patients are asked by those treating them to serve as their research subjects. It is desirable to delegate the negotiations concerning consent to another health professional who has no direct link to the future medical management of the patient.

Continuing Consent

Continuing consent must be elicited during the progress of the research. Subjects must be informed of the duration of their involvement in the study and must be free to leave the study at any time without prejudice to their rights. Research must not become dependent on the continued participation of any particular subject.

Gene Therapy Involving Children

Damage from genetic diseases is often progressive, cumulative, and fatal at an early age. Ideally, people should be treated as soon as a diagnosis is made to maximize the potential for therapeutic benefit. A delay in treatment will cause greater harm through the irreversible accumulation of effects of the disease. However, the younger the subjects, the less able they are to consent. Children cannot provide legally or ethically valid consent: their parents or guardians must provide proxy consent, and their decision must be based on the same information that would be given to a competent prospective research subject. In-depth counselling should be provided to ensure full understanding of the risk of new mutations, the possible effects on the germ line, the relative risks and benefits of alternative therapies, and the reversibility of any side-effects.

Even if a child is not capable of consenting to gene therapy, the wish of the child should be respected. According to the MRC Guidelines,

> A concept has developed that a child incapable of giving legally and ethically acceptable consent may give an "assent" which is significant in respecting a level of autonomy. Related to this concept is the recognition that a child, whose consent or assent to participate in research is questionable, may nevertheless have the power to decline invasive involvement with conclusive effect. Parental consent may be a necessary condition of engaging the child in research, but it is not necessarily a sufficient condition; the child's negative preferences in such cases should be respected.[23]

Gene Therapy on Fetuses

In the future, severe diseases of early childhood may be able to be treated during fetal development to avoid irreversible damage. Any discussion must consider the risks and benefits of the therapy for the mother and the fetus. The possibility of affecting the germ cells also must be considered when determining the time of treatment; the gonads must be fully formed.

Confidentiality

Generally, confidentiality cannot be breached without the consent of the subject. Access to personally identifying information and its use in research must be guarded. Information obtained during somatic cell gene therapy trials may be prejudicial to the patient or the family, and therefore must be reported in a manner that conceals the identity of the patient. No one outside the research team should be permitted to handle the data. Identifying information should be disclosed only with the authorization of the subject.

The anonymity of the patient may be difficult to maintain because of the widespread interest in gene therapy among the public, scientific, religious, and government communities. The publicity potential is great, and it may be difficult to ensure privacy to the subjects. The risk of media exposure should be part of the process of informed consent.

Allocation of Resources

Gene therapy will probably not be applicable to a large number of patients, because diseases for which gene therapy is contemplated are quite rare. They include single-gene recessive disorders that affect an accessible tissue or organ. ADA deficiency has been reported in only 40 to 50 patients worldwide. Another candidate, purine-nucleoside phosphorylase deficiency, affects only six families worldwide.[24] Initially, the procedures will be expensive because of the sophisticated laboratory techniques required. Some people question allocating resources to the development of such expensive therapies when social programs such as child care, which could benefit many more people, need support. This choice is artificial; in our system, curtailing the support of research in this area does not guarantee that resources will be diverted to social programs. The initial cost of gene therapy will be high, but as technology progresses the cost of individual treatments is likely to decrease — gene therapy would probably be less expensive than bone marrow replacement, for example. Research activities associated with the development of gene therapy increase the understanding of genetics, developmental biology, and mechanisms by which genes exert their control over life processes. Some of the new knowledge gained may be used to produce better standards of health care and bring other benefits. The social cost of prohibiting the funding of research in a given area, or even the feasibility of prohibition, must also be considered when allocating resources.

Gene Insertion for Enhancement of Characteristics

Concern has been expressed that if somatic cell gene therapy is shown to be safe and effective, and becomes more common, the techniques might be used to enhance certain desirable human characteristics. Enhancement engineering involves the insertion of a gene to enhance normal characteristics of a person (e.g., the placement of additional growth hormone genes into a normal infant to increase the size of the child). When the growth hormone gene was inserted into mouse eggs, there was a great increase in size of the resulting mice.[25] However, chronic exposure to high levels of growth hormone results in the clinical condition referred to as gigantism. In humans, the condition is associated with such problems as enlarged organs, bone and soft tissue deformities, and multiple endocrine function disturbances. The normal genome is a result of millennia of selection by environmental forces. It is highly improbable that any "normal" gene can be improved, as selective forces have been working on improvement for millions of years. Any alteration or addition is likely to have deleterious, not beneficial, results. Any gene acts on the background of many other genes that also have evolved over millennia.

The insertion of a gene to alter, selectively, a characteristic such as growth would affect the entire organism by endangering the overall balance of individual cells and organs; this could disturb the child's physiological systems. More serious consequences, such as the altering of regulatory pathways, could also occur. The results of enhancement engineering are too uncertain to risk inserting a gene for "improvement" into a healthy person. Furthermore, "normal" traits such as longevity, intelligence, beauty, or vigour are multifactorial, involving the complex interplay of many genes and environmental factors. No one gene plays a major part in enhancing such characteristics. It is highly unlikely that any such genes will ever be mapped, much less become amenable to enhancement.

Even if enhancement engineering were feasible and safe, it would not be acceptable ethically because it does not involve the treatment of disease. Apart from the ethically complex question of who would decide which characteristics are normal and which are superior, the use of enhancement engineering (if it became possible) could lead to an increase in inequality and discrimination in society. If certain characteristics were frequently selected for, those without those characteristics could be seen as inferior. Gene therapy is being developed for and should be reserved only for the treatment of serious disorders that have no equally effective alternative therapy. This applies to germ line as well as somatic gene therapy.

Legal Issues

Regulation of Gene Therapy

Whether gene therapy should be regulated by guidelines or by legislation is an issue for consideration. Although legislation might arguably have more force, it might not effectively address relevant ethical issues. One argument against the use of legislation is that it prescribes standard responses to anticipated situations. The field of gene therapy is changing quickly, and legislation is not responsive to such rapid change. The ethical assessment of research proposals will raise many issues, including risk-to-benefit evaluations for specific cases that cannot be standardized. Particular factors will have a different weight in different circumstances.

Also, it is desirable to promote ethical awareness to encourage researchers to respond to changing social views and new ethical issues; this may not be accomplished by legislation. Mere conformity to the law will not necessarily promote awareness of ethical values; instead, awareness will be developed through the careful consideration of options available, the resolution of dilemmas, and the exercise of reasoned choice. The use of guidelines, instead of legislation, will help to promote thoughtful decision making by proposing criteria and procedures for the exercise of choice. Researchers will achieve awareness and understanding of ethical values rather than adhere blindly to the law.

It will also be important to have nationwide standards or guidelines. Because the research proposals will affect health, hospitals, and universities, they will fall within provincial jurisdiction. The use of federal guidelines would promote nationwide harmonization, rather than differences between provinces.

Review Boards

In the United States, under the Department of Health and Human Services regulations for the protection of human research subjects, every human gene therapy protocol must be reviewed by the Institutional Review Board at the institution of the investigator. In addition, any federally funded gene therapy experiment involving recombinant DNA must be approved by the NIH. The NIH requires experiments involving the transfer of recombinant DNA into human subjects to be reviewed by the Institutes' RAC. The RAC considers each proposal on a case-by-case basis, and the proposal is reviewed again by the RAC's Subcommittee on Human Gene Therapy. The RAC recommendations on each proposal are forwarded to the director of the NIH who either approves the proposal or suggests alterations. Final review by the RAC (in public session) is preceded by seven levels of committee review at the NIH and the Food and Drug Administration.[26]

In Canada, the view of the MRC Standing Committee on Ethics in Experimentation is that all gene therapy techniques used in human subjects fall within the context of clinical research. Thus, they require approval of a Research Ethics Board (REB), as defined in the MRC Guidelines.[27] The requirements of the MRC for ethics review include a local review and a national review. The local review would allow for local awareness and resolution of ethical issues, and would address the needs and interests of communities that may differ across the country. Local institutions may not have sufficient members with the experience and knowledge to review the protocol, whereas the national review board would have more access to experts. In addition, it is likely that local experts would be involved with the proposed research, and the national review would help to achieve uniformity in the application of proposed guidelines and allow progress in the field to be shared more readily. In the MRC Guidelines of 1990,[28] the Working Group recommended a two-tier process of review: initial review by a local REB, which, if positive, would allow the proposal to be forwarded to a national review committee. The MRC is currently considering a national committee to review clinical proposals. It would be important to have people from many fields on such a committee.

Legal Liability

There is no reason to suppose that the legal issues raised by gene therapy would differ from those relating to other types of biomedical experimentation.

Current Research

Research in the United States

On 19 January 1989, the first federal approval for gene transfer into humans was given in the United States. Dr. Steven Rosenberg at the National Cancer Institute injected five patients having advanced melanomas with their own cells, genetically altered tumour-infiltrating lymphocytes (TILs), which specifically kill the tumour cells.   The TILs carried a retrovirus-mediated bacterial gene for neomycin resistance as a marker to allow the study of where the TIL cells go and how they survive in vivo. The results were promising.   The genetically altered cells remained in circulation for at least three weeks and up to two months, and were recovered from tumour deposits in three of five patients. No live virus was detected in the patients, and no ill effects from the experiment were observed.[29]   The results provide the first clinical study of retrovirus-mediated gene transfer in humans. The information gained from these studies may lead to improved cancer treatments.

The first gene therapy involving human subjects began in September 1990. The key researchers in the experiment are Dr. Michael Blaese of the U.S. National Cancer Institute and Drs. W. French Anderson and Kenneth Culver of the National Heart, Lung, and Blood Institute. The researchers removed T cells from a four-year-old child who has ADA deficiency. The T cells were infected *in vitro* with a normal ADA gene inserted in a retroviral vector, then injected back into the child during a blood transfusion. The experiment was done using the child's T cells, which have a finite life span; the inserted gene will not remain permanently in the child, but will be lost as these cells die. After six infusions over 200 days, the patient's ADA activity had increased to 20 percent of normal and the clinical signs had improved. A second patient in this project began treatment in January 1991 and is being closely monitored.

A second human gene therapy clinical protocol received final approval in January 1991. This protocol, by Dr. Steven Rosenberg, involves removing the patient's TIL cells, inserting a gene for a tumour necrosis factor (TNF), and returning the cells to the patient, who has a malignant melanoma. TNF has been demonstrated to cause the regression of several murine cancers.[30] By inserting the gene coding for TNF into TILs, the TILs can then bring the TNF directly to the tumour cells where it can be concentrated to kill them.

Two other gene marker proposals have received approval with stipulations by the Subcommittee on Human Gene Therapy and are being considered by the RAC. The first was presented by Dr. Malcolm Brenner in Memphis. This protocol involves the insertion of a marker gene into bone marrow cells to study paediatric acute myelogenous leukemia. The second proposal, by Dr. Michael Lotze of the University of Pittsburgh School of Medicine, is a study marking TILs, which is similar to that of Dr. Steven Rosenberg. Two additional marking protocols, in adult leukemia and paediatric neuroblastoma, were deferred pending the submission of additional pre-clinical data.

Research in Canada

Several research centres across Canada are involved in the study of gene therapy and its potential clinical use. Groups at the Royal Victoria Hospital in Montreal, the Mount Sinai Hospital Research Institute and The Hospital for Sick Children Research Institute in Toronto, and the Terry Fox Laboratory in Vancouver are investigating protocols using retrovirus-mediated gene transfer into haematopoietic stem cells.[31] These stem cells are pluripotent primitive cells, which reside in bone marrow, from which differentiated blood cells arise. They are being studied for the following reasons: well-developed procedures for bone marrow transplantation exist; haematopoietic cells are found in large numbers and are widely distributed; and many diseases affect haematopoietic cells. Another advantage is that transfer of the normal gene into a pluripotent stem cell could result in the continued presence of the gene in all haematopoietic lineages for the life of the animal, thereby providing long-term therapy. This contrasts with gene transfer into a differentiated cell type that results in expression of the gene in a restricted class of haematopoietic cells for a limited time so that .repeated treatments would be necessary. Clinical applications of this research are expected within the next few years.

One project under way is gene insertion into stem cells for use against HIV, the virus responsible for AIDS. HIV is a retrovirus that infects and destroys white cells in the immune system, the body's defensive network. With the immune system weakened, the body becomes vulnerable to infection, cancer, and neurologic disorders that healthy (uninfected) persons could normally combat. Dr. Sadhna Joshi at the University of Toronto is developing ways of blocking HIV infection through genetic alteration of white cells (lymphocytes). One method is to change genetically or eliminate the HIV attachment site on lymphocytes, the CD4 receptor. Another approach is to turn ordinary cells into HIV fighters by inserting a gene for the CD4 receptor into the cells such that they produce soluble CD4 protein. This protein coats the virus, making it unable to bind to the lymphocytes; this prevents infection of the cells. Dr. Joshi has had positive results in cell lines, is currently doing animal studies, and expects to begin human clinical trials in one year.[32]

In addition to retrovirus-mediated gene therapy, physical methods of DNA transfer are being researched (see Chemical and Physical Treatments). One such technique, being examined by Dr. Armand Keating at the Toronto General Hospital, is the use of electroporation, which involves exposing a cell suspension to a brief electric pulse that causes areas of reversible cell membrane breakdown. DNA present in the surrounding medium passes passively through the transiently formed membrane pores into the cell. This is the most efficient physical method of DNA transfer[33] and avoids the danger of using viral vectors. A physical method is being used currently by a Toronto research group to transfer the factor 9 blood coagulation gene into bone marrow cells to treat haemophilia B. Animal studies involving this method have been completed in mice, and a clinical protocol for human gene therapy soon will be submitted to the national review board.[34]

Germ Line Gene Therapy

Germ line gene therapy is the modification of reproductive cells in such a way that the therapeutic gene is inserted directly into the egg, sperm, or the early embryo, thus affecting the developing gonadal cells. If inserted at an early enough stage of development of an embryo, the gene is integrated not only into cells of the organism as they divide, but into the chromosomes of the germ cells. Consequently, copies of the DNA sequence are present in the cells of the resulting developing embryo, including its own embryonic reproductive cells, and the genetic correction is passed on to the children of the patient. This would eliminate the genetic disease in the offspring of the patient, instead of in one person as in somatic cell gene therapy. Also, it may be useful in situations where somatic cell gene therapy is not effective, such as when the cells or tissues to be treated are inaccessible, when several organs need to be treated simultaneously, or when gene therapy is required immediately after fertilization to prevent irreversible damage during fetal development. The possibility raises new ethical and technical issues in addition to those already discussed in relation to somatic cell gene therapy.

Technical Aspects

Theoretically, germ line gene therapy would be technically much more difficult than somatic cell gene therapy. The gene insertion can be directed at either the gametes or at the early stages of the developing embryo.

Apart from the fact that donor insemination would be infinitely simpler, sperm would be difficult to alter genetically because they are small and difficult to penetrate, and millions are required for insemination. Although only one sperm fertilizes the egg, every sperm would have to be genetically altered, as it is not known which one will be successful. Even if *in vitro* techniques could assist some sperm to fertilize the egg, confirming that every sperm used carried the genetic correction would be a problem. It may be more efficient to alter sperm by treating the testicular cells that produce them, because such cells are larger and easier to manipulate. However, this would not lead to genetic correction in all sperm by current techniques. Substantial increases in technologic knowledge are required before gene insertion could be contemplated on sperm or their precursor cells.

Theoretically, a second approach could be to genetically alter the ova, which are much larger than sperm. The fertilized ovum is available during the procedures used for *in vitro* fertilization or uterine lavage (which is not the preferred method of obtaining donor eggs),[35] which allows recovery of the human embryo from the oviducts or uterine cavity at approximately the 200-cell blastocyst stage or earlier.[36] In either case, methods would be required to confirm that the desired alterations had occurred in the embryos to be used. These cannot be done on the egg itself, and testing the polar body would not be informative. It could be done by sampling the tissue of the early embryo using one of two techniques. The first procedure would involve the removal of one or two cells from the eight-cell embryo after *in vitro* fertilization.[37] The second method would require removal of a few cells from the blastocyst that has been obtained for biopsy by uterine lavage. This technique has been successful in animal models,[38] but the risk and efficiency have not yet been evaluated adequately for routine use in humans. Once obtained, the blastocysts could then be analyzed for the presence of the inserted gene before the embryo was implanted.

Germ line gene therapy has raised several technical issues. Although germ line transmission and expression of inserted genes have been obtained in mice,[39] the failure rate is high; most eggs are so damaged by the microinjection and transfer procedures that they do not develop into live offspring. In addition, even if germ line gene therapy were safe, its effectiveness would have to be determined by diagnosis *in vitro* before the implantation of the embryo. The success rates of *in vitro* fertilization and implantation are low, and often repeated attempts are required. A third issue is that it is not yet feasible to target, unerringly, the inserted gene to a specific chromosomal site, nor is it likely to be soon. The consequences of random insertion would not cause as much concern in somatic cells, because it would affect only a single target cell or tissue; in germ line therapy the corrective gene would be incorporated into every cell of the developing embryo. This presents a greater statistical likelihood of problems. It would have to be shown that the inserted gene did not cause adverse developmental effects (which it has been shown to do in transgenic animals) and does not cause chromosomal aberrations or cause cancer to develop in subsequent generations. Current and future increases in knowledge on homologous recombination and targeting may resolve these aspects. A fourth issue to be addressed in any analysis of technical feasibility is the current inability to have reliable, time-specific expression of the inserted gene.

It may soon be possible to diagnose genetic abnormalities *in vitro* at an early stage of embryogenesis, as described previously, so that only unaffected embryos would be implanted. Most couples are likely to regard this as less dangerous than having an embryo implanted that has been genetically altered. Methods are being developed to separate the first polar body from unfertilized oocytes to allow for identification of eggs carrying defective genes.[40] Only those eggs without the defective gene would be used for *in vitro* fertilization. The selection of normal embryos or oocytes would be less hazardous than genetically manipulating an abnormal embryo and returning it to the mother for further development. The only case in which couples could not produce normal embryos without genetic manipulation is when both parents are homozygous for a recessive disorder that does not prevent childbearing. Such disorders are likely to be relatively mild (e.g., deafness). Thus, the number of clinical situations to which germ line gene therapy would be applicable seems extremely small.

It is possible to introduce a normal gene into a strain of mice to correct the disorder caused by a defective gene; DNA containing the corrective gene is injected into the nucleus of a sperm after it enters the egg at fertilization. In a small proportion, the normal DNA is incorporated into the sperm DNA and then into those embryos resulting, including their gonads (trans-fection). The resulting mice then may transmit the normal gene to half of their offspring. Only a small proportion are corrected, and this approach would not be acceptable for human application.

The current method of gene insertion used in somatic cell gene correction also would not be useful for germ cells, because the defective gene is not removed and could reappear in subsequent generations.

Any feasible application to humans would require a method that ensured that the defective gene was removed or altered to the normal state. In addition, for post-natal use, the corrective DNA would have to reach *all* of the germ cells, which seems highly unlikely, since current rates of transfection are very low. For treatment of the early embryo, assurance would have to be given that the treatment altered all of the cells of the embryo, some of which would give rise to the gonads. This also seems unlikely because preimplantation diagnosis, with selection of unaffected embryos for transfer, would (if it becomes practicable) seem to be preferable.

Ethical Aspects

Germ line gene therapy can be considered from several points of view. Will it ever be feasible? What are the possible consequences for future generations? What moral issues will arise? Should such techniques even be considered for human beings?

Concern over the consequences of germ line correction would be (1) that it would produce changes in the genetic material that would be passed on to future generations, and could affect the human gene pool; and (2) subsequent generations could be exposed to risks that could not be foreseen by the results of testing in experimental animals.

To alter the prevalence of a specific gene in the population germ line, gene correction would have to be practised widely for many generations. To eliminate a mutant recessive gene completely, it would be necessary to treat not only the homozygous individuals with the disorder but the many more heterozygous carriers. It seems unrealistic to expect pressure to be exerted for such a draconian approach. For dominant disorders, treatment of all carriers (an unrealistic possibility) would reduce the disease frequency to twice the mutation rate, but most serious dominant disorders are already infrequent. In either case, implantation of embryos without the disease gene is likely to be a more relevant option.

Of lesser concern is that germ line therapy, if it became common, would decrease genetic diversity. A few recessive diseases are more common because of the advantage they confer on those who carry only one copy of the aberrant gene (heterozygotes). For example, people who carry one copy of the sickle cell anaemia gene are better able to combat malarial infections. If the gene could be eliminated, would the harm caused (in malarial regions) by reducing resistance to malaria outweigh the benefit resulting from removing the burden of sickle cell disease? It seems likely that the potential benefits of avoiding a genetic disease would, in most environments, outweigh the risk of slightly decreasing genetic diversity.

Arguments about the morality of germ cell gene therapy stem largely from the idea that it would be an unacceptable, arrogant tampering with our germ plasm ("playing God") in ways that could have unforeseen consequences for future generations. (Archbishop Gregorios commented that if playing God meant tampering with Her/His design for the world then the objection would apply also to building a dam, or shaving.[41])

One philosopher[42] declared that it is a matter of moral judgment; that there is a categoric borderline dividing the permissible from the prohibited, and that humans must under no condition whatsoever tamper with their nature. He added that this is not an argument, but an assertion of conviction; a consequential argument is not valid since to know the consequences of an experiment requires doing it.

More specifically, it is argued that one should not tamper with genes that might be passed to the next generation unless one could be sure that no consequent harm would come to any future recipient of the altered gene. A total absence of risk could never be ensured, and the risk-benefit calculations used to justify (or not) new treatments for patients in the current generation would not be appropriate when the risks, possibly unforeseen, apply to future generations.

Some ethical, religious, and public policy bodies have concluded that somatic genetic manipulation for the purpose of ameliorating disease should be pursued, but did not endorse germ cell genetic manipulation. These include the World Council of Churches; the Parliamentary Assembly of the Council of Europe; the U.S. Presidential Commission for the Study of Ethical Problems in Medicine and Biomedical Research; the Office of Technology Assessment; the National Council of Churches; the medical research councils of Canada and Australia; and the governments of Denmark and the Federal Republic of Germany.[43] The RAC Subcommittee on Human Gene Therapy declared in 1990 that "the RAC and its Subcommittee will not at present entertain proposals for germ cell alteration." The Declaration of Inuyama adds, however, that although the modification of human germ cells is not at present in prospect, such therapy might be the only means of treating certain conditions (it is not clear what these conditions might be) so continued discussion of both its technical and its ethical aspects is essential.[44]

Conclusion

It is doubtful that techniques for germ cell gene correction that could be feasible to apply to humans will be developed in the foreseeable future. If they ever are developed, they should not be applied without assurance of their efficacy and safety. Most bodies that have made pronouncements on the subject have not endorsed germ cell modification in humans as an appropriate procedure, for both technical and ethical reasons.[45] On the other hand, some argue that it would be unwise to foreclose, through international pronouncements, the possibilities for germ line genetic correction. Predictions have been in error before, and the field is changing fast. Recommendations should be made in the context of "our present state of knowledge," and guidelines should have some resilience to adapt to changing situations. Above all, there should be continued vigorous discussion of these issues in forums where the public, ethicists, and scientists can exchange views and work toward a common understanding of the problems.

Notes

1. P.A. Baird et al., "Genetic Disorders in Children and Young Adults: A Population Study," *American Journal of Human Genetics* 42 (1988): 677-93.

2. U.S. Congress, Office of Technology Assessment, *Human Gene Therapy: Background Paper* (Washington, DC: Office of Technology Assessment, 1984), 2.

3. M.A. Frohman and G.R. Martin, "Cut, Paste, and Save: New Approaches to Altering Specific Genes in Mice," *Cell* 56 (27 January 1989): 145-47.

4. M. Holloway, "Neural Vector," *Scientific American* 264 (January 1991): 32.

5. M.A. Rosenfeld et al., "Adenovirus-Mediated Transfer of a Recombinant Alpha$_1$-Antitrypsin Gene to the Lung Epithelium In Vivo," *Science* 252 (1991): 431-34.

6. J.A. Wolff et al., "Direct Gene Transfer into Mouse Muscle In Vivo," *Science* 247 (1990): 1465-68.

7. K. Yagi, "A Gene Transfer Experiment," in *Genetics, Ethics and Human Values: Human Genome Mapping, Genetic Screening and Gene Therapy*, ed. Z. Bankowski and A.M. Capron (Geneva: Council for International Organizations of Medical Sciences, 1991), 139-42.

8. F.H. Gage et al., "Grafting Genetically Modified Cells to the Brain: Possibilities for the Future," *Neuroscience* 23 (1987): 795-807.

9. J.A. Wolff et al., "Grafting Fibroblasts Genetically Modified to Produce L-Dopa in a Rat Model of Parkinson Disease," *Proceedings of the National Academy of Sciences of the United States of America* 86 (1989): 9011-14.

10. M.B. Rosenberg et al., "Grafting Genetically Modified Cells to the Damaged Brain: Restorative Effects of NGF Expression," *Science* 242 (1988): 1575-78.

11. O. Smithies et al., "Insertion of DNA Sequences into the Human Chromosomal ß-Globin Locus by Homologous Recombination," *Nature* 317 (1985): 230-34.

12. K.R. Thomas and M.R. Capecchi, "Targeted Disruption of the Murine *int-1* Proto-Oncogene Resulting in Severe Abnormalities in Midbrain and Cerebellar Development," *Nature* 346 (1990): 847-50.

13. P.W. Kantoff et al., "*In Utero* Gene Transfer and Expression: A Sheep Transplantation Model," *Blood* 73 (1989): 1066-73.

14. Office of Technology Assessment, *Human Gene Therapy;* H.M. Temin, "Safety Considerations in Somatic Gene Therapy of Human Disease with Retrovirus Vectors," *Human Gene Therapy* 1 (1990): 111-23.

15. R. Jaenisch, "Transgenic Animals," *Science* 240 (1988): 1468-74.

16. Temin, "Safety Considerations in Somatic Gene Therapy."

17. J.P. Dougherty and H.M. Temin, "Determination of the Rate of Base-Pair Substitution and Insertion Mutations in Retrovirus Replication," *Journal of Virology* 62 (1988): 2817-22.

18. K. Cornetta et al., "Amphotropic Murine Leukemia Retrovirus Is Not an Acute Pathogen for Primates," *Human Gene Therapy* 1 (1990): 15-30.

19. S.A. Rosenberg et al., "Gene Transfer into Humans — Immunotherapy of Patients with Advanced Melanoma, Using Tumor-Infiltrating Lymphocytes Modified by Retroviral Gene Transduction," *New England Journal of Medicine* 323 (1990): 570-78.

20. United States, National Institutes of Health, Subcommittee on Human Gene Therapy, "Revised Points to Consider Document," *Human Gene Therapy* 1 (1990): 93-103.

21. W.F. Anderson, R.M. Blaese, and K. Culver, "The ADA Human Gene Therapy Clinical Protocol," *Human Gene Therapy* 1 (1990): 331-62.

22. Medical Research Council of Canada, *Guidelines on Research Involving Human Subjects* (Ottawa: Medical Research Council, 1987), 21-23.

23. Ibid., 29.

24. Office of Technology Assessment, *Human Gene Therapy.*

25. R.D. Palmiter et al., "Dramatic Growth of Mice that Develop from Eggs Microinjected with Metallothionein-Growth Hormone Fusion Genes," *Nature* 300 (1982): 611-15.

26. J. Wyngaarden, "Keynote Address," in *Genetics, Ethics and Human Values: Human Genome Mapping, Genetic Screening and Gene Therapy*, ed. Z. Bankowski and A.M. Capron (Geneva: Council for International Organizations of Medical Sciences, 1991), 16-20.

27. Medical Research Council, *Guidelines on Research Involving Human Subjects.*

28. Medical Research Council of Canada, *Guidelines for Research on Somatic Cell Gene Therapy in Humans* (Ottawa: Medical Research Council, 1990).

29. Rosenberg et al., "Gene Transfer into Humans."

30. E.A. Carswell et al., "An Endotoxin-Induced Serum Factor that Causes Necrosis of Tumors," *Proceedings of the National Academy of Sciences of the United States of America* 72 (1975): 3666-70.

31. D. Cournoyer et al., "Gene Transfer of Adenosine Deaminase into Primitive Human Hematopoietic Progenitor Cells," *Human Gene Therapy* 2 (1991): 203-13; P. Laneuville et al., "High-Efficiency Gene Transfer and Expression in Normal Human Hematopoietic Cells with Retrovirus Vectors," *Blood* 71 (1988): 811-14; P.F.D. Hughes et al., "High-Efficiency Gene Transfer to Human Hematopoietic Cells Maintained in Long-Term Marrow Culture," *Blood* 74 (1989): 1915-22.

32. Personal communication with Dr. Sadhna Joshi.

33. A. Keating et al., "Effect of Different Promoters on Expression of Genes Introduced into Hematopoietic and Marrow Stromal Cells by Electroporation," *Experimental Hematology* 18 (1990): 99-102.

34. Personal communication with Dr. Armand Keating.

35. Canadian Fertility and Andrology Society and Society of Obstetricians and Gynaecologists of Canada, *Ethical Considerations of the New Reproductive Technologies* (Toronto: Ribosome Communications, 1990), 24.

36. J.E. Buster and S.A. Carson, "Genetic Diagnosis of the Preimplantation Embryo," *American Journal of Medical Genetics* 34 (1989): 211-16.

37. A.H. Handyside et al., "Biopsy of Human Preimplantation Embryos and Sexing by DNA Amplification," *Lancet* (18 February 1989): 347-49.

38. M. Monk et al., "Pre-Implantation Diagnosis of HPRT-Deficient Male and Carrier Female Mouse Embryos by Trophectoderm Biopsy," *Human Reproduction* 3 (1988): 377-81.

39. Palmiter et al., "Dramatic Growth of Mice."

40. M. Monk and C. Holding, "Amplification of a ß-Haemoglobin Sequence in Individual Human Oocytes and Polar Bodies," *Lancet* (28 April 1990): 985-88.

41. P. Gregorios, "Ethical Reflections on Human Gene Therapy: Towards the Formulation of a Few Questions and Some Answers," in *Genetics, Ethics and Human Values: Human Genome Mapping, Genetic Screening and Gene Therapy*, ed. Z. Bankowski and A.M. Capron (Geneva: Council for International Organizations of Medical Sciences, 1991), 143-53.

42. W. Ch. Zimmerli in discussion with B.D. Davis, "Limits to Genetic Intervention in Humans," in *Human Genetic Information: Science, Laws and Ethics*, ed. D. Chadwick, G. Bock, and J. Whelan, Ciba Foundation Symposium 149 (Chichester: John Wiley and Sons, 1990), 90-91.

43. T. Friedmann, "Progress Toward Human Gene Therapy," *Science* 244 (1989): 1275-81.

44. Z. Bankowski and A.M. Capron, eds., *Genetics, Ethics and Human Values: Human Genome Mapping, Genetic Screening and Gene Therapy* (Geneva: Council for International Organizations of Medical Sciences, 1991). Countries that have said "yes" to somatic cell therapy: The national commissions in Canada, Germany, Switzerland, and the United States have approved the possibility of genetic diagnosis and (when possible) somatic cell therapy; CANADA: Medical Research Council of Canada, *Guidelines for Research on Somatic Cell Gene Therapy in Humans*, 1990; GERMANY: Report of the Enquete Commission to the Bundestag of the Federal Republic of Germany, *Prospects and Risks of Gene Technology*, 1987, in "A Report from Germany," *Bioethics* 2 (1988): 254-63; SWITZERLAND: Commission d'experts pour la génétique humaine et la médecine de la reproduction, *Rapport au Département fédéral de l'Intérieur et au Département de la Justice et Police*, 1988, takes the position that somatic cell therapy should be limited to cases of grave hereditary disorders only; UNITED STATES: the President's Commission for the Study of Ethical Problems in Medicine and Biomedical and Behavioral Research, *Splicing Life: A Report on the Social and Ethical Issues of Genetic Engineering with*

Human Beings, 1982; and the 1983 report of that same commission on *Screening and Counseling for Genetic Conditions;* see also "Gene Therapy in Man. Recommendations of European Medical Research Councils," *Lancet* (4 June 1988): 1271-72: "Only somatic cell gene therapy resulting in non-heritable changes to particular body tissues should be contemplated"; SPAIN: Law n° 35/1988 on Techniques of Assisted Reproduction of 24 November 1988 and O.J. n° 283 of November 1988; COUNCIL OF EUROPE: *Recommendation 934 (1982) on Genetic Engineering; Recommendation 1046 (1986) on the Use of Human Embryos and Foetuses for Diagnostic, Therapeutic, Scientific, Industrial and Commercial Purposes; Recommendation 1100 (1989), on the Use of Human Embryos and Foetuses in Scientific Research;* EUROPEAN COMMUNITIES: European Parliament, *Resolution on the ethical and legal problems of genetic engineering* (16 March 1989).

Countries that have said "no" to germ line alteration: DENMARK, Law n° 353 of June 1987 on the Establishment of an Ethical Council and the Regulation of Certain Forms of Biomedical Research, while awaiting legislation; FRANCE, Conseil d'État, *Sciences de la vie: De l'éthique au droit,* 1988 takes the position that all germ line therapy alterations should be prohibited. It also recommended prohibiting genetic diagnosis of preimplantation embryos through the method of embryo biopsy. This position of the Conseil d'État is similar to that taken by the Comité national d'Éthique, *Rapport C.E.,* "Avis relatif aux recherches sur les embryons humains et leur utilisation à des fins médicales et scientifiques" (15 December 1986) as reiterated in "Avis relatif à la thérapie génique" (19 December 1990); GERMANY: Working Group on In Vitro Fertilisation, Genom Analysis and Gene Therapy, *Report,* 1985. Since germ line research would involve the use of embryos and their possible destruction in experiments, it was not justified. The commission recommended the prohibition of any germ line experiments or treatments. This position was reaffirmed in the recent report of the Enquete Commission to the Bundestag of the Federal Republic of Germany, *Prospects and Risks of Gene Technology,* 1987, as reported in "A Report from Germany," *Bioethics* 2 (1988): 254-63, which accepted the philosophical base of the natural development of human beings as the core of their humanity and would totally prohibit even therapeutic experimentation on the human germ line; NORWAY: "Act n° 628, 1987, Relating to Artificial Procreation." See also "Gene Therapy in Man. Recommendations of European Medical Research Councils," *Lancet* (4 June 1988): 1271-72: "Germline Therapy, for the Introduction of Heritable Genetic Modifications, Is Not Acceptable." SWITZERLAND: Commission d'experts pour la génétique humaine et la médecine de la reproduction, *Rapport au Département fédéral de l'Intérieur et du Département de la Justice et Police,* 1988, at 97 takes the position that genetic therapy (germ line) on gametes or embryos is to be prohibited as well as all non-therapeutic genetic manipulations on the human person. The opinion of this commission is particularly interesting as it is based on the Council of Europe's equation between the right to dignity and the inheritance of a genetic pattern as found in Recommendation 934 (1982) on Genetic Engineering.

45. Friedmann, "Progress Toward Human Gene Therapy."

Bibliography

Anderson, W.F., R.M. Blaese, and K. Culver. "The ADA Human Gene Therapy Clinical Protocol." *Human Gene Therapy* 1 (1990): 331-62.

Baird, P.A., et al. "Genetic Disorders in Children and Young Adults: A Population Study." *American Journal of Human Genetics* 42 (1988): 677-93.

Bankowski, Z., and A.M. Capron, eds. *Genetics, Ethics and Human Values: Human Genome Mapping, Genetic Screening and Gene Therapy.* Geneva: Council for International Organizations of Medical Sciences, 1991.

Buster, J.E., and S.A. Carson. "Genetic Diagnosis of the Preimplantation Embryo." *American Journal of Medical Genetics* 34 (1989): 211-16.

Canadian Fertility and Andrology Society and Society of Obstetricians and Gynaecologists of Canada. *Ethical Considerations of the New Reproductive Technologies.* Toronto: Ribosome Communications, 1990.

Carswell, E.A., et al. "An Endotoxin-Induced Serum Factor that Causes Necrosis of Tumors." *Proceedings of the National Academy of Sciences of the United States of America* 72 (1975): 3666-70.

Cornetta, K., et al. "Amphotropic Murine Leukemia Retrovirus Is Not an Acute Pathogen for Primates." *Human Gene Therapy* 1 (1990): 15-30.

Cournoyer, D., et al. "Gene Transfer of Adenosine Deaminase into Primitive Human Hematopoietic Progenitor Cells." *Human Gene Therapy* 2 (1991): 203-13.

Davis, B.D. "Limits to Genetic Intervention in Humans: Somatic and Germline." In *Human Genetic Information: Science, Law and Ethics*, ed. D. Chadwick, G. Bock, and J. Whelan. Ciba Foundation Symposium 149. Chichester: John Wiley and Sons, 1990.

Dougherty, J.P., and H.M. Temin. "Determination of the Rate of Base-Pair Substitution and Insertion Mutations in Retrovirus Replication." *Journal of Virology* 62 (1988): 2817-22.

Federal Republic of Germany. Enquete Commission to the Bundestag. *Prospects and Risks of Gene Technology.* In "A Report from Germany." *Bioethics* 2 (1988): 254-63.

Federal Republic of Germany. Working Group on In Vitro Fertilisation, Genom Analysis and Gene Therapy. *Report.* Bonn: 1985. (Benda Report)

France. Comité national d'éthique. *Avis relatif aux recherches sur les embryons humains et leur utilisation à des fins médicales et scientifiques.* Paris: 1986.

France. Conseil d'État. *Sciences de la vie: De l'éthique au droit.* Paris: La Documentation française, 1988.

Friedmann, T. "Progress Toward Human Gene Therapy." *Science* 244 (1989): 1275-81.

Frohman, M.A., and G.R. Martin. "Cut, Paste, and Save: New Approaches to Altering Specific Genes in Mice." *Cell* 56 (27 January 1989): 145-47.

Gage, F.H., et al. "Grafting Genetically Modified Cells to the Brain: Possibilities for the Future." *Neuroscience* 23 (1987): 795-807.

"Gene Therapy in Man. Recommendations of European Medical Research Councils." *Lancet* (4 June 1988): 1271-72.

Gregorios, P. "Ethical Reflections on Human Gene Therapy: Towards the Formulation of a Few Questions and Some Answers." In *Genetics, Ethics and Human Values: Human Genome Mapping, Genetic Screening and Gene Therapy*, ed. Z. Bankowski and A.M. Capron. Geneva: Council for International Organizations of Medical Sciences, 1991.

Handyside, A.H., et al. "Biopsy of Human Preimplantation Embryos and Sexing by DNA Amplification." *Lancet* (18 February 1989): 347-49.

Holloway, M. "Neural Vector." *Scientific American* 264 (January 1991): 32.

Hughes, P.F.D., et al. "High-Efficiency Gene Transfer to Human Hematopoietic Cells Maintained in Long-Term Marrow Culture." *Blood* 74 (1989): 1915-22.

Jaenisch, R. "Transgenic Animals." *Science* 240 (1988): 1468-74.

Kantoff, P.W., et al. "In Utero Gene Transfer and Expression: A Sheep Transplantation Model." *Blood* 73 (1989): 1066-73.

Keating, A., et al. "Effect of Different Promoters on Expression of Genes Introduced into Hematopoietic and Marrow Stromal Cells by Electroporation." *Experimental Hematology* 18 (1990): 99-102.

Laneuville, P., et al. "High-Efficiency Gene Transfer and Expression in Normal Human Hematopoietic Cells with Retrovirus Vectors." *Blood* 71 (1988): 811-14.

Medical Research Council of Canada. *Guidelines for Research on Somatic Cell Gene Therapy in Humans*. Ottawa: Medical Research Council, 1990.

—. *Guidelines on Research Involving Human Subjects*. Ottawa: Medical Research Council, 1987.

Monk, M., and C. Holding. "Amplification of a β-Haemoglobin Sequence in Individual Human Oocytes and Polar Bodies." *Lancet* (28 April 1990): 985-88.

Monk, M., et al. "Pre-Implantation Diagnosis of HPRT-Deficient Male and Carrier Female Mouse Embryos by Trophectoderm Biopsy." *Human Reproduction* 3 (1988): 377-81.

Palmiter, R.D., et al. "Dramatic Growth of Mice that Develop from Eggs Microinjected with Metallothionein-Growth Hormone Fusion Genes." *Nature* 300 (1982): 611-15.

Rosenberg, M.B., et al. "Grafting Genetically Modified Cells to the Damaged Brain: Restorative Effects of NGF Expression." *Science* 242 (1988): 1575-78.

Rosenberg, S.A., et al. "Gene Transfer into Humans — Immunotherapy of Patients with Advanced Melanoma, Using Tumor-Infiltrating Lymphocytes Modified by Retroviral Gene Transduction." *New England Journal of Medicine* 323 (1990): 570-78.

Rosenfeld, M.A., et al. "Adenovirus-Mediated Transfer of a Recombinant Alpha$_1$-Antitrypsin Gene to the Lung Epithelium In Vivo." *Science* 252 (1991): 431-34.

Smithies, O., et al. "Insertion of DNA Sequences into the Human Chromosomal β-Globin Locus by Homologous Recombination." *Nature* 317 (1985): 230-34.

Switzerland. Commission d'experts pour la génétique humaine et la médecine de la reproduction. *Rapport au Département fédéral de l'Intérieur et au Département de la Justice et Police.* Berne: 1988.

Temin, H.M. "Safety Considerations in Somatic Gene Therapy of Human Disease with Retrovirus Vectors." *Human Gene Therapy* 1 (1990): 111-23.

Thomas, K.R., and M.R. Capecchi. "Targeted Disruption of the Murine *int-1* Proto-Oncogene Resulting in Severe Abnormalities in Midbrain and Cerebellar Development." *Nature* 346 (1990): 847-50.

United States. Congress. Office of Technology Assessment. *Human Gene Therapy: Background Paper.* Washington, DC: Office of Technology Assessment, 1984.

United States. National Institutes of Health. Subcommittee on Human Gene Therapy. "Revised Points to Consider Document." *Human Gene Therapy* 1 (1990): 93-103.

United States. President's Commission for the Study of Ethical Problems in Medicine and Biomedical and Behavioral Research. *Screening and Counseling for Genetic Conditions.* Washington, DC: The Commission, 1983.

—. *Splicing Life: A Report on the Social and Ethical Issues of Genetic Engineering with Human Beings.* Washington, DC: The Commission, 1982.

Wolff, J.A., et al. "Direct Gene Transfer into Mouse Muscle *In Vivo.*" *Science* 247 (1990): 1465-68.

—. "Grafting Fibroblasts Genetically Modified to Produce L-Dopa in a Rat Model of Parkinson Disease." *Proceedings of the National Academy of Sciences of the United States of America* 86 (1989): 9011-14.

Wyngaarden, J. "Keynote Address." In *Genetics, Ethics and Human Values: Human Genome Mapping, Genetic Screening and Gene Therapy,* ed. Z. Bankowski and A.M. Capron. Geneva: Council for International Organizations of Medical Sciences, 1991.

Yagi, K. "A Gene Transfer Experiment." In *Genetics, Ethics and Human Values: Human Genome Mapping, Genetic Screening and Gene Therapy,* ed. Z. Bankowski and A.M. Capron. Geneva: Council for International Organizations of Medical Sciences, 1991.

Contributors

Shelin Adam, M.Sc., University of British Columbia; National Coordinator, the Canadian Collaborative Study on Predictive Testing for Huntington Disease.

Michael Cooke, M.A.

F. Clarke Fraser, O.C., Ph.D., M.D., FRCPC, FCCMG.

Michael R. Hayden, MB, ChB, DCh, Ph.D., FRCPC, Professor, Medical Genetics; Director, the Canadian Collaborative Study on Predictive Testing for Huntington Disease.

Z.G. Miller, M.H.A., M.Sc.

Lynn Prior, M.Sc.

Martin Thomas, Ph.D., Department of Political Science, York University, Toronto.

Mandate

(approved by Her Excellency the Governor General
on the 25th day of October, 1989)

The Committee of the Privy Council, on the recommendation of the Prime Minister, advise that a Commission do issue under Part I of the Inquiries Act and under the Great Seal of Canada appointing The Royal Commission on New Reproductive Technologies to inquire into and report on current and potential medical and scientific developments related to new reproductive technologies, considering in particular their social, ethical, health, research, legal and economic implications and the public interest, recommending what policies and safeguards should be applied, and examining in particular,

(a)   implications of new reproductive technologies for women's reproductive health and well-being;

(b)   the causes, treatment and prevention of male and female infertility;

(c)   reversals of sterilization procedures, artificial insemination, *in vitro* fertilization, embryo transfers, prenatal screening and diagnostic techniques, genetic manipulation and therapeutic interventions to correct genetic anomalies, sex selection techniques, embryo experimentation and fetal tissue transplants;

(d)   social and legal arrangements, such as surrogate childbearing, judicial interventions during gestation and birth, and "ownership" of ova, sperm, embryos and fetal tissue;

(e)   the status and rights of people using or contributing to reproductive services, such as access to procedures, "rights" to parenthood, informed consent, status of gamete donors and confidentiality, and the impact of these services on all concerned parties, particularly the children; and

(f)   the economic ramifications of these technologies, such as the commercial marketing of ova, sperm and embryos, the application of patent law, and the funding of research and procedures including infertility treatment.

The Research Volumes

Volume 1: New Reproductive Technologies: Ethical Aspects

Volume 2: Social Values and Attitudes Surrounding New Reproductive Technologies

Volume 3: Overview of Legal Issues in New Reproductive Technologies

Volume 4: Legal and Ethical Issues in New Reproductive Technologies: Pregnancy and Parenthood

Juridical Interference with Gestation and Birth	S. Rodgers
Reproductive Hazards in the Workplace: Legal Issues of Regulation, Enforcement, and Redress	J. Fudge/E. Tucker
The Challenge of the New Reproductive Technologies to Family Law	E. Sloss/R. Mykitiuk
"Surrogate Motherhood": Legal and Ethical Analysis	J.R. Guichon
Surrogate Parenting: Bibliography	J. Kitts

Volume 5: New Reproductive Technologies and the Science, Industry, Education, and Social Welfare Systems in Canada

Discovery, Community, and Profit: An Overview of the Science and Technology System	L. Edwards, with the assistance of R. Voyer
An Overview of Select Social and Economic Forces Influencing the Development of *In Vitro* Fertilization and Related Assisted Reproductive Techniques	A. Rochon Ford
Commercial Involvement in New Reproductive Technologies: An Overview	J. Rowlands/ N. Saby/J. Smith
The Role of the Biotechnology Industry in the Development of Clinical Diagnostic Materials for Prenatal Diagnosis	G. Chaloner-Larsson/ F. Haynes/C. Merritt
Report on a Survey of Members of the Pharmaceutical Manufacturers Association of Canada and Biotechnology Companies	SPR Associates Inc.
Canada's School Systems: An Overview of Their Potential Role in Promoting Reproductive Health and Understanding of New Reproductive Technologies	Shannon and McCall Consulting Ltd.
Social Welfare and New Reproductive Technologies: An Overview	S. Torjman

Volume 6: The Prevalence of Infertility in Canada

Volume 7: Understanding Infertility: Risk Factors Affecting Fertility

Volume 8: Prevention of Infertility

Volume 9: Treatment of Infertility: Assisted Reproductive Technologies

Volume 10: Treatment of Infertility: Current Practices and Psychosocial Implications

Volume 11: New Reproductive Technologies and the Health Care System: The Case for Evidence-Based Medicine

Volume 12: Prenatal Diagnosis: Background and Impact on Individuals

Volume 13: Current Practice of Prenatal Diagnosis in Canada

Volume 14: Technologies of Sex Selection and Prenatal Diagnosis

Volume 15: Background and Current Practice of Fetal Tissue and Embryo Research in Canada

ommission Organization

Commissioners

Patricia Baird
Chairperson
Vancouver, British Columbia

Grace Jantzen
London, United Kingdom

Bartha Maria Knoppers
Montreal, Quebec

Susan E.M. McCutcheon
Toronto, Ontario

Suzanne Rozell Scorsone
Toronto, Ontario

Staff

John Sinclair
Executive Director

Mimsie Rodrigue
Executive Director (from July 1993)

Research & Evaluation

Sylvia Gold
Director

Nancy Miller Chénier
Deputy Director
Causes and Prevention of Infertility

Janet Hatcher Roberts
Deputy Director
Assisted Human Reproduction

F. Clarke Fraser
Deputy Director
Prenatal Diagnosis and Genetics

Burleigh Trevor Deutsch
Deputy Director
Embryo and Fetal Tissue Research

Consultations & Coordination

Dann M. Michols
Director

Mimsie Rodrigue
Deputy Director
Coordination

Anne Marie Smart
Deputy Director
Communications

Judith Nolté
Deputy Director
Analysis

Denise Cole
Deputy Director
Consultations

Mary Ann Allen
Director
Administration and Security

Gary Paradis
Deputy Director
Finance